MW01096391

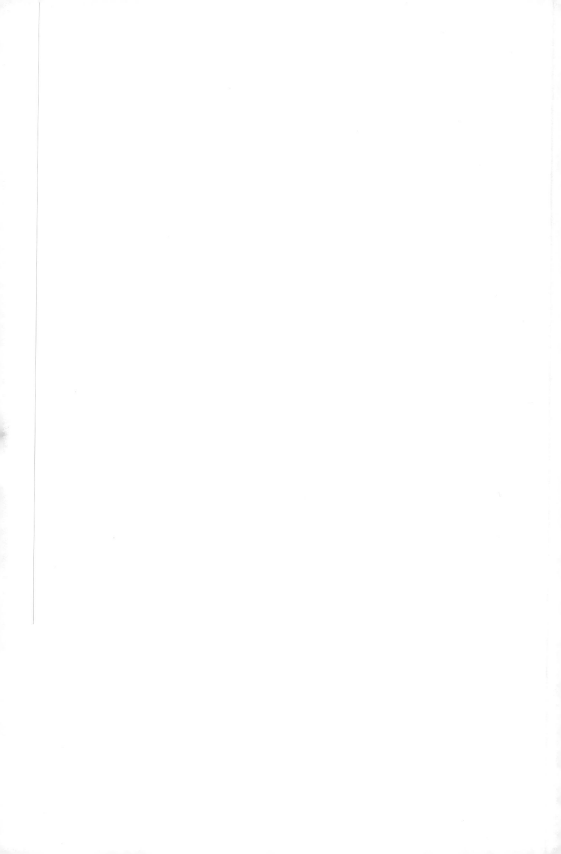

Contemporary Health Issues on Marijuana

Contemporary Health Issues
on Marijuana

Edited by
Kevin A. Sabet and Ken C. Winters

OXFORD
UNIVERSITY PRESS

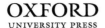

Oxford University Press is a department of the University of Oxford. It furthers
the University's objective of excellence in research, scholarship, and education
by publishing worldwide. Oxford is a registered trade mark of Oxford University
Press in the UK and certain other countries.

Published in the United States of America by Oxford University Press
198 Madison Avenue, New York, NY 10016, United States of America.

© Oxford University Press 2018

All rights reserved. No part of this publication may be reproduced, stored in
a retrieval system, or transmitted, in any form or by any means, without the
prior permission in writing of Oxford University Press, or as expressly permitted
by law, by license, or under terms agreed with the appropriate reproduction
rights organization. Inquiries concerning reproduction outside the scope of the
above should be sent to the Rights Department, Oxford University Press, at the
address above.

You must not circulate this work in any other form
and you must impose this same condition on any acquirer.

Library of Congress Cataloging-in-Publication Data
Names: Sabet, Kevin A. (Kevin Abraham), 1979– editor. |
Winters, Ken C., editor.
Title: Contemporary health issues on marijuana /
edited by Kevin A. Sabet and Ken C. Winters.
Description: New York, NY : Oxford University Press, [2018]
Identifiers: LCCN 2017058870 | ISBN 9780190263072 (hardcover) |
ISBN 9780190671860 (epub)
Subjects: LCSH: Marijuana—Health aspects. | Marijuana abuse—Treatment.
Classification: LCC RC568.C2 C65 2018 | DDC 615.3/23648—dc23
LC record available at https://lccn.loc.gov/2017058870

9 8 7 6 5 4 3 2 1

Printed by Sheridan Books, Inc., United States of America

CONTENTS

Preface vii
Ken C. Winters and Kevin A. Sabet
Contributors xi

Introduction 1
   Nicholas Chadi, Sharon Levy, Rajiv Radhakrishnan, Mohini Ranganathan, and Aaron S. B. Weiner

1. Recent Epidemiological Trends in Marijuana Use 14
   Linda B. Cottler and Chukwuemeka N. Okafor

2. International Trends in Cannabis Use 39
   James C. Anthony, Omayma Alshaarawy, and Catalina Lopez-Quintero

3. Clinical Characteristics of Cannabis Use Disorder 72
   Tammy A. Chung and Ken C. Winters

4. Effects of Adolescent Cannabis Use on Brain Structure and
   Function: Current Findings and Recommendations for Future Research 91
   Randi Melissa Schuster, Jodi Gilman, and A. Eden Evins

5. The Impact of Marijuana on Mental Health 122
   Christine L. Miller

6. Impact of Marijuana Smoking on Lung Health 165
   Donald P. Tashkin

7. Marijuana-Impaired Driving: A Path through the Controversies 183
   Robert L. DuPont, Erin A. Holmes, Stephen K. Talpins, and J. Michael Walsh

8. Risk Factors for Adolescent Marijuana Use 219
   Richard F. Catalano, Elizabeth C. Speaker, Martie L. Skinner, Jennifer A. Bailey, Ge Hong, Kevin P. Haggerty, Katarina Guttmannova, and Erin N. Harrop

9. Status Update on the Treatment of Cannabis Use Disorder 236
   Alan J. Budney, Catherine Stanger, Ashley A. Knapp, and Denise D. Walker

10. What Is the Evidence of Marijuana as Medicine? 256
    Kevin A. Sabet, David Atkinson, and Shayda M. Sabet

11. Policy Implications 295
    Kevin A. Sabet and Ken C. Winters

Index 307

Marijuana is probably the most commonly used illicit drug worldwide. In the United States, approximately 13% of individuals 12 years of age or older reported using this drug in 2014, with the rate at about 32% among persons aged 18 to 25 years (Azofeifa et al., 2016). In total, this represents 2.5 million persons and an average of approximately 7,000 new users each day. Older teen use has especially increased: High school senior use of marijuana is at a near 20-year high, and levels of first-time marijuana use in college have grown to the highest levels recorded in the past three decades. In 2015, about one in five college students became a first-time marijuana user. And while the prevalence rates of almost every category of substance has fallen, marijuana use among 8th, 10th, and 12th graders combined have increased in the past decade (University of Michigan, 2017). Also, the prevalence of perceived *great risk* from smoking marijuana once or twice a week and once a month decreased, and the prevalence of perceived *no risk* increased (Azofeifa et al., 2016), and it is becoming a popular notion that it should be made legal. As of early 2017, 29 states in the United States and the District of Columbia either allow medical or recreational use of the drug (see https://learnaboutsam.org/legalization-map/). Increased access to and legalization of medical marijuana will likely impact the prevalence and intensity/frequency of marijuana use and alter perceptions of harm through expanded availability, increased commercialization, and decreased restrictiveness around the drug (National Academies of Sciences, Engineering, and Medicine, 2017). Data from the largest student survey of drug use in 2016 found that marijuana rates were higher in states with loose laws and that students in states with medical/legal marijuana were more likely to use edible marijuana often found in candies or drinks (National Institute on Drug Abuse, 2016).

As policy shifts gain favor toward the medicalization and legalization of marijuana, several complex health, social, and legal issues become prominent. The science is stronger for some areas than others, but overall the field is still relatively young. The body of research is evocative but not equivocal. The most research has focused on the link between marijuana use and negative health effects, and the evidence varies as a function of the age of the user, whether use is occasional or regular, and health domain. Anecdotal reports exist by individuals

suffering from chronic pain and a variety of chronic illnesses that using marijuana improved their conditions. The possible medical value of elements of the
marijuana plant is the focus of several pharmacological investigations.

A scholarly book on marijuana and its health and social impacts is important
for several reasons. First, the goal of this edited book is to provide an up-to-
date source on marijuana that is empirically based on relevant to researchers,
clinicians, and policymakers. In this light, the book strives to accomplish the
following objectives: (a) challenge misconceptions and myths that create barriers
to informed and balanced perspectives and derail rational approaches to prevention and treatment approaches; (b) offer a benchmark reference for researchers
who seek a source for the current status of research on marijuana and insights
for what future directions can guide additional research; and (c) provide a
balanced view of the health impacts and potential benefits of medical marijuana
to policymakers so that legislation about legalization can be informed by science
and not public opinion or economic interests. Second, the aim of this edited book
is to highlight new and meaningful theory and empirical pertaining to studies
on marijuana use trends and to provide an overview of several health domains,
including the drug's impact on cognitive and neurological functioning, its medical effects, and treatment approaches for those with a cannabis use disorder.

The book's invited authors, all of whom are prominent in the field of substance abuse, provide a review of marijuana research in their area of expertise. We emphasized to each author that their chapter 'follow the data,' provide
balanced conclusions, and be relevant to a wide-ranging readership. Viewing
marijuana from multiple perspectives, the book serves as a scholarly source on
the myriad health issues that pertain to marijuana use. The book leads-off with
two chapters that present the latest epidemiology data, one focusing on U.S. data
(Cottler & Okafor), and the other on international trends (Anthony, Alshaarawy,
& Lopez-Quintero). The diagnostic characteristics of cannabis use disorders for
adults and adolescents are addressed in the next chapter (Chung & Winters).
The next section of the book focuses on particular health domains: brain structure and functioning (Schuster, Gilman & Evins); mental health (Miller); lung
functioning (Tashkin); and effects on driving (DuPont, Holmes, Talpins, &
Walsh). Additional chapters provide summaries of these key areas: psychosocial
risk factors (Catalano, Speaker, Skinner, Bailey, Hong, Haggerty, Guttmannova,
& Harrop); treatment (Budney, Stanger, Knapp, & Walker), and medical marijuana (Sabet, Atkinson, & Sabet). A concluding chapter (Sabet & Winters) will
sum up the various key points raised in the previous chapters, highlight where
the weight of science provides compelling evidence with respect to various
health issues, discuss policy implications in terms of medical and recreational
marijuana legislation, and highlight future directions as we move forward in an
ever-changing health, policy and legal environment.

The scientific debate and media coverage surrounding marijuana's health
effects and medical benefits has accelerated of late. This trend is characterized
by increased attention at the National Institute on Drug Abuse to fund research,
a growing trend for libertarian and economic interests to advance the argument

that marijuana should be legal for recreational purposes, and a partisan debate about how to harness marijuana's potential medical properties. Marijuana is a prominent topic when it comes to the pros and cons to health, in the last few decades there seems to be a widening gap between science's views on marijuana's potential for harm and popular opinion.

The editors hope that *Contemporary Health Issues on Marijuana* will offer a science-based and balanced resource to researchers, healthcare professionals, and government policymakers. With a sound foothold on the state of knowledge about the health issues surrounding marijuana, the drug's status with communities and its role in the medical field can move forward in a positive way.

REFERENCES

Azofeifa, A., Mattson, M. E., Schauer, G., McAfee, T., Grant, A., & Lyerla, R. (2016). National estimates of marijuana use and related indicators: National survey on drug use and health, United States, 2002–2014. *MMWR Surveillance Summary, 65*(SS-11), 1–25.

National Academies of Sciences, Engineering, and Medicine. (2017). *The health effects of cannabis and cannabinoids: The current state of evidence and recommendations for research.* Washington, DC: Author.

National Institute on Drug Abuse. (2016). *NIH Monitoring the Future survey shows use of most illicit substances down, but past year marijuana use relatively stable.* Retrieved from https://www.drugabuse.gov/news-events/news-releases/2016/12/teen-substance-use-shows-promising-decline

University of Michigan (2017). Monitoring the Future, 2017 Press Releases. http://www.monitoringthefuture.org/pressreleases/17drugpr.pdf and http://ns.umich.edu/new/releases/24773-first-time-marijuana-use-in-college-at-highest-level-in-three-decades

K.C.W.

K.A.S.

CONTRIBUTORS

Omayma Alshaarawy, PhD
Postdoctoral Fellow
Department of Epidemiology and
  Biostatistics
Michigan State University

James C. Anthony, MSc, PhD
Professor
Department of Epidemiology and
  Biostatistics
Michigan State University

David Atkinson, MD
Assistant Professor
Department of Psychiatry
University of Texas Southwestern,
  Medical Center

Jennifer A. Bailey, PhD
Social Development Research Group
School of Social Work
University of Washington

Alan J. Budney, PhD
Professor of Psychiatry
Department of Psychiatry
Geisel School of Medicine
Dartmouth College

Richard F. Catalano, PhD
Social Development Research Group
School of Social Work
University of Washington

Nicholas Chadi, MD
Division of Developmental Medicine
Division of Adolescent/Young Adult
  Medicine
Boston Children's Hospital
Department of Pediatrics
Harvard Medical School

Tammy A. Chung, PhD
Associate Professor of Psychiatry and
  Epidemiology
Department of Psychiatry
University of Pittsburgh

Linda B. Cottler, PhD, MPH
Dean's Professor and Founding Chair
Department of Epidemiology
University of Florida

Robert L. Dupont, MD
President
Institute for Behavior and Health
Rockville, Maryland

A. Eden Evins, MD, MPH
Director
Massachusetts General Hospital
  Center for Addiction Medicine
Cox Family Professor of Psychiatry
Harvard Medical School

Jodi Gilman, PhD
Assistant Professor
Center for Addiction Medicine
Harvard Medical School/
  Massachusetts General Hospital

Katarina Guttmannova, PhD
Social Development Research Group
School of Social Work
University of Washington

Kevin P. Haggerty, PhD
Social Development Research Group
School of Social Work
University of Washington

Erin N. Harrop, MSW
Social Development Research Group
School of Social Work
University of Washington

Erin A. Holmes, MA
Director
Traffic Safety and Technical Writer
  for Criminal Justice Programs
Foundation for Advancing Alcohol
  Responsibility

Ge Hong, PhD
Washington State Department of
  Social and Health Services
Olympia, Washington

Ashley A. Knapp, PhD
Postdoctoral Fellow
Department of Psychiatry
Geisel School of Medicine
Dartmouth College

Sharon Levy, MD, MPH
Division of Developmental Medicine
Boston Children's Hospital
Department of Pediatrics
Harvard Medical School

Catalina Lopez-Quintero, MD, PhD
Postdoctoral Associate
Center for Research on U.S. Latino
  HIV/AIDS and Drug Abuse
Florida International University

Christine L. Miller, PhD
President and Founder
MillerBio, Baltimore, MD

**Chukwuemeka N. Okafor,
PhD, MPH**
Postdoctoral Fellow
CHIPTS and The Center for
  Behavioral and Addiction Medicine
University of California, Los Angeles

Rajiv Radhakrishnan, MBBS, MD
Department of Psychiatry
Yale University School of Medicine

Mohini Ranganathan, MD
Department of Psychiatry
Yale University School of Medicine

Kevin A. Sabet, PhD
Affiliated Fellow
Yale University
Director
Drug Policy Institute

Shayda M. Sabet, MPA
Research Associate
International Initiative for Impact
  Evaluation (3ie)

Randi Melissa Schuster, PhD
Post-Doctoral Research Fellow
Center for Addiction Medicine
Harvard Medical School/
  Massachusetts General Hospital

Martie L. Skinner, PhD
Social Development Research Group
School of Social Work
University of Washington

Elizabeth C. Speaker, MS
Washington State Department of
  Social and Health Services
Olympia, Washington

Catherine Stanger, PhD
Associate Professor Psychiatry
Department of Psychiatry
Geisel School of Medicine
Dartmouth College

Stephen K. Talpins, JD
Partner
Rumberger, Kirk & Caldwell
Miami, FL

Donald P. Tashkin, MD
Emeritus Professor of Medicine
Department of Medicine
David Geffen School of Medicine
University of California, Los Angeles

Denise D. Walker, PhD
Research Associate Professor
School of Social Work
University of Washington

J. Michael Walsh, PhD
President, The Walsh Group

Aaron S. B. Weiner, PhD
Addiction Services
Linden Oaks Behavioral Health
Naperville, IL

Ken C. Winters, PhD
Senior Scientist, Oregon Research
  Institute & Adjunct Faculty,
  Department of Psychology,
  University of Minnesota,
  Minneapolis

Introduction

NICHOLAS CHADI, SHARON LEVY,
RAJIV RADHAKRISHNAN, MOHINI RANGANATHAN,
AND AARON S. B. WEINER

The psychoactive and medicinal properties of marijuana have been reported for thousands of years. It wasn't until the early 1900s that marijuana became a prohibited substance and that laws restricting the use and sale of marijuana products started being enforced (Pain, 2015). In the past two decades, a steady movement towards legalization of marijuana for "medical" or "adult/recreational" use has been gathering steam. In the United States, California was the first state to legalize "medical marijuana" in 1996, followed closely by a growing number of states and countries. With changing marijuana laws, the nature of the substance as well as its perception in the public eye have been changing rapidly (Albertson, Chenoweth, Colby, & Sutter, 2016; Richter & Levy, 2014). For instance, the potency of smoked marijuana has increased three- to fivefold since the 1970s, while perceived riskiness associated with the regular use of marijuana has been steadily decreasing among adolescents (ElSohly et al., 2016; Johnston, O'Malley, Miech, Bachman, & Schulenberg, 2017). At the same time, a rapidly evolving multimillion dollar marijuana industry has come to life, and as a result a plethora of marijuana-infused products including marijuana-infused "edibles" and highly concentrated oils and resins have become much more readily available (Friese, Slater, Annechino, & Battle, 2016).

The long-term health risks and potential benefits of marijuana use remain poorly understood, and there is a pressing need for high-quality research to identify the long-term effects of marijuana use in different populations, especially in children and adolescents (Calabria, Degenhardt, Hall, & Lynskey, 2010; Rieder, 2016). In the United States, marijuana remains a controlled substance by federal law, but the shift toward legalization of marijuana for "medical use" at the state level is well on its way. This introduction provides an overview of recent trends in marijuana use and policies in addition to discussing some basic concepts about "medical marijuana." We also discuss some of the risks and potential uses of cannabinoids in the field of medicine and health.

MARIJUANA: THE BASICS

The term *marijuana* historically has referred to the dried leaves, stems, and flowers from the marijuana sativa or indica plants (Radwan et al., 2009). Several other cannabinoid-containing products, including edible and topical preparations and high-potency marijuana concentrates such as oils and resins, are technically referred to as marijuana-infused products, though are also referred to simply as "marijuana." As policy has been liberalized, the word *marijuana* has taken on new meanings. In the vernacular, marijuana has become an umbrella term referring to products ranging from plant material to highly concentrated oils and resins to edible products infused with cannabinoid-containing plant extracts, while "medical marijuana" (a phrase coined by industry) is sometimes used to refer to products ranging from FDA-approved cannabinoid preparations to crude extracts from the marijuana plant. The imprecision surrounding these terms can lead to substantial confusion around marijuana policy, which is generally determined by ballot initiatives. As such, it remains unclear whether voters understand the range or products under discussion for legalization when they go to the voting booth and the practical implications of these laws, if adopted (MacCoun, Pacula, Chriqui, Harris, & Reuter, 2009).

The marijuana plant contains more than 100 cannabinoid molecules that can bind to the body's cannabinoid receptors and mimic chemical messengers naturally produced by the body (Mackie, 2008). Delta-9-tetrahydrocannabinol (THC) and cannabidiol (CBD) are two exogenous cannabinoids found in marijuana that are thought to have the most biological activity in humans and have been the subject of the most study (Babson, Sottile, & Morabito, 2017). THC is the main psychoactive component of marijuana and is primarily responsible for its psychoactive and pleasurable effects as well as many of its side effects (Volkow et al., 2016). CBD has been found to carry neuroprotective and anti-inflammatory properties without psychoactive effects and is of significant interest as a potential therapy for the treatment of seizures (Campbell, Phillips, & Manasco, 2017). Over the past several decades marijuana plants have been selectively bred to increase content of THC and/or CBD, while extracts and marijuana-infused products yield varying concentrations of THC and CBD depending on method of preparation.

Several endogenous cannabinoid ligands have been discovered; the best described of which is called anandamide (Mechoulam & Parker, 2013). Exogenous cannabinoids mimic anandamide and can bind cannabinoid receptors. THC has a much stronger affinity for the receptor than anandamide, and consumption of THC overwhelms the endocannabinoid system, resulting in the psychoactive effects described by marijuana users: a calming, yet euphoric sensation, decreased coordination, and altered perceptions, which may be pleasant but can also include hallucinations and paranoia (Johns, 2001). Cannabinoids when bound to receptors depress cells and prevent the secretion of neurotransmitters, including dopamine and serotonin, from pre-synaptic cells (Bloomfield, Ashok, Volkow, & Howes, 2016). They are particularly abundant in the prefrontal cortex of the brain, thought to be the seat of executive functioning; the nucleus accumbens, also known as the reward center of the brain, which explains the addictive potential of marijuana (Simpson & Magid, 2016); and in areas involved in coordination, learning, memory formation, and executive functioning (Mackie, 2008).

IMPACTS OF MARIJUANA POLICIES ON YOUTH

There is compelling evidence that marijuana use is harmful to the developing adolescent brain. Thus, a question of significant interest to scientists, policymakers, and the public is the impact of changing marijuana policy on adolescent marijuana use rates. Unfortunately, the impact of changing policy can be difficult to discern. The largest source of data comes from several nationally representative cross-sectional surveys that track youth use rates over time, though survey questions may miss nuanced findings (such as amounts, types of products, and nuanced measures of frequency of use). Also missing from these surveys are markers of harm such as associated accidents, injuries, or subclinical symptoms such as hallucinations or delusions that may not otherwise come to attention (Levy & Weitzman, 2016). It can be difficult to determine the exact geographical area of impact of a new policy: while laws typically are statewide, some localities may opt out of certain provisions creating differing environments that can impact even relatively small areas differently. Alternatively, the impact of a law may not respect state boundaries particularly near state borders (Hao & Cowan, 2017). Medical and adult use laws vary substantially from state to state and efforts to cluster them together have significant limitations. Finally, new laws can take years to impact behavior; it can take months to write and implement regulations and years for distribution systems and marketing efforts to mature (Pacula & Smart, 2017).

According to new data from the National Survey on Drug Use and Health, the average rate of regular teen marijuana use in the legalized states of Alaska, Colorado, Oregon, and Washington is 30% higher than the US rate as a whole (Behavioral Health Statistics and Quality, 2017). Almost one third of all 18- to 25-year-olds in legal states used marijuana in the past month, up from around one fifth ten years ago. As of 2017, Colorado is the top state in the United States for first-time marijuana users, and its rate of first-time users has more than doubled in the last decade. In that state, use among people 18 and over has also increased, as well as use among young adults, up from 37% in 2005 (Behavioral Health Statistics and Quality, 2017).

The Nation's 2017 annual survey of students by the University of Michigan reported today marijuana use among 8th, 10th, and 12th grades was significantly higher than 2016, marking first significant increase in seven years (Meich et al., 2017). The survey also found that students in medical marijuana law states vaped marijuana at higher rates than students in other states and consumed pot edibles (that can come in candies, sodas, or ice creams) at double the rate than in nonmedical marijuana law states. Virtually all other substances are at their lowest point in the history of the survey. The survey also showed that daily marijuana use among 12th graders is at 5.9%, compared to a low of 1.9% in 1991. It is now more popular than daily cigarette use, which is down to 4.2% compared to its peak of 24.6% in 1997 (Meich et al., 2017). These data are a significant concern as health risks of marijuana use are dose-dependent and accumulate over time (Coffey & Patton, 2016).

One finding has been consistent: marijuana legalization has been associated with decreased perception of risk by older adolescents (Johnston et al., 2017). Perceived riskiness of marijuana, which is inversely correlated with marijuana use, is at its lowest in more than three decades, with less than one third of high school seniors considering daily use of marijuana to pose a health risk (Miech et al., 2017). Concurrently, rates of marijuana use have risen sharply in states that have legalized marijuana for adult use, as might be predicted. For instance, in Colorado, where marijuana was legalized for adult use in 2012, the number of high school junior and senior students who had used marijuana in the past 30 days increased 19 percent and 14 percent, respectively from 2013 to 2015 (Rocky Mountain High Intensity Drug Trafficking Area, 2016). This is a significant concern as health risks of marijuana use are dose-dependent and accumulate over time (Ammerman, Ryan, & Adelman, 2015; Coffey & Patton, 2016).

MARIJUANA'S IMPACT ON COGNITIVE FUNCTION AND MENTAL HEALTH

The effects of marijuana on cognition and its impact on the symptom expression and course of mental illness have been extensively studied using epidemiological as well as experimental paradigms (Ranganathan, Skosnik, & D'Souza, 2016). Marijuana is associated with cognitive deficits acutely, during the period of intoxication as well as chronically following recurrent use. A number of randomized control trials with THC and CBD have demonstrated that THC acutely produces deficits in attention, verbal learning, working memory, and electrophysiological indices of information processing (Radhakrishnan, Wilkinson, & D'Souza, 2014; Sherif, Radhakrishnan, D'Souza, & Ranganathan, 2016). The data with CBD are limited but suggest that it may protect against some of the cognitive deficits induced by THC. Worse cognitive performance has also been reported with chronic exposure among heavy marijuana users (Bolla, Brown, Eldreth, Tate, & Cadet, 2002; Broyd, van Hell, Beale, Yucel, & Solowij, 2016; Pope, Gruber, Hudson, Huestis, & Yurgelun-Todd, 2001; Solowij et al., 2002).

The question of whether these cognitive deficits resolve with abstinence, however, remains less clear. While some studies found that the cognitive deficits resolved or improved with one to three months of abstinence (Fried, Watkinson, & Gray, 2005; Pope et al., 2001), others have reported persistent deficits despite prolonged periods of abstinence (McHale & Hunt, 2008; Thames, Arbid, & Sayegh, 2014). Factors that may contribute to these discrepant findings include age at onset of marijuana use, premorbid intelligence quotient (IQ) or cognitive function, the dose (i.e., amount of marijuana use), the variable content of THC versus CBD in the marijuana, and individual genetic vulnerability (Colizzi & Bhattacharyya, 2017; Cosker et al., 2017; Ruiz-Contreras et al., 2014). Perhaps even more concerning are the effects of marijuana exposure in adolescents. It is increasingly well-recognized that adolescence is a critical period of neurodevelopment (Juraska & Willing, 2017), and epidemiological studies, both cross-sectional and longitudinal, have revealed that adolescent marijuana use is associated with a 5.5 to 7.3 point lower IQ (Meier et al., 2017), lower educational attainment (Fergusson, Boden, & Horwood, 2015; Melchior et al., 2017), poorer academic performance (Meier, Hill, Small, & Luthar, 2015), higher school dropout rates (Homel, Thompson, & Leadbeater, 2014), increased risk of unemployment (Rodwell et al., 2017), and increased risk of psychiatric disorders as young adults (Duperrouzel et al., 2017; Marwaha, Winsper, Bebbington, & Smith, 2017). Longitudinal studies of cognition among adolescent marijuana users demonstrated in particular significant impairments in verbal memory, working memory, and executive function even at two- and three-year follow-up (Becker et al., 2017; Jacobus et al., 2015). These data are particularly concerning given the high rates of marijuana use in this population.

Epidemiological studies have also consistently noted an associated between marijuana use and psychotic disorders including schizophrenia (Marconi, Di Forti, Lewis, Murray, & Vassos, 2016; Radhakrishnan et al., 2014). A meta-analysis of 18 studies, enrolling 66,816 individuals, found an increased risk (odds ratio: 3.90) for the development of schizophrenia and other psychosis-related outcomes among heavy marijuana users (Marconi et al., 2016). Marijuana use is recognized as a "component cause" of schizophrenia, in that it is neither necessary nor sufficient to result in schizophrenia but contributes to overall increased risk. Recent studies also suggest that marijuana use in adolescence may increase the risk of bipolar disorder in a dose-dependent fashion (Gibbs et al., 2015; Marwaha et al., 2017). In both these disorders, continued marijuana use has been associated with a worse course of illness, greater number of hospitalizations, and overall poorer outcomes (Kvitland et al., 2015; Ringen et al., 2016; Romer Thomsen et al., 2017).

In summary, converging data demonstrate that marijuana exposure is associated with short and longer-term cognitive deficits, as well as an increased risk for and a worse course of illness in schizophrenia and bipolar disorder. Adolescents may be particularly vulnerable both to long-term cognitive deficits that persist after cessation of marijuana use with significant psychosocial consequences as well as a greater risk of serious mental illness associated with marijuana exposure. Given the high rates of marijuana use among adolescents, further studies need to be conducted to better understand the factors that may contribute to this

increased vulnerability and to direct targeted suitable interventions to those at
highest risk.

MARIJUANA AS MEDICINE: FACTS AND CONTROVERSIES

Further complicating the current mainstream perception of marijuana
are the possible therapeutic applications for cannabis and cannabinoids.
Cannabis impacts human physiology in myriad ways, but the most promising for therapeutic value is through interaction with the endocannabinoid
system. Endocannabinoids (such as anandamide, 2-Arachidonoyl glycerol, O-
Arachidonoyl ethanolamine, and N-Arachidonoyl dopamine) have been associated with modulation of numerous conditions, including energy metabolism
(such as appetite regulation) pain and inflammation, central nervous system
disorders (such as neurotoxicity, stroke, multiple sclerosis, Parkinson's disease,
Huntington's disease, amyotrophic lateral sclerosis, and epilepsy), psychiatric
conditions (including schizophrenia, anxiety, and depression), nausea and em-
esis, other drug addiction (including opioids, nicotine, alcohol, and cocaine),
cardiovascular disorders (including hypertension), eye disorders (such as glaucoma), cancer, gastrointestinal disorders (such as inflammatory bowel disease),
acute and chronic liver disease, musculoskeletal disorders, and reproductive
functioning (Pacher, Bátkai, & Kunos, 2006).

The previous list is broad but should not be misconstrued as a list of conditions
in which consumption of nonendogenous cannabinoids (such as smoking marijuana or using cannabidiol tinctures) are medically therapeutic or beneficial.
The endocannabinoid system's influence in these areas is promising, but our
ability to impact it to achieve consistent medical results is a separate area of empirical inquiry. As an example, although smoked marijuana has been found to
reduce intraocular pressure in humans with glaucoma (Green, 1998), the duration of the effect is brief and does not provide any enduring benefit. This,
along with marijuana's overall risk/benefit profile, led the American Glaucoma
Society (Jampel, 2009) to "preclude recommending this drug in any form for the
treatment of glaucoma at the present time."

Research into effective therapeutic uses for consumed marijuana and cannabinoid products is ongoing and is supported by federal funding organizations such as The National Institutes of Health (NIH). However, agencies such
as NIH note that funding is more often directed towards research examining
individual cannabinoid products rather than smoked marijuana, as smoked marijuana carries increased risk to the lungs, the potential for addiction, and a vast
number of cannabinoids and other compounds that create possible confounds
when interpreting study results (NIH, 2016).

Despite the endocannabinoid system's involvement in numerous health-
related concerns, empirical support for cannabis and cannabinoids in similarly
impacting these conditions has thus far been limited. Currently, extant literature

indicates substantial support for the use of smoked marijuana for temporary relief of pain and specific cannabinoids for treatment of chemotherapy-induced nausea and vomiting (oral cannabinoids) and multiple sclerosis spasticity symptoms (National Academies of Sciences, Engineering, and Medicine [NAS], 2017). Moderate evidence exists supporting the use of certain cannabinoids for short-term sleep outcomes related to certain medical conditions. Beyond these conditions, support for the use of marijuana and cannabinoid products for therapeutic benefit is limited at best and insufficient to form any conclusions in other cases (NAS, 2017). This limited support is largely unknown to the public, however, and is further obfuscated by state-supported medical marijuana programs, which authorize the use of smoked marijuana for the treatment of numerous physiological and psychological conditions that are often largely unsupported by published scientific and medical literature (Belendiuk, Baldini, & Bonn-Miller, 2015).

ACCURATE INTERPRETATION OF PUBLISHED DATA ON MEDICAL MARIJUANA

Although further study is warranted regarding the therapeutic applications of cannabis and cannabinoids, careful interpretation of new data is imperative to accurately understanding the possible benefits of these products and how to accurately represent these data to the public. It is recommended to be mindful of the following four points regarding the therapeutic value of marijuana:

Cannabis versus Cannabinoid

When being represented to the general public, the distinction between the therapeutic value of cannabis and cannabinoids is not often clear. This is a critical discrimination, however, as smoked marijuana is often perceived as having therapeutic effects, despite the majority of research being conducted on isolated cannabinoids.

Palliative versus Curative

When a state approves marijuana for the treatment of a health condition, there can be an assumption by the public that marijuana will actually treat that illness, providing curative effects or enduring gains. However, this is not generally the case: cannabis or cannabinoids may positively impact certain symptoms of the diagnosis in question but are not in themselves curative agents and generally must be consumed on a regular basis due to a relatively short duration of therapeutic action.

Strength and Quality of Evidence

The results and conclusions of newly published scientific studies can often be overstated by media outlets—essentially as new facts rather than new data to consider as broader conclusions are formulated. These types of news stories rarely highlight study limitations (e.g., quasi-experimental designs, selection biases, or small sample sizes) and also rarely emphasize that findings must be replicated before they can be regarded as empirically supported. As an example, extensive media coverage surrounding the case of Charlotte Figi, a child whose reported 300 seizures per day were reduced to 2-3 times per month after regular consumption of cannabidiol oil with food (Young, 2013), fueled public perception that marijuana can be used to effectively treat seizures. However, published research of clinical trials has produced no reliable evidence that cannabis or cannabinoids can be used to effectively treat seizures, leading the NAS (2017) to categorize seizures in the "no sufficient evidence to support or refute the conclusion that cannabis or cannabinoids are an effective treatment" category.

"Medical" versus "Therapeutic"

Lastly, there is often confusion in the general public about whether marijuana is "medicine." A pharmaceutical "medicine" is a controlled, tested, and standardized substance. Medicines in the United States are tightly regulated, requiring completion of the Food and Drug Administration (FDA) multiphase approval process. Prescriptions are for a specific drug, dosage, and administration frequency. "Medical marijuana" is something of a misnomer, as marijuana has many strains and variants, has not been approved by the FDA to treat any condition, and is not prescribed, produced, nor dispensed like a pharmaceutical medicine. True cannabinoid medicines include dronabinol (brand name: Marinol, FDA-approved), nabixmols (brand name: Sativex, undergoing the FDA approval process), and an oral solution of cannabidiol (brand name: Epidiolex, undergoing the FDA approval process).

CONCLUDING THOUGHTS

Marijuana continues to have a significant place in the social and cultural discussion of policy in America. There are fervent arguments on many sides regarding the legalization of marijuana. There is a growing scientific body of work to support the view that marijuana is not a harmless drug. This appears particularly the case for those who begin use during adolescence and use heavily over the course of time. Also, while extant science does not justify the claims by many that the marijuana plant has miracle curative properties (NAS, 2017), there may be elements of the plant that have some medical promise (e.g., cannabidiol).

In this light, research needs to continue to explore marijuana's possible harms and benefits. The range of expert scholars who contributed to this book seek to help in this effort for science to clarify the many complex issues surrounding marijuana.

REFERENCES

Albertson, T. E., Chenoweth, J. A., Colby, D. K., & Sutter, M. E. (2016). The changing drug culture: Medical and recreational marijuana. *FP Essent, 441*, 11–17.

Ammerman, S., Ryan, S., & Adelman, W. P. (2015). The impact of marijuana policies on youth: Clinical, research, and legal update. *Pediatrics, 135*(3), e769–e785. http://dx.doi.org/10.1542/peds.2014-4147

Babson, K. A., Sottile, J., & Morabito, D. (2017). Cannabis, cannabinoids, and sleep: A review of the literature. *Current Psychiatry Reports, 19*(4), 23. http://dx.doi.org/10.1007/s11920-017-0775-9

Becker, M. P., Collins, P. F., Schultz, A., Urosevic, S., Schmaling, B., & Luciana, M. (2017). Longitudinal changes in cognition in young adult cannabis users. *Journal of Clinical and Experimental Neuropsychology*, 1–15. http://dx.doi.org/10.1080/13803395.2017.1385729

Bloomfield, M. A. P., Ashok, A. H., Volkow, N. D., & Howes, O. D. (2016). The effects of Δ9-tetrahydrocannabinol on the dopamine system. *Nature, 539*(7629), 369–377. http://dx.doi.org/10.1038/nature20153

Bolla, K. I., Brown, K., Eldreth, D., Tate, K., & Cadet, J. L. (2002). Dose-related neurocognitive effects of marijuana use. *Neurology, 59*(9), 1337–1343. http://dx.doi.org/10.1212/01.WNL.0000031422.66442.49

Broyd, S. J., van Hell, H. H., Beale, C., Yucel, M., & Solowij, N. (2016). Acute and chronic effects of cannabinoids on human cognition: A systematic review. *Biologicall Psychiatry, 79*(7), 557–567. http://dx.doi.org/10.1016/j.biopsych.2015.12.002

Calabria, B., Degenhardt, L., Hall, W., & Lynskey, M. (2010). Does cannabis use increase the risk of death? Systematic review of epidemiological evidence on adverse effects of cannabis use. *Drug and Alcohol Review, 29*(3), 318–330. http://dx.doi.org/10.1111/j.1465-3362.2009.00149.x

Campbell, C. T., Phillips, M. S., & Manasco, K. (2017). Cannabinoids in pediatrics. *Journal of Pediatric Pharmacology and Therapeutics, 22*(3), 176–185. http://dx.doi.org/10.5863/1551-6776-22.3.176

Center for Behavioral Health Statistics and Quality. (2017). *2016 National Survey on Drug Use and Health: Detailed tables*. Rockville, MD: Substance Abuse and Mental Health Services Administration.

Chadi, N., & Levy, S. (2017). Understanding the highs and lows of adolescent marijuana use. *Pediatrics, 140*(6). http://dx.doi.org/10.1542/peds.2017-3164

Coffey, C., & Patton, G. C. (2016). Cannabis use in adolescence and young adulthood: A review of findings from the Victorian Adolescent Health Cohort Study. *Canadian Journal of Psychiatry, 61*(6), 318–327. http://dx.doi.org/10.1177/0706743716645289

Colizzi, M., & Bhattacharyya, S. (2017). Does cannabis composition matter? Differential effects of delta-9-tetrahydrocannabinol and cannabidiol on human cognition. *Current Addiction Reports, 4*(2), 62–74. http://dx.doi.org/10.1007/s40429-017-0142-2

Cosker, E., Schwitzer, T., Ramoz, N., Ligier, F., Lalanne, L., Gorwood, P., . . . Laprevote, V. (2017). The effect of interactions between genetics and cannabis use on neurocognition: A review. *Progress in Neuropsychopharmacology & Biological Psychiatry*. http://dx.doi.org/10.1016/j.pnpbp.2017.11.024

Duperrouzel, J., Hawes, S. W., Lopez-Quintero, C., Pacheco-Colon, I., Comer, J., & Gonzalez, R. (2017). The association between adolescent cannabis use and anxiety: A parallel process analysis. *Addictive Behaviors, 78*, 107–113. http://dx.doi.org/10.1016/j.addbeh.2017.11.005

ElSohly, M. A., Mehmedic, Z., Foster, S., Gon, C., Chandra, S., & Church, J. C. (2016). Changes in cannabis potency over the last 2 decades (1995–2014): Analysis of current data in the United States. *Biological Psychiatry, 79*(7), 613–619. http://dx.doi.org/10.1016/j.biopsych.2016.01.004

Fergusson, D. M., Boden, J. M., & Horwood, L. J. (2015). Psychosocial sequelae of cannabis use and implications for policy: Findings from the Christchurch Health and Development Study. *Social Psychiatry and Psychiatric Epidemiology, 50*(9), 1317–1326. http://dx.doi.org/10.1007/s00127-015-1070-x

Fried, P. A., Watkinson, B., & Gray, R. (2005). Neurocognitive consequences of marihuana: A comparison with pre-drug performance. *Neurotoxicology and Teratology, 27*(2), 231–239. http://dx.doi.org/10.1016/j.ntt.2004.11.003

Friese, B., Slater, M. D., Annechino, R., & Battle, R. S. (2016). Teen use of marijuana edibles: A Focus group study of an emerging issue. *Journal of Primary Prevention, 37*(3), 303–309. http://dx.doi.org/10.1007/s10935-016-0432-9

Gibbs, M., Winsper, C., Marwaha, S., Gilbert, E., Broome, M., & Singh, S. P. (2015). Cannabis use and mania symptoms: A systematic review and meta-analysis. *Journal of Affective Disorders, 171*, 39–47. http://dx.doi.org/10.1016/j.jad.2014.09.016

Green, K. (1998). Marijuana smoking vs cannabinoids for glaucoma therapy. *Archives of Ophthalmology, 116*, 1433–1437. http://dx.doi.org/10.1001/archopht.116.11.1433

Hao, Z., & Cowan, B. (2017). The cross-border spillover effects of recreational marijuana legalization. NBER Working Paper no. 23426. http://dx.doi.org/10.3386/w23426

Hasin, D. S., Wall, M., Keyes, K. M., Cerda, M., Schulenberg, J., O'Malley, P. M., . . . Feng, T. (2015). Medical marijuana laws and adolescent marijuana use in the USA from 1991 to 2014: Results from annual, repeated cross-sectional surveys. *Lancet Psychiatry, 2*(7), 601–608. http://dx.doi.org/10.1016/s2215-0366(15)00217-5

Homel, J., Thompson, K., & Leadbeater, B. (2014). Trajectories of marijuana use in youth ages 15-25: Implications for postsecondary education experiences. *Journal of Studies on Alcohol and Drugs, 75*(4), 674-683. http://dx.doi.org/10.15288/jsad.2014.75.674

Jacobus, J., Squeglia, L. M., Infante, M. A., Castro, N., Brumback, T., Meruelo, A. D., & Tapert, S. F. (2015). Neuropsychological performance in adolescent marijuana users with co-occurring alcohol use: A three-year longitudinal study. *Neuropsychology, 29*(6), 829–843. http://dx.doi.org/10.1037/neu0000203

Jampel, H. (2009). *Position statement on marijuana and the treatment of glaucoma*. Retrieved from http://www.americanglaucomasociety.net/patients/position_statements/marijuana_glaucoma

Johns, A. (2001). Psychiatric effects of cannabis. *British Journal of Psychiatry, 178*(2), 116–22. http://dx.doi.org/10.1192/bjp.178.2.116

Johnston, L., O'Malley, P., Miech, R., Bachman, J., & Schulenberg, J. (2017). *Monitoring the Future national survey results on drug use, 1975–2016: Overview, key findings on adolescent drug use. Monitoring the Future: National survey results on drug use.* Ann Arbor: Institute for Social Research, University of Michigan.

Juraska, J. M., & Willing, J. (2017). Pubertal onset as a critical transition for neural development and cognition. *Brain Research, 1654*(Pt B), 87–94. http://dx.doi.org/ 10.1016/j.brainres.2016.04.012

Kvitland, L. R., Melle, I., Aminoff, S. R., Demmo, C., Lagerberg, T. V., Andreassen, O. A., & Ringen, P. A. (2015). Continued cannabis use at one year follow up is associated with elevated mood and lower global functioning in bipolar I disorder. *BMC Psychiatry, 15*, 11. http://dx.doi.org/10.1186/s12888-015-0389-x

Levy, S., & Weitzman, E. R. (2016). Building a learning marijuana surveillance system. *JAMA Pediatrics, 170*(3), 193–194. http://dx.doi.org/10.1001/ jamapediatrics.2015.3489

MacCoun, R., Pacula, R. L., Chriqui, J., Harris, K., & Reuter, P. (2009). Do citizens know whether their state has decriminalized marijuana? Assessing the perceptual component of deterrence theory. *Review of Law & Economics, 5*(1), 347–371. http:// dx.doi.org/10.2202/1555-5879.1227

Mackie, K. (2008). Cannabinoid receptors: Where they are and what they do. *Journal of Neuroendocrinology, 20*(Suppl 1), 10–14. http://dx.doi.org/doi.org/10.1111/ j.1365-2826.2008.01671.x

Marconi, A., Di Forti, M., Lewis, C. M., Murray, R. M., & Vassos, E. (2016). Meta-analysis of the association between the level of cannabis use and risk of psychosis. *Schizophrenia Bulletin, 42*(5), 1262–1269. http://dx.doi.org/10.1093/schbul/sbw003

Marwaha, S., Winsper, C., Bebbington, P., & Smith, D. (2017). Cannabis use and hypomania in young people: A prospective analysis. *Schizophrenia Bulletin*, sbx158. http://dx.doi.org/10.1093/schbul/sbx158

McHale, S., & Hunt, N. (2008). Executive function deficits in short-term abstinent cannabis users. *Human Psychopharmacology, 23*(5), 409–415. http://dx.doi.org/10.1002/ hup.941

Mechoulam, R., & Parker, L. A. (2013). The endocannabinoid system and the brain. *Annual Review of Psychology, 64*(1), 21–47. http://dx.doi.org/10.1146/ annurev-psych-113011-143739

Meier, M. H., Caspi, A., Danese, A., Fisher, H. L., Houts, R., Arseneault, L., & Moffitt, T. E. (2017). Associations between adolescent cannabis use and neuropsychological decline: A longitudinal co-twin control study. *Addiction, 113*(2), 257–265. http:// dx.doi.org/10.1111/add.13946

Meier, M. H., Hill, M. L., Small, P. J., & Luthar, S. S. (2015). Associations of adolescent cannabis use with academic performance and mental health: A longitudinal study of upper middle class youth. *Drug and Alcohol Dependence, 156*, 207–212. http:// dx.doi.org/10.1016/j.drugalcdep.2015.09.010

Melchior, M., Bolze, C., Fombonne, E., Surkan, P. J., Pryor, L., & Jauffret-Roustide, M. (2017). Early cannabis initiation and educational attainment: is the association causal? Data from the French TEMPO study. *International Journal of Epidemiology, 46*(5), 1641–1650. http://dx.doi.org/10.1093/ije/dyx065

Miech, R. A., Schulenberg, J. E., Johnston, L. D., Bachman, J. G., O'Malley, P. M., & Patrick, M. E. (2017). National adolescent drug trends in 2017: Findings released. Ann Arbor, MI: Monitoring the Future.

National Academies of Sciences, Engineering and Medicine. (2017). The health effects of cannabis and cannabinoids: The current state of evidence and

recommendations for research. Retrieved from https://www.nap.edu/catalog/24625/
the-health-effects-of-cannabis-and-cannabinoids-the-current-state

National Institutes of Health. (2016). NIDA research on marijuana and
cannabinoids. Retrieved from https://www.drugabuse.gov/drugs-abuse/marijuana/
nida-research-marijuana-cannabinoids

Pacher, P., Bátkai, S., & Kunos, G. (2006). The endocannabinoid system as an emerging
target of pharmacotherapy. *Pharmacology Review, 58*(3), 389-462. http://dx.doi.org/
10.1124/pr.58.3.2

Pacula, R. L., & Smart, R. (2017). Medical marijuana and marijuana legalization.
Annual Review of Clinical Psychology, 13, 397–419. http://dx.doi.org/10.1146/
annurev-clinpsy-032816-045128

Pain, S. (2015). A potted history. *Nature, 525*(7570), S10–S11. https://doi.org/10.1038/
525S10a

Pope, H. G., Jr., Gruber, A. J., Hudson, J. I., Huestis, M. A., & Yurgelun-Todd, D. (2001).
Neuropsychological performance in long-term cannabis users. *Archives of General
Psychiatry, 58*(10), 909–915. http://dx.doi.org/10.1001/archpsyc.58.10.909

Radwan, M. M., ElSohly, M. A., Slade, D., Ahmed, S. A., Khan, I. A., & Ross, S. A.
(2009). Biologically active cannabinoids from high-potency cannabis sativa. *Journal
of Natural Products, 72*(5), 906–911. http://dx.doi.org/10.1021/np900067k

Radhakrishnan, R., Wilkinson, S. T., & D'Souza, D. C. (2014). Gone to pot: A review of
the association between cannabis and psychosis. *Frontiers in Psychiatry, 5*, 54. http://
dx.doi.org/10.3389/fpsyt.2014.00054

Ranganathan, M., Skosnik, P. D., & D'Souza, D. C. (2016). Marijuana and
madness: Associations between cannabinoids and psychosis. *Biological Psychiatry,
79*(7), 511–513. http://dx.doi.org/10.1016/j.biopsych.2016.02.007

Richter, K. P., & Levy, S. (2014). Big Marijuana: Lessons from Big Tobacco. *New England
Journal of Medicine, 371*(5), 399–401. http://dx.doi.org/10.1056/NEJMp1406074

Rieder, M. J. (2016). Is the medical use of cannabis a therapeutic option for children?
Pediatric Child Health, 21(1), 31–34.

Ringen, P. A., Nesvag, R., Helle, S., Lagerberg, T. V., Lange, E. H., Loberg, E. M., . . .
Melle, I. (2016). Premorbid cannabis use is associated with more symptoms and
poorer functioning in schizophrenia spectrum disorder. *Psychological Medicine,
46*(15), 3127–3136. http://dx.doi.org/10.1017/S0033291716001999

Rocky Mountain High Intensity Drug Trafficking Area. (2016). Colorado youth marijuana use: Up—down—flat? Examine the data and you decide! Retrieved from
http://www.rmhidta.org/html/FINAL Denver Post HKCS Response (3).pdf

Rodwell, L., Romaniuk, H., Nilsen, W., Carlin, J. B., Lee, K. J., & Patton, G. C. (2017).
Adolescent mental health and behavioural predictors of being NEET: A prospec-
tive study of young adults not in employment, education, or training. *Psychological
Medicine*, 1–11. http://dx.doi.org/10.1017/S0033291717002434

Romer Thomsen, K., Thylstrup, B., Pedersen, M. M., Pedersen, M. U., Simonsen, E., &
Hesse, M. (2017). Drug-related predictors of readmission for schizophrenia among
patients admitted to treatment for drug use disorders. *Schizophrenia Research.*
http://dx.doi.org/10.1016/j.schres.2017.09.026

Ruiz-Contreras, A. E., Carrillo-Sanchez, K., Ortega-Mora, I., Barrera-Tlapa,
M. A., Roman-Lopez, T. V., Rosas-Escobar, C. B., . . . Prospero-Garcia, O. (2014).
Performance in working memory and attentional control is associated with the

rs2180619 SNP in the CNR1 gene. *Genes, Brain and Behavior, 13*(2), 173–178. http://dx.doi.org/10.1111/gbb.12097

Sherif, M., Radhakrishnan, R., D'Souza, D. C., & Ranganathan, M. (2016). Human laboratory studies on cannabinoids and psychosis. *Biological Psychiatry, 79*(7), 526–538. http://dx.doi.org/10.1016/j.biopsych.2016.01.011

Simpson, A. K., & Magid, V. (2016). Cannabis use disorder in adolescence. *Child Adolescent Psychiatric Clinics of North America, 25*(3), 431–443. http://dx.doi.org/10.1016/j.chc.2016.03.003

Solowij, N., Stephens, R. S., Roffman, R. A., Babor, T., Kadden, R., Miller, M., . . . Vendetti, J. (2002). Cognitive functioning of long-term heavy cannabis users seeking treatment. *JAMA, 287*(9), 1123–1131. http://dx.doi.org/10.1001/jama.287.9.1123

Substance Abuse and Mental Health Services Administration. (2017). Key substance use and mental health indicators in the United States: Results from the 2016 National Survey on Drug Use and Health. (N.S.H.-52) (HHS Publication No. SMA 17-5044, Ed.). Rockville, MD: Center for Behavioral Health Statistics and Quality, Substance Abuse and Mental Health Services Administration.

Thames, A. D., Arbid, N., & Sayegh, P. (2014). Cannabis use and neurocognitive functioning in a non-clinical sample of users. *Addictive Behaviors, 39*(5), 994–999. http://dx.doi.org/10.1016/j.addbeh.2014.01.019

The National Academies of Sciences Engineering and Medicine. (2017). *The health effects of cannabis and cannabinoids: The current state of evidence and recommendations for research: Health and Medicine Division.* Retrieved from http://nationalacademies.org/hmd/Reports/2017/health-effects-of-cannabis-and-cannabinoids.aspx

Young, S. (2013, August 7). *Marijuana stops child's severe seizures.* Retrieved from http://www.cnn.com/2013/08/07/health/charlotte-child-medical-marijuana/index.html

1

Recent Epidemiological Trends in Marijuana Use

LINDA B. COTTLER AND
CHUKWUEMEKA N. OKAFOR

INTRODUCTION

Marijuana contains over 400 chemical compounds, including 80 compounds that are unique to the plant and are termed *cannabinoids* (Gaoni & Mechoulam, 1964; Mechoulam & Gaoni, 1967). The best known of these cannabinoids is delta-9-tetrahydrocannabinol (THC), probably because it is one of the most abundant in the marijuana plant and is responsible for the psychoactive effects of marijuana (ElSohly & Slade, 2005). Other cannabinoids, including cannabidiol, have also been identified in the marijuana plant (Mechoulam & Shvo, 1963) and have been found to have differing effects to THC's psychoactive properties (Morgan, Schafer, Freeman, & Curran, 2010). Marijuana is most frequently smoked either in the form of cigarettes or joints (i.e., dried marijuana leaves rolled up in a cigarette wrapper) or blunts (marijuana rolled in tobacco wrapper from a cigar) or with the use of water pipes, other variations of pipes, and vaporizers (devices used to vaporize the active constituents of the plant for inhalation). Marijuana leaves, stems, and buds can also be brewed and consumed as a tea or ingested as edibles (e.g., baked products such as brownies, cookies, etc.) as well as made into candies. Alternate routes of administration include topicals made from marijuana oils (e.g., lotions, balms, or salves) and wax made by collecting resins from the flowering tops.

The majority of the effects of cannabinoids including THC are proposed to be mediated through their actions at specific receptor sites: cannabinoid receptors CB1 (Devane, Dysarz, Johnson, Melvin, & Howlett, 1988) and CB2 (Munro, Thomas, & Abu-Shaar, 1993). CB1 receptors have been found to be abundant in the brain with high concentrations in the basal ganglia (including the globus pallidus and substantia nigra), cerebellum, and cerebral cortex and moderate concentrations in the amygdala and hippocampus (Glass, Dragunow, & Faull, 1997; Herkenham et al., 1990). These areas of the brain are involved in a number of cognitive functions including motor and psychomotor functions, learning, memory, and executive functioning. Furthermore, CB1 receptors have also been found in regions of the brain's reward circuits including the ventral tegmental area (VTA) and nucleus accumbens, and their actions in these regions have been proposed as a mechanism linked to the neuropathophsysiology of problematic use and use disorders including addiction (Volkow, Wang, et al., 2014). On the other hand, CB2 receptors are present mostly in cells and tissues of the immune system (Galiègue et al., 1995; Munro et al., 1993) as well as in the central nervous system. It has been proposed that CB2 receptors are part of a protective system in the mammalian body (Pacher & Mechoulam, 2011). Cannabidiol has been linked to a number of therapeutic benefits including analgesic, anxiolytic, and potent anti-inflammatory effects and are proposed to confer beneficial effects in a number of conditions including HIV/AIDS, cancer, multiple sclerosis, and seizures (Rom & Persidsky, 2013).

Although marijuana and its constituents may have some therapeutic benefits, its use has been associated with broad adverse health outcomes including cognitive impairment, reduced intelligent quotient, addiction, cardiovascular and respiratory problems, and motor vehicle crashes (Compton, Weiss, & Wargo, in press; Volkow, Baler, Compton, & Weiss, 2014). Of particular interest is marijuana use among adolescents, as there is emerging evidence that regular marijuana use in this age group may have profound detrimental effects on the developing brain (Lisdahl, Gilbart, Wright, & Shollenbarger, 2013; Lisdahl, Wright, Medina-Kirchner, Maple, & Shollenbarger, 2014; Schuster, Gilman, & Eden, in press). Therefore, monitoring indicators, trends, and patterns of marijuana use is important for predicting future rates of marijuana use, identifying subgroups with consistently high rates of use, which can then be targeted for intervention programs to prevent or delay marijuana use, subsequently reducing adverse health outcomes of marijuana use.

DATA SOURCES

This chapter includes data gathered from a variety of national surveys conducted in the United States that have assessed marijuana and other drug use among adolescents and adults, including the National Survey on Drug Use and Health (NSDUH), Monitoring the Future (MTF), Youth Risk Behavior Surveillance System (YRBSS), and the National Monitoring of Adolescent Prescription Stimulant Study (N-MAPSS). Details of each data source are described in the following discussion.

National Survey on Drug Use

The NSDUH is an annual survey of a representative sample of the civilian, noninstitutionalized population 12 years of age and older in the United States

(Center for Behavioral Health Statistics and Quality, 2015). The NSDUH is the primary source of statistical information on the use of illicit drugs, alcohol, and tobacco by the U.S. population. A random sample of households across the United States is selected after which an interviewer visits the household, and residents in the household are asked to participate by completing a face-to-face interview. Participation is voluntary, and the information is confidential; once an individual is selected to participate, no one else can take his or her place. The NSDUH survey is sponsored by the Substance Abuse and Mental Health Services Administration (SAMHSA) of the U.S. Department of Health and Human Services and is planned and managed by the SAMHSA's center for Behavioral Health Statistics and Quality. Data are collected using audio computer-assisted self-interviewing, and respondents are given a $30 incentive payment for participation. The total target sample size of 67,500 participants is allocated equally across the three age groups: 12 to 17, 18 to 25, and 26 years of age and older. The NSDUH sample frame includes residents in noninstitutionalized group quarters, residents of the 50 states and the District of Columbia, and civilians living on military bases. The sample excludes persons with no fixed household address and long-term residents of institutional group quarters (e.g., prison, nursing home).

Youth Risk Behavior Surveillance System

The YRBSS was initiated in 1990 by the Centers for Disease Control and Prevention to monitor health risk behaviors, including marijuana use, among students in the United States (Kann et al., 2014). Although the YRBSS is conducted at the state, local, and territorial level, a national survey is also conducted and that is what is highlighted here. The national YRBSS has a sampling frame of all regular public and private schools in at least one of grades 9 to 12 in the 50 states and the District of Columbia. Participants are selected using a three-stage cluster sample design to produce a nationally representative sample of students in grades 9 to 12 who attend public and private schools. In the first stage of sampling, sampling units consisted of subareas of large-sized counties or groups of smaller-sized counties. In the second stage of sampling, public and private schools with any of the grades 9 to 12 were sampled with a probability proportional to the school's enrollment. In the final stage of sampling, one or two randomly selected classes from either a required subject (e.g., social studies) or a required period (e.g., second period) in each of grades 9 to 12 were selected. All students in a randomly selected class are eligible to participate. The survey includes procedures to oversample black or African American, Hispanic, and Latinx students to enable separate analysis of these subgroups. Schools that declined to participate in the original sample were not replaced. Students confidentially complete self-administered, paper-and-pencil questionnaires and record their answers directly in the questionnaire booklet or on a separate computer-scannable answer sheet.

Monitoring the Future

MTF is an ongoing annual survey of 8th, 10th, and 12th graders designed to study changes in the beliefs, values, attitudes, and behaviors of young people in the United States (Johnston, O'Malley, Bachman, Schulenberg, & Miech, 2014). MTF is a repeated series of surveys in which participants are presented with the same set of questions over a period of years to understand how behaviors change over time. The survey began in 1975 with 12th-grade students only, and each year about 16,000 students participate from approximately 133 public and private high schools in the United States. Beginning in 1991, similar surveys of nationally representative samples of 8th and 10th graders have been conducted annually; the 8th-grade samples contain about 18,000 students in about 150 schools, and the 10th-grade samples contain about 17,000 students in about 140 schools. Beginning with the class of 1976, a randomly selected sample from each senior class has been followed-up every other year after high school on a continuing basis. These respondents receive a mail questionnaire at their home, which they complete and return to MTF. The data from students are collected during the spring of each year. Each year's data collection of about 50,000 students takes place in approximately 420 public and private high schools and middle schools selected to provide an accurate representative cross-section of students throughout the coterminous United States at each grade level. The MTF uses a three-stage random sampling procedure: in the first stage geographic areas within the United States are randomly selected, followed by the selection (with probability proportionate to size) of one or more schools in each geographic area in the second stage, and in the third stage, classes are selected for each school. In schools with fewer than 350 students, all students may be selected to participate. In larger schools, a subset of students is selected by randomly sampling entire classrooms. The MTF biannual questionnaires are administered in classrooms during a normal class period. Follow-up questionnaires are mailed to respondents with a return self-addressed, stamped envelope and a small monetary remuneration.

National Monitoring of Adolescent Prescription Stimulants

N-MAPSS was initiated in 2008 to detect current levels of nonmedical use of prescription stimulants among preteens and adolescents. A detailed description of methods of the N-MAPSS has been published elsewhere (Cottler, Striley, & Lasopa, 2013). N-MAPSS utilized the entertainment venue intercept method to comprehensively and inclusively reach youth where they were likely to be to achieve representativeness, accomplished by sending recruiter interviewers to carefully selected venues (shopping malls, movie theaters, sports and recreation centers, libraries, arcades, skate parks, and parks) to locate a diverse and representative sample of youth. Eligibility criteria for the N-MAPSS include youth aged 10 to 18 years of age residing in specific urban, suburban, or rural

ZIP codes from one of the following 10 cities across the United States: Boston, New York City; Philadelphia; Tampa, Florida; Cincinnati, Ohio; Houston, Texas; Saint Louis, Missouri; Denver, Colorado; Los Angeles; and Seattle, Washington. Recruiter interviewers approached youth at the venues. The N-MAPSS research team adapted survey questions from the Substance Abuse Module and the Washington University Risk Behavior Assessment on quantity and frequency, route of administration, reasons, and source of use. The 20-min assessment, conducted in private, was divided into two parts. After Part 1 was completed, mostly on demographics and dosage and pill recognition, respondents completed Part 2, in which information on lifetime and last 30-day use of a variety of pre-scription stimulants as well as other licit and illicit substances was assessed. The study was carried out in four cross sections of data collection—the waves were fall 2008, spring 2009, fall 2010 and spring 2011—and therefore marijuana use data for this period is covered in this chapter.

PREVALENCE OF MARIJUANA USE

Lifetime Prevalence

Lifetime prevalence refers to use of marijuana at least once in the respondent's lifetime, which also includes use of marijuana in the past 30 days and past 12 months. Lifetime prevalence of marijuana has limited utility as a measure-ment indicator of the level of marijuana use in the population and, as such, is not commonly reported in the extant literature. However, it must be noted that when past 30-day or past 12-month use rates are reported as a dichotomous variable, persons who used in their lifetime but did not in the past 30 days are categorized as nonusers.

ADOLESCENTS

Table 1.1 displays the lifetime prevalence of marijuana use by two different use groups: adolescents 12 to 17 years of age and adults 18 years of age and older. In 2014, according to data from the NSDUH (Center for Behavioral Health Statistics and Quality, 2015), the prevalence of lifetime marijuana use was 16.4% in adolescents. Among this age group, the rates were similar for males (16.7%) and females (16.2%). By racial/ethnic status, the rate was highest among American Indians or Alaskan Natives (23.7%) and lowest among Asians (7.7%). When considering geographic region, the rates were highest in the West (18.8%) and lowest in Midwest (15.6%) and the South (15.3%).

ADULTS

In 2014, approximately 47.1% of adults 18 years of age and older reported ever using marijuana in their lifetime, according to the NSDUH survey (Table 1.1). The rates were higher among males (53.1%) than for females (41.4%). By ra-cial/ethnic status, the prevalence rate was highest among American Indians or

Table 1.1 LIFETIME PREVALENCE OF MARIJUANA USE AMONG ADOLESCENTS AND ADULTS, BY SELECTED DEMOGRAPHIC CHARACTERISTICS—NATIONAL SURVEY ON DRUG USE AND HEALTH 2014: UNITED STATES

Characteristics	12 to 17 Years of Age (%; 95 CI)	18 Years of Age and Older (%; 95 CI)
Overall	16.4 (15.6–17.2)	47.1 (46.4–47.8)
GENDER		
Male	16.7 (15.7–17.7)	53.1 (52.1–54.1)
Female	16.2 (15.2–17.2)	41.4 (40.5–42.3)
RACE/ETHNICITY		
Non-Hispanic White	16.1 (15.1–17.1)	52.1 (51.2–52.9)
Black or African American	17.9 (15.9–19.9)	45.7 (43.8–47.6)
Asian	7.7 (5.2–10.2)	18.7 (16.2–21.3)
American Indian or Alaskan Native	23.7 (15.2–32.2)	57.8 (49.9–65.2)
Native Hawaiian or Other Pacific Islander[a]		52.9 (42.3–63.5)
Hispanic	18.0 (16.3–19.7)	34.4 (32.7–36.1)
EDUCATION		
< High school	N/A	36.1 (34.2–37.9)
High School Graduate	N/A	45.5 (44.4–46.7)
Some College	N/A	52.5 (51.3–53.7)
College Graduate	N/A	48.6 (47.3–49.9)
CURRENT EMPLOYMENT		
Full-Time	N/A	53.3 (52.4–54.2)
Part-Time	N/A	49.4 (47.7–51.1)
Unemployed	N/A	56.5 (53.9–59.1)
Other	N/A	34.3 (33.0–35.6)
GEOGRAPHIC DIVISION		
Northeast	16.3 (14.7–17.9)	49.7 (48.1–51.3)
Midwest	15.6 (14.1–17.1)	49.0 (47.5–50.5)
South	15.3 (14.1–16.5)	43.7 (42.6–44.8)
West	18.8 (16.9–20.6)	48.8 (47.1–50.5)

NOTE: Based on response to the question: "How long has it been since you last used marijuana or hashish?" Responses of "within the past 30 days" were classified as "yes." CI = confidence interval. N/A = not applicable. Data from Center for Behavioral Health Statistics and Quality (2015).

[a]Low precision; no estimate reported.

Alaska Natives (57.8%) followed by Non-Hispanic, Whites (52.1%) and Native Hawaiians or Other Pacific Islanders (52.9%), Blacks or African Americans (45.7%), and Hispanics (34.4%); Asians had the lowest rate (18.7%). Across educational attainment, adults who had some college education had the highest rate (52.5%), followed by those who were college graduates (48.6%); those with less than a high school education had the lowest rate (36.1%). By employment status, the rates were higher among those who were unemployed (56.5%) compared to those with a full-time job (53.3%). The pattern of rates across geographic region of the United States indicates that the rates were highest among adults residing in the Northeast (49.7%) and Midwest (49.0%).

Past 12-Month Prevalence

Past 12-month prevalence estimates indicate use of marijuana in the 12 months prior to the interview, and therefore this indicator of use also includes respondents who used marijuana in the 30 days prior to the interview.

ADOLESCENTS

Among adolescents 12 to 17 years of age in the United States, past 12-month prevalence of marijuana use in 2014 was 13.1%, according to data from the NSDUH (Table 1.2). The rates were similar for males (13.2%) and females (13.0%), and rates were highest among American Indians and Alaskan Natives (20.2%), followed by Hispanics (14.1%). Furthermore, the rates were similar for Non-Hispanic, Whites (13.2%) and Blacks or African Americans (13.6%); Asians had the lowest rates (6.2%; Table 1.2), and those who resided in the West had the highest rate (15.9%). Across U.S. states when using estimates from 2013 and 2014, Colorado had the highest rate (20.8%), followed by the District of Columbia (19.4%).

ADULTS

Among adults 18 years of age and older, past 12-month prevalence of marijuana use was 13.3% according to the 2014 NSDUH report (Table 1.2). Males had higher rates (16.9%) than females (9.9%). The rates were highest among American Indians and Alaskan Natives (17.9%) followed by Black or African Americans (16.0%), Non-Hispanic, Whites (13.8%), and Hispanics (10.9%); Asians had the lowest rate (5.2%). The rates by educational attainment indicate that individuals who had some college degree had the highest rate (16.0%). The rates of past 12-month marijuana use was highest among those who were unemployed (24.1%) and among those who lived in the West (15.5%). By states, the rates were highest in District of Columbia (21.8%) in 2013 and 2014, followed by Colorado (20.7%) and Vermont (20.1%). Furthermore, in a recent study using data from the National Epidemiologic Survey on Alcohol and Related Conditions found past 12-month prevalence of marijuana use of 9.5% among adults 18 years of age and older in 2012–2013, which was a significant increase from the 4.1% reported in 2001–2002. The study also noted significant increases

Table 1.2 PAST 12-MONTH PREVALENCE OF MARIJUANA USE AMONG ADOLESCENTS AND ADULTS, BY SELECTED DEMOGRAPHIC CHARACTERISTICS— NATIONAL SURVEY ON DRUG USE AND HEALTH 2014: UNITED STATES

Characteristics	12 to 17 Years of Age (%; 95 CI)	18 Years of Age and Older (%; 95 CI)
Overall	13.1 (12.4–13.8)	13.3 (12.9–13.7)
GENDER		
Male	13.2 (12.3–14.1)	16.9 (16.2–17.6)
Female	13.0 (12.1–13.9)	9.9 (9.4–10.4)
RACE/ETHNICITY		
Non-Hispanic Whites	13.2 (12.3–14.1)	13.8 (13.3–14.3)
Black or African American	13.6 (11.9–15.3)	16.0 (14.8–17.2)
Asian	6.2 (3.9–8.5)	5.2 (4.1–6.3)
American Indian or Alaskan Native	20.2 (11.6–28.8)	17.9 (13.7–22.1)
Native Hawaiian or Other Pacific Islander[a]		
Hispanic	14.1 (12.6–15.6)	10.9 (9.9–11.9)
EDUCATION		
< High school	N/A	13.3 (12.2–14.4)
High School Graduate	N/A	13.3 (12.6–14.0)
Some College	N/A	16.0 (15.1–16.9)
College Graduate	N/A	10.7 (9.9–11.4)
CURRENT EMPLOYMENT		
Full-Time	N/A	13.7 (13.1–14.3)
Part-Time	N/A	18.3 (17.1–19.5)
Unemployed	N/A	24.1 (22.2–25.9)
Other	N/A	8.6 (7.9–9.3)
GEOGRAPHIC DIVISION		
Northeast	14.0 (12.5–15.5)	14.9 (13.9–15.9)
Midwest	11.8 (10.4–13.2)	12.5 (11.7–13.3)
South	11.7 (10.7–12.7)	11.5 (10.9–12.1)
West	15.9 (14.3–17.5)	15.5 (14.4–16.6)

NOTE: Based on response to the question: "How long has it been since you last used marijuana or hashish?" Responses of "within the past 30 days" were classified as "yes." CI = confidence interval. N/A = not applicable. Data from Center for Behavioral Health Statistics and Quality (2015).

[a]Low precision; no estimate reported.

in past-year prevalence when comparing 2001–2002 and 2013–2013 in several subgroups including women, blacks, Hispanics, and those residing in the South (Hasin, Wall, et al., 2015).

Past 30-Day Prevalence

Past 30-day prevalence of marijuana use has become the most frequently cited indicator of marijuana use in the United States today. NSDUH defines current marijuana use as any past-month (or past 30-day) use of marijuana. NSDUH measures current marijuana use with "How long has it been since you last used marijuana or hashish?" with response options within the past 30 days, more than 30 days but within the past 12 months, or more than 12 months ago.

ADOLESCENTS

According to data from the 2014 NSDUH report, the prevalence of past 30-day marijuana use among adolescents 12 to 17years of age was 7.4%, which was higher for males, 7.9%, than for females, 6.8% (Table 1.3). Among adolescents, by racial/ethnic status, the rate was highest among American Indian or Alaska Natives (9.4%), whereas the rate was comparable among Hispanics (7.9%), non-Hispanic whites (7.7%), and blacks or African Americans (6.9%); lowest rate was among Asians (2.5%). Finally, by geographic division, the prevalence rate of past 30-day marijuana use was highest in the West (9.7%) and Northeast (7.9%). By state, using data for 2013 and 2014, the rates were highest in Colorado (12.5%), followed by Vermont (11.4%).

ADULTS

The prevalence of past 30-day marijuana use among adults 18 years of age and older based on NSDUH data was 8.5% (Table 1.3). The rates were higher among males (11.3%) than among females (5.9%). By racial/ethnic status, the prevalence rate was highest among American Indians or Alaskan Natives (12.1%) and Native Hawaiians or Other Pacific Islanders (12.9%), followed by Blacks or African Americans (10.8%), Non-Hispanic, Whites (8.8%), and Hispanics (6.5%) whereas Asians had the lowest rate (2.8%). Adults who had some college degree had the highest rate (10.2%), and those who were college graduates had the lowest rate (5.8%). By current employment, the rate was highest among the unemployed (15.3%), followed by individuals reporting part-time employment (11.3%); the rate was 8.7% among those with full-time employment. By geographic location, the rates were highest in the West (10.3%) and lowest in the South (7.2%) and Midwest (7.8%). By state, using combined 2013 and 2014 data, the rates were again highest in Colorado (15.7%)—representing a statistically significant increase from the estimates in combined 2012 and 2013 data (12.8%, $p < 0.005$).

Table 1.3 Past 30-Day Prevalence of Marijuana Use among Adolescents
and Adults, by Selected Demographic Characteristics—National
Survey on Drug Use and Health 2014: United States

Characteristics	12 to 17 Years of Age (%; 95 CI)	18 Years of Age and Older (%; 95 CI)
Overall	7.4 (6.9–7.9)	8.5 (8.2–8.8)
GENDER		
Male	7.9 (7.1–8.7)	11.3 (10.8–11.8)
Female	6.8 (6.1–7.5)	5.9 (5.5–6.3)
RACE/ETHNICITY		
Non-Hispanic White	7.7 (6.9–8.4)	8.8 (8.4–9.2)
Black or African American	6.9 (5.6–8.2)	10.8 (9.8–11.8)
Asian	2.5 (1.1–3.9)	2.8 (2.1–3.5)
American Indian or Alaskan Native	9.4 (3.8–14.9)	12.1 (8.1–16.1)
Native Hawaiian or Other Pacific Islander[a]		12.9 (6.6–19.2)
Hispanic	7.9 (6.7–9.1)	6.5 (5.8–7.2)
EDUCATION		
< High school	N/A	9.1 (8.3–9.9)
High School Graduate	N/A	9.3 (8.7–9.9)
Some College	N/A	10.2 (9.5–10.9)
College Graduate	N/A	5.9 (5.4–6.4)
CURRENT EMPLOYMENT		
Full-Time	N/A	8.7 (8.2–9.2)
Part-Time	N/A	11.3 (10.3–12.3)
Unemployed	N/A	15.3 (13.8–16.8)
Other	N/A	5.8 (5.3–6.3)
GEOGRAPHIC DIVISION		
Northeast	7.9 (6.8–9.0)	9.6 (8.7–10.5)
Midwest	6.2 (5.3–7.1)	7.8 (7.2–8.4)
South	6.5 (5.7–7.3)	7.2 (6.7–7.7)
West	9.7 (8.3–11.1)	10.3 (9.4–11.2)

NOTES: Based on response to the question: "How long has it been since you last used marijuana or hashish?" Responses of "within the past 30 days" were classified as "yes." CI = confidence interval. N/A = not applicable. Data from Center for Behavioral Health Statistics and Quality (2015).

[a]Low precision; no estimate reported.

Comparisons of Prevalence Rates of Marijuana Use

Overall, the prevalence estimates reported in this chapter have relied heavily on data from the NSDUH, and therefore it is important to make comparisons between these estimates with data from other sources, including the YRBSS and MTF. However, the comparison of estimates of rates between NSDUH and YRBSS and MTF may not be straightforward as the methods/designs for each of these surveys differed substantially, as we previously noted. Let us examine these differences in more detail. While the NSDUH conducts yearly surveys, the YRBSS interviews respondents every other year. The MTF collects information from students in 8th, 10th, and 12th grades, and the YRBSS interviews students in the 9th through 12th grades. The NSDUH collects information from respondents 12 years of age and older. Thus, there are substantial differences in the ages covered in each survey. In addition, not all surveys collect information on all indicators of marijuana use such as frequency measures or dependence or abuse. Notwithstanding, it is still useful to compare these surveys to understand whether there are consistent patterns of marijuana use across the age groups. Here, we focus on the comparison of estimates among adolescents (or among those with an age range close to 12 to 17 years of age) as they represent those with the most similar ages covered across the three surveys. For the MTF, data on 8th and 10th graders are combined using simple average computations, and data from the YRBSS include respondents in 9th through 12th grade.

COMPARISONS FOR PAST 12-MONTH PREVALENCE
First, it is noteworthy that, historically, the rates reported in the MTF and YRBSS are higher than those in the NSDUH (e.g., Substance Abuse and Mental Health Services Administration, 2013). The overall past 12-month prevalence of marijuana use among adolescents in the MTF was 19.5%, which was substantially higher than the estimate reported by the NSDUH (13.1%; Table 1.4). Past 12-month prevalence of marijuana use was higher in males (20.1%) than in females (18.5%) in the MTF whereas the estimates reported in the NSDUH showed that the rates were similar by gender (males, 13.2; females, 13.0%). Furthermore, when comparing across racial/ethnic groups in which data are available for both surveys, both surveys suggest that the rates are highest among Hispanics (MTF, 24.3%; NSDUH, 14.1%), followed by Blacks (MTF, 21.9%; NSDUH, 13.6%; Table 1.4).

COMPARISONS FOR PAST 30-DAY PREVALENCE
The overall past 30-day prevalence of marijuana use among adolescents was 7.1%, 23.4%, and 11.5% in the NSDUH, YRBSS, and MTF respectively (Table 1.4). Once again, the rates in the YRBSS and MTF are higher than in the NSDUH. All three surveys show higher rates among males compared with females. When comparing across racial/ethnic groups in which data are available for all three surveys (i.e.,

Table 1.4 Comparisons of NSDUH, YRBSS, and MTF Past 12-Month and
Past 30-Day Prevalence of Marijuana Use among Adolescents
(12–17 Years of Age), 2014 United States

Characteristics	Past 12-Month Prevalence			Past 30-Day Prevalence		
	NSDUH	YRBSS[a]	MTF[b]	NSDUH	YRBSS[a]	MTF[b]
	%	%	%	%	%	%
Overall	13.1	–	19.5	7.1	23.4	11.5
GENDER						
Male	13.2	–	20.1	7.9	25.0	12.5
Female	13.0	–	18.5	6.2	21.9	10.8
RACE/ETHNICITY						
White	13.2	–	17.8	7.1	20.4	10.5
Black	13.6	–	21.9	7.4	28.9	13.4
Asian	6.2	–	–[c]	3.6	16.4	–[c]
Hispanic	14.1	–	24.3	9.1	27.6	14.2
American Indian or Alaskan Native	20.2	–	–[c]	–[d]	35.5	–[c]
Native Hawaiian or Other Pacific Islander	–[d]	–	–[c]	7.2	23.4	–[c]

NOTES: NSDUH = National Survey on Drug Use and Health. YRBSS = Youth Risk Behavior Surveillance System. MTF = Monitoring the Future.

[a]Includes data from 2013 among adolescents in grades 9 through 12 (Kann et al., 2014).

[b]Data for respondents in grades 8 and 10 combined using simple averages (Johnston et al., 2014).

[c]Estimates not reported in the MTF.

[d]Low precision; estimate not provided.

Whites, Blacks and Hispanics), estimates from the MTF and NSDUH show that the rates are highest among Hispanic adolescents (MTF, 14.2%; NSDUH, 9.1%), whereas the rates are highest among blacks or African American adolescents in the YRBSS (28.9%). However, all three surveys indicate that non-Hispanic white adolescents have the lowest rates (MTF, 10.5%; NSDUH, 7.1%; YRBSS, 20.4%). Furthermore, as shown in Table 1.5, estimates from the N-MAPSS survey of adolescents 12 to 17 years of age also corroborates data from the MTF and NSDUH in which Hispanics had the highest rates of past 30-day marijuana use, although the data presented for the N-MAPSS was collected in 2011. In addition, the rates from N-MAPSS were slightly higher for Non-Hispanic, Whites (18.7%) than for Blacks or African Americans (17.2%).

Table 1.5 PREVALENCE OF PAST 30-DAY MARIJUANA USE AMONG ADOLESCENTS
BY SELECTED DEMOGRAPHIC CHARACTERISTICS: NATIONAL MONITORING
OF ADOLESCENT PRESCRIPTION STIMULANTS STUDY 2011: UNITED STATES

Characteristics	12 to 17 Years of Age (%; 95 CI)
Overall	18.0 (16.4–20.0)
GENDER	
Male	22.2 (19.6–24.8)
Female	14.4 (12.4–16.4)
RACE/ETHNICITY	
Non-Hispanic White	18.7 (16.0–21.4)
Black or African American	17.2 (13.8–20.6)
Asian	8.9 (4.7–13.1)
Hispanic	20.7 (16.9–24.6)
Other[a]	19.8 (14.9–24.8)
GEOGRAPHIC DIVISION[b]	
Northeast	20.1 (17.0–23.3)
Midwest	12.6 (9.7–15.5)
South	13.7 (10.3–17.0)
West	24.2 (20.6–27.8)

NOTES: Based on responses to the question "In the last 30 days, how many days did you use marijuana?" CI = confidence level. Data from Cottler et al. (2013).

[a]Includes Alaskan Native/Eskimo, American Indian, Middle Eastern, Pacific Islander, and biracial or multiracial.

[b]Data include three cities in the Northeast (Philadelphia, New York City, and Boston), two cities in the Midwest (Saint Louis, Missouri, and Cincinnati, Ohio), two cities in the South (Tampa, Florida, and Houston, Texas), and three cities in the West (Los Angeles; Seattle, Washington; and Denver).

INITIATION OF MARIJUANA USE

Initiation of marijuana or new use refers to the use of marijuana for the first time. In the NSDUH, initiation estimates are based on questions about the age at first use of marijuana, year and month of first use for recent initiates (i.e., used marijuana for the first time in the past year), and the respondent's date of birth, as well as the interview date. For these estimates, respondents who are immigrants are included notwithstanding of whether their first use occurred inside or outside the United State. Table 1.6 displays the number (in thousands) and percentage of past year initiates among persons at risk for initiation (risk is defined as persons who did not use marijuana in their lifetime or used marijuana for the first time in the past year). In 2014, approximately 1.2 million adolescents

Table 1.6 PAST 12-MONTH INITIATION OF MARIJUANA USE AMONG ADOLESCENTS
AND ADULTS FROM THE NATIONAL SURVEY ON DRUG USE AND HEALTH
2014: UNITED STATES

Characteristics	Number of Past Year Initiates (in thousands)	Percentage of Past Year Initiates among Persons at Risk for Initiation[a]
Age group	N	(%; 95 CI)
Overall (12–25)	2,298	5.8 (5.4–6.2)
12–17	1,203	5.5 (5.0–5.9)
12–13	133	1.7 (1.2–2.2)
14–15	461	5.9 (5.1–6.7)
16–17	609	9.5 (8.3–10.7)
18–25	1,094	6.2 (5.5–6.9)
18–20	755	9.7 (8.4–11.0)
21–25	340	3.4 (2.8–4.0)
GENDER		
Male	1,226	1.9 (1.7–2.1)
Female	1,342	1.6 (1.5–1.7)

NOTE: CI = confidence interval. Data from Center for Behavioral Health Statistics and
Quality (2015).

[a]At risk for initiation is defined as persons who have not use marijuana in their
lifetime or used marijuana for the first time in the past year.

12 to 17 years of age used marijuana for the first time, which represents 5.5% of
adolescents at risk for initiation within the past year. Within age groups among
adolescents 12 to 17 years of age, the rate of initiation of marijuana use increased
with age, with rates of 1.7%, 5.9%, and 9.5% among children 12 to 13, 14 to 15,
and 16 to 17 years of age, respectively (Table 1.6). Among adults 18 to 25 years
of age, approximately 1 million used marijuana for the first time within the past
year, which represents 6.2% of the adults at risk for initiation. Overall, the percentage initiating marijuana for the first time in the past year by gender was similar (male, 1.9%; females, 1.6%).

Trends over Time Prevalence of Past 30-Day
Marijuana Use

To understand how rates of marijuana use may have changed in recent years,
we utilized data on past 30-day prevalence of marijuana use from the NSDUH
for the period 2002–2014. This trend in rates is displayed in Figure 1.1 for both
adolescents 12 to 17 years of age and adults 18 years of age and older. Here, the

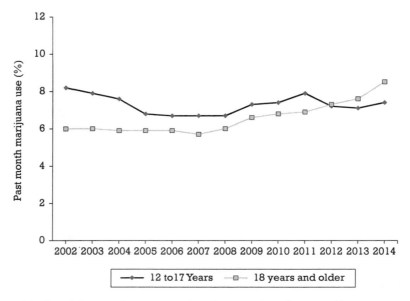

Figure 1.1 Trends in prevalence proportions for recently active cannabis use among adolescents and adults (past 30 days): National Survey on Drug Use and Health, United States, 2002 to 2014.

NOTE: Based on response to the question: "How long has it been since you last used marijuana or hashish?" Respondents indicating "within the past 30 days" were classified as "yes."

SOURCE: 2014 NSDUH: Substance Abuse And Mental Health Services Administration (United States, 2015)

trends in rates among adolescents indicate a small decline in the past 30-day prevalence of marijuana from 8.2% in 2002 to 6.7% in 2006; rates then remained steady until 2009 when prevalence increased slightly to 7.3%. However, following 2011 when the rates reached 7.9%, the rates declined modestly. Among adults aged 18 years of age and older, the rates were approximately 6% in 2002 and remained steady until 2008 when the rates began to increase modestly and consistently until 2014 when the rate reached 8.5%. Past 30-day prevalence differed by gender as shown in Figure 1.2 for adolescents and adults. Across the period examined (i.e., 2002–2014), the prevalence rate of past 30-day marijuana use was consistently higher for male than for female adolescents 12 to 17 years of age. In addition, in both male and female adolescents 12 to 17 years of age, there was a modest decline in rates from 2002 to 2006, after which the rates began to increase steadily (2007–2008 onward); this increase was slightly sharper for males than for females (Figure 1.2). Similarly, among adults 18 years of age and older, the rates were consistently higher for males than for females across the period examined, although the difference among adults 18 years of age and older was smaller than that among adolescents 12 to 17 years of age. The trend in rates across the period for both males and females of this age group remained steady from 2002 to 2007

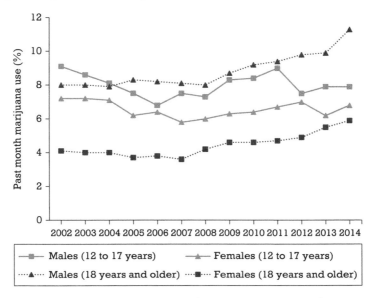

Figure 1.2 Trends in prevalence proportions for recently active cannabis use among adolescents and adults, by gender (past 30 days): National Survey on Drug Use and Health, United States: 2002 to 2014.

NOTE: Based on response to the question: "How long has it been since you last used marijuana or hashish?" Respondents indicating "within the past 30 days" were classified as "yes."

SOURCE: Data from 2014 National Survey on Drug Use and Health (United States, 2015).

and then increased steadily from 2008 to 2013. By racial/ethnic status, the trends in past 30-day marijuana use show that rates were highest among American Indians or Alaskan Natives across nearly all the period covered. From 2008 to 2009, the rates began to increase among Blacks or African Americans, Hispanics, and non-Hispanic whites; American Indians or Alaskan Natives experienced a steady rise in rates from 2011 to 2014. The rates among Asians remained steady across the period covered (Figure 1.3). Comparisons of trends in past 30-day marijuana use among adolescents across the three surveys—the NSDUH, MTF, and N-MAPSS—during the period 2002–2014 are displayed in Figure 1.4. The trends indicate a modest decline in use rates from 2002 to 2008 in both the NSDUH and MTF (data for these periods were not available in the N-MAPSS). However, the trends indicate a small increase in use rates from 2009 onward in all three surveys.

Prevalence of Heavy Marijuana Use

Heavy marijuana use is an important measure used to describe marijuana use because simply monitoring past 12-month or past 30-day use may obscure information about those who use heavily, as heavy use has been the measure most

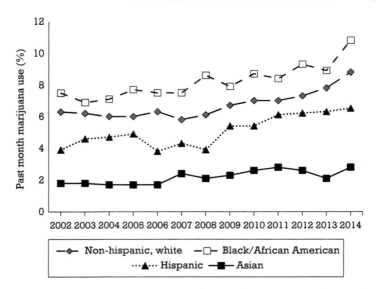

Figure 1.3 Trends in prevalence proportions for recently active cannabis use among
adults 18 years of age and older, by race/ethnicity (past 30 days): National Survey on
Drug Use and Health, United States, 2002 to 2014.
NOTE: Data on other racial/ethnic categories were not consistently reported over
the period. Based on responses to the question "How long has it been since you last
used marijuana or hashish?" Respondents indicating "within the past 30 days" were
classified as "yes."
SOURCE: Data from 2014 National Survey on Drug Use and Health (United States, 2015).

predictive of some of the deleterious health effects associated with marijuana use
(Brook, Lee, Finch, Seltzer, & Brook, 2013; Fergusson & Boden, 2008). Daily or
near-daily marijuana use is a frequently reported measure of heavy marijuana
use (Caulkins, Kilmer, Reuter, & Midgette, 2015). In the NSDUH, daily or near-
daily marijuana use is defined as using marijuana for 20 or more days in the
past 30 days. Figure 1.5 displays the trends in daily or near-daily marijuana use
among adolescents 12 to 17 years of age and adults 26 years of age and older
(estimates for adults 18 years of age are not reported). In 2014, data from the
NSDUH indicates that 21.8% of adolescents 12 to 17 years of age or approximately 400,000 who used marijuana in the past 30 days used it daily or near
daily. Overall, the trends in the rate of daily or near daily use among adolescents
have remained relatively consistent since 2007, until 2014 when there was a nearly
4% decline. However, across the same time period, the rates of heavy use among
adults 26 years of age and older have increased: from 30% in 2002 to 43.0% in
2014 (Figure 1.5). Furthermore, Caulkins et al. (2016), using NSDUH data, recently showed that heavy marijuana use in adults 18 years of age and older has
increased since 1992 and that there are about seven times as many heavy marijuana users in 2013 as there were in 1992 (Caulkins, Kilmer, & Kleiman, 2016).

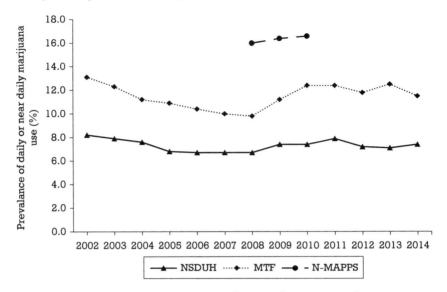

Figure 1.4 Trends in prevalence proportions for recently active cannabis use among adolescents in the United States (past 12 months), based on National Surveys on Drug Use and Health (NSDUH), Monitoring the Future (MTF), and National Monitoring of Adolescent Prescription Stimulant Study (N-MAPSS) in the United States: 2002 to 2014.

NOTE: Data from NSDUH estimates based on responses to the question about recency of use "How long has it been since you last used marijuana or hashish?" Respondents indicating "within the past 12 months" were classified as past-year users. MTF estimates are based on response to the question "During the past 12-months, on how many occasions (if any) have you used marijuana?" Respondents indicating "1 to 2 occasions or more" were classified as past-year users.

SOURCE: Data from United States (2015), Johnston et al. (2014), and Cottler et al. (2013).

Prevalence of Marijuana Abuse and Dependence

Marijuana abuse, as defined by the *Diagnostic and Statistical Manual of Mental Disorders*, fourth edition (DSM–IV; American Psychiatric Association, 1994) is defined as repeated use of marijuana under hazardous conditions in addition to a maladaptive pattern of use leading to clinically significant impairment or distress in social, occupational, or educational functioning and legal problems at any time in the same 12-month period. Marijuana dependence in the DSM–IV is defined as a pattern of use associated with increased tolerance and compulsive use despite the physical and psychological problems caused by it use. NSDUH asked questions about symptoms consistent with the DSM–IV if respondents indicated marijuana use six or more days in the past 12 months. In 2014, data from NSDUH showed that 20% of adolescents 12 to 17 years of age who were past 12-month users met criteria for a marijuana abuse or dependence (Figure 1.6). Among adults 18 to 25 years of age, prevalence of marijuana abuse or dependence

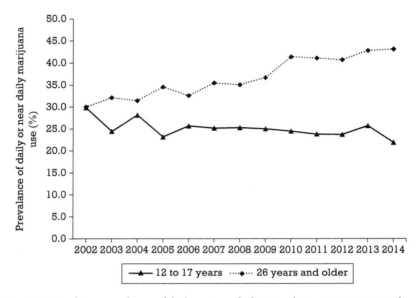

Figure 1.5 Trends in prevalence of daily or near daily cannabis use among recently active cannabis users (past 30 days), by age group: National Survey on Drug Use and Health, United States, 2002 to 2014.
NOTE: Daily or near daily used defined as use for 20 or more days in the past 30 days.
SOURCE: Data from United States (2015).

in the past 12 months was lower (15.2%). Figure 1.6 indicates that from 2002 to 2014, the rates of marijuana abuse or dependence were higher among adolescents 12 to 17 years of age than among adults 18 to 25 years of age and older. The overall trend suggests that the rates of marijuana abuse or dependence declined in both age groups: from 27% in 2002 to 20% in 2014 among adolescents aged 12 to 17 years of age and from 20% in 2002 to 15% in 2014 among adults 18 to 25 years of age. Here, we focus on presenting estimates of a marijuana abuse or disorder among users as it can be misleading to discuss use disorders among persons who have never used. To underscore this point, a recent study using data from National Epidemiologic Survey on Alcohol and Related Conditions found that the overall prevalence of a marijuana use disorder (either abuse or dependence) among adults 18 years and older doubled from 1.5% in 2001–2002 to 2.9% in 2012–2013. However, prevalence of a marijuana use disorder among marijuana users decreased significantly from 2001–2002 (35.6%) to 2012–2013 (30.6%; Hasin, Wall, et al., 2015), consistent with data reported here from the NSDUH.

Medical Marijuana Use

As of mid-2016 when this chapter was written, 25 U.S. states and the District of Columbia had passed medical marijuana legislation, with other states considering

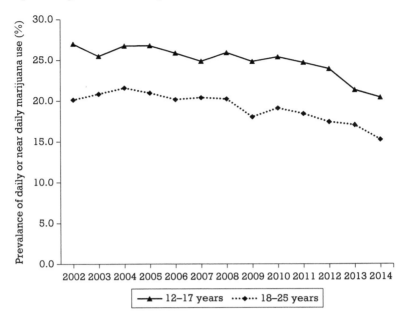

Figure 1.6 Trends in prevalence proportions for cannabis use disorders found among recently active cannabis users (past 12 months), by age group: National Surveys on Drug Use and Health, United States, 2002 to 2014.
NOTE: Cannabis use disorder assessment is based on definitions found in the fourth edition of the *Diagnostic and Statistical Manual of Mental Disorders* (American Psychiatric Association, 1994).
SOURCE: Data United States (2015).

such legislation. While the medical marijuana legislations vary substantially by state (Bestrashniy & Winters, 2015), all contain provisions that allow the medical use of marijuana in patients with qualifying clinical conditions, despite the U.S. Drug Enforcement Agency's current classification of marijuana as an illegal Schedule 1 substance. Under this classification, marijuana is regarded as having no acceptable medicinal use with a high potential for addiction with long-term use.

California was the first U.S. state to have passed a proposition (in 1996) allowing for the medical use of marijuana. In a recent study that utilized the California Behavioral Risk Factor Surveillance System, medical marijuana use was defined as use for a serious health condition. Overall, the study found that approximately 5% of adults in California reported ever using medical marijuana. Prevalence of medical marijuana use was highest among those 18 to 24 years old (9.3%) and lowest among those 65 years of age or more (2%). Also, prevalence was higher among males (5.7%) than among females (4.6%) and higher among non-Hispanic whites (7.4%) than African Americans (5.1%), Asians, (4.1%), and Hispanics or Latinx (3.3%). In addition, prevalence of use was higher among those with a high school diploma or GED (6.6%) than those with less education (5.4%) and those with at least some college (4.6%). Finally, the most commonly reported reasons for medical marijuana use were chronic pain (31%), followed by arthritis (11%), migraines (8%), and cancer (7%).

Attitudes and Perceptions toward Marijuana Use

The recent changes in state laws allowing the use of marijuana for medical and recreational reasons may suggest that such shifts may play a role in influencing adolescent's attitudes and perceptions of harm related to marijuana use, which may lead to increased rates of marijuana use among adolescents. The data examining the issue of attitude changes have produced mixed findings. In a recent report of youths in California's Monitoring the Future Survey, between 2012 and 2013, 12th graders in California as compared to 12th graders in other states were 20% less likely to perceive that regular marijuana use was a great health risk and 20% less likely to strongly disapprove of regular marijuana use (Miech et al., 2015). Another report that examined changes in attitudes of marijuana use among American youths found a significant increase in the proportion of adolescents 12 to 14 years of age reporting "strong disapproval" of marijuana use initiation over the past decade (74.4% in 2002 to 78.9% in 2013; Salas-Wright, Vaughn, Todic, Córdova, & Perron, 2015). In addition, among adolescents 15 to 17 years of age, Salas-Wright et al. found that, between 2002 and 2008, the proportion reporting disapproval increased from 49.4% in 2002 to 55.6% in 2008, but decreased thereafter to 49.9% disapproval in 2013. Two states that recently passed recreational laws—Washington and Colorado—were the focus of a recent analysis (Cerdá et al., 2017). Among 8th and 10th graders, perceived harmfulness of marijuana use decreased, and marijuana use increased following legalization of recreational marijuana use in Washington; in contrast, Colorado students in these grades did not exhibit any differential change in perceived harmfulness or past-month adolescent marijuana use following legalization. College students have also received research attention on this topic. Among the seven large public universities located in states that passed legal recreational marijuana prior to 2015 and that participated in the national Healthy Minds Survey, rates of marijuana use increased from pre- to post-2015 at six of the seven universities, a trend that was significant overall (Kerr et al., 2017).

What about changes in marijuana use among youth in the context of state medical marijuana laws? Whether such laws are associated with increased rates of marijuana use in adolescents in the United States is a topic of ongoing debate in the research community. A myriad of studies have been published supporting medical marijuana legalization as a risk factor for increased adolescent marijuana use (Cerdá, Wall, Keyes, Galea, & Hasin, 2012; Wen, Hockenberry, & Cummings, 2015). Other studies either indicate no effect (Anderson, Hansen, & Rees, 2015; Lynne-Landsman, Livingston, & Wagenaar, 2013) or a decrease in rates of adolescent marijuana use following passing state medical marijuana laws (Harper, Strumpf, & Kaufman, 2012). However, a recent study utilizing a large sample of over 1 million adolescents from the Monitoring the Future Survey from over 48 U.S. states across 24 years (1991–2014) represents the strongest evidence regarding this topic (Hasin, Wall, et al., 2015). Although the authors found that states that had ever passed a medical marijuana law up to the year 2014 had higher rates of adolescent marijuana use (particularly among 12th graders), they found no evidence that the rates increased after state medical marijuana laws were passed. Interestingly, the study also found a decrease in rates of marijuana use among 8th graders in states that had passed a medical marijuana law.

CONCLUDING REMARKS AND IMPLICATIONS

In this chapter, we have described recent epidemiologic trends in marijuana use among U.S. adolescents and adults. Data from large national surveys conducted in the United States on rates of marijuana use have documented trends in marijuana use. Based on the most rigorous survey of nation trends across all age groups (NSDUH), the data indicate increases in past 30-day prevalence among adults 18 years of age and older in recent years, whereas the rates among adolescents 12 to17 years of age have remained steady. Heavy marijuana use (defined as daily or near-daily use) among past 30-day users increased in recent years, with adults 26 years of age and older experiencing the sharpest rate of increases. Prevalence of marijuana abuse or dependence among adolescents and adults examined in this chapter has remained relatively steady. These data provide insights into subgroups of the population in which interventions to prevent, delay, or reduce marijuana use may need to focus. These data also underscore the importance of continued monitoring of rates of marijuana use especially at a time of state policy shifts regarding legalization of marijuana for medical or recreational purposes. However, it is important to note that the data used in this chapter rely heavily on national surveys, which may sometimes belie local trends. This is important given that marijuana policy experimentation is occurring at the local/state level, and therefore data on rates of marijuana use collected at the local level are needed. Also, the impact of policy shifts on behavior may not occur right away, and thus extant data may not reflect subsequent trends.

ACKNOWLEDGMENTS

This chapter was prepared grants from the National Institute of Health, National Institute on Drug Abuse awards RO1-DA20791 and T32DA035167 to L. B Cottler and F31DA03981 to Chukwuemeka Okafor. The National Monitoring of Adolescent of Adolescent Prescription Stimulants Study (N-MAPSS) was implemented by Washington University in St. Louis and the University of Florida under contract from Pinney Associates, Inc., with funding provided by Shire Development LLC and Noven Therapeutics. The content of this chapter is solely the responsibility of the authors and does not necessarily represent the views of the National Institute of Health.

REFERENCES

American Psychiatric Association. (1994). *Diagnostic and statistical manual of mental disorders* (4th ed.). Washington, DC: Author.

Anderson, D. M., Hansen, B., & Rees, D. I. (2015). Medical marijuana laws and teen marijuana use. *American Law and Economics Review, 17*, 495–528. http://dx.doi.org/10.1093/aler/ahv002

Bestrashniy, J., & Winters, K. C. (2015). Variability in medical marijuana laws in the United States. *Psychology of Addictive Behaviors, 29*, 639–642. http://dx.doi.org/10.1037/adb0000111

Caulkins, J. P., Kilmer, B., & Kleiman, M. (2016). *Marijuana legalization: What everyone needs to know.* Oxford: Oxford University Press.

Caulkins, J. P., Kilmer, B., Reuter, P. H., & Midgette, G. (2015). Cocaine's fall and marijuana's rise: Questions and insights based on new estimates of consumption and expenditures in US drug markets. *Addiction, 110*, 728–736. http://dx.doi.org/10.1111/add.12628

Center for Behavioral Health Statistics and Quality. (2015). *Behavioral health trends in the United States: Results from the 2014 National Survey on Drug Use and Health.* HHS Publication No. SMA 15-4927, NSDUH Series H-50. Rockville, MD: Author. Retrieved from https://www.samhsa.gov/data/sites/default/files/NSDUH-FRR1-2014/NSDUH-FRR1-2014.pdf

Cerdá, M., Wall, M., Feng, T., Keyes, K. M., Sarvet, A., Schulenberg, J., . . . & Hasin, D. S. (2016). Association of state recreational marijuana laws with adolescent marijuana use. *JAMA Pediatrics, 171*, 142–149. http://dx.doi.org/10.1001/jamapediatrics.2016.3624

Cerdá, M., Wall, M., Keyes, K. M., Galea, S., & Hasin, D. (2012). Medical marijuana laws in 50 states: Investigating the relationship between state legalization of medical marijuana and marijuana use, abuse and dependence. *Drug and Alcohol Dependence, 120*(1–3), 22–27. http://dx.doi.org/10.1016/j.drugalcdep.2011.06.011

Compton, W. M., Weiss, S. R. B., & Wargo, E. M. (in press). Introduction. In K. Sabet & K. C. Winters (Eds.), *Contemporary health issues on marijuana.* New York: Oxford University Press.

Cottler, L. B., Striley, C. W., & Lasopa, S. O. (2013). Assessing prescription stimulant use, misuse, and diversion among youth 10–18 years of age. *Current Opinion in Psychiatry, 26*, 511–519. http://dx.doi.org/10.1097/YCO.0b013e3283642cb6

Devane, W. A., Dysarz, F. A., Johnson, M. R., Melvin, L. S., & Howlett, A. C. (1988). Determination and characterization of a cannabinoid receptor in rat brain. *Molecular Pharmacology, 34*, 605–613.

ElSohly, M. A., & Slade, D. (2005). Chemical constituents of marijuana: The complex mixture of natural cannabinoids. *Life Sciences, 78*, 539–548. http://dx.doi.org/10.1016/j.lfs.2005.09.011

Fergusson, D. M., & Boden, J. M. (2008). Cannabis use and later life outcomes. *Addiction, 103*, 969–976; discussion: 977–978. http://dx.doi.org/10.1111/j.1360-0443.2008.02221.x

Galiègue, S., Mary, S., Marchand, J., Dussossoy, D., Carrière, D., Carayon, P., . . . Casellas, P. (1995). Expression of central and peripheral cannabinoid receptors in human immune tissues and leukocyte subpopulations. *European Journal of Biochemistry, 232*, 54–61.

Gaoni, Y., & Mechoulam, R. (1964). Isolation, structure, and partial synthesis of an active constituent of hashish. *Journal of the American Chemical Society, 86*, 1646–1647. http://dx.doi.org/10.1021/ja01062a046

Glass, M., Dragunow, M., & Faull, R. L. (1997). Cannabinoid receptors in the human brain: a detailed anatomical and quantitative autoradiographic study in the fetal, neonatal and adult human brain. *Neuroscience, 77*, 299–318.

Government of Canada. (2012). *Alcohol and Drug Use Monitoring Survey*. Retrieved from https://www.canada.ca/en/health-canada/services/health-concerns/drug-prevention-treatment/canadian-alcohol-drug-use-monitoring-survey.html

Harper, S., Strumpf, E. C., & Kaufman, J. S. (2012). Do medical marijuana laws increase marijuana use? Replication study and extension. *Annals of Epidemiology, 22*, 207–212. http://dx.doi.org/10.1016/j.annepidem.2011.12.002

Hasin. D. S., Saha, T. D., Kerridge, B. T., et al. (2015). Prevalence of marijuana use disorders in the United States between 2001–2002 and 2012–2013. *JAMA Psychiatry, 72*, 1235–1242. http://dx.doi.org/10.1001/jamapsychiatry.2015.1858

Hasin, D. S., Wall, M., Keyes, K. M., Cerdá, M., Schulenberg, J., O'Malley, P. M., . . . Feng, T. (2015). Medical marijuana laws and adolescent marijuana use in the USA from 1991 to 2014: Results from annual, repeated cross-sectional surveys. *The Lancet Psychiatry, 2*, 601–608. http://dx.doi.org/10.1016/S2215-0366(15)00217-5

Herkenham, M., Lynn, A. B., Little, M. D., Johnson, M. R., Melvin, L. S., Costa, B. R. de, & Rice, K. C. (1990). Cannabinoid receptor localization in brain. *Proceedings of the National Academy of Sciences, 87*, 1932–1936.

Johnston, L. D., O'Malley, P. M., Bachman, J. G., Schulenberg, J. E., & Miech, R. A. (2014). *Monitoring the Future national survey results on drug use, 1975–2013: Vol. 1. Secondary school students*. Ann Arbor: Institute for Social Research, University of Michigan.

Kann, L., Kinchen, S., Shanklin, S. L., Flint, K. H., Hawkins, J., Harris, W. A., . . . & Whittle, L. (2014). Youth Risk Behavior Surveillance—United States, 2013. *Morbidity and Mortality Weekly Report*, 63(Suppl. 4): 1–168.

Kerr, D. C., Bae, H., Phibbs, S., & Kern, A. C. (2017). Changes in undergraduates' marijuana, heavy alcohol, and cigarette use following legalization of recreational marijuana use in Oregon. *Addiction, 112*, 1992–2001. http://dx.doi.org/10.1111/add.13906

Lisdahl, K. M., Gilbart, E. R., Wright, N. E., & Shollenbarger, S. (2013). Dare to delay? The impacts of adolescent alcohol and marijuana use onset on cognition, brain structure, and function. *Frontiers in Psychiatry, 4*, art. 53. http://dx.doi.org/10.3389/fpsyt.2013.00053

Lisdahl, K. M., Wright, N. E., Medina-Kirchner, C., Maple, K. E., & Shollenbarger, S. (2014). Considering cannabis: The effects of regular cannabis use on neurocognition in adolescents and young adults. *Current Addiction Reports, 1*, 144–156. http://dx.doi.org/10.1007/s40429-014-0019-6

Lynne-Landsman, S. D., Livingston, M. D., & Wagenaar, A. C. (2013). Effects of state medical marijuana laws on adolescent marijuana use. *American Journal of Public Health, 103*, 1500–1506. http://dx.doi.org/10.2105/AJPH.2012.301117

Mechoulam, R., & Gaoni, Y. (1967). The absolute configuration of delta-1-tetrahydrocannabinol, the major active constituent of hashish. *Tetrahedron Letters, 12*, 1109–1111.

Mechoulam, R., & Shvo, Y. (1963). Hashish—I : The structure of cannabidiol. *Tetrahedron, 19*, 2073–2078. http://dx.doi.org/10.1016/0040-4020(63)85022-X

Miech, R. A., Johnston, L., O'Malley, P. M., Bachman, J. G., Schulenberg, J., & Patrick, M. E. (2015). Trends in use of marijuana and attitudes toward marijuana among youth before and after decriminalization: The case of California 2007–2013. *International Journal on Drug Policy, 26*, 336–344. http://dx.doi.org/10.1016/j.drugpo.2015.01.009

Morgan, C. J. A., Schafer, G., Freeman, T. P., & Curran, H. V. (2010). Impact of cannabidiol on the acute memory and psychotomimetic effects of smoked cannabis: Naturalistic study: Naturalistic study [corrected]. *British Journal of Psychiatry: Journal of Mental Science, 197*, 285–290. http://dx.doi.org/10.1192/bjp.bp.110.077503

Munro, S., Thomas, K. L., & Abu-Shaar, M. (1993). Molecular characterization of a peripheral receptor for cannabinoids. *Nature, 365*(6441), 61–65. http://dx.doi.org/10.1038/365061a0

Pacher, P., & Mechoulam, R. (2011). Is lipid signaling through cannabinoid 2 receptors part of a protective system? *Progress in Lipid Research, 50*, 193–211. http://dx.doi.org/10.1016/j.plipres.2011.01.001

Rom, S., & Persidsky, Y. (2013). Cannabinoid receptor 2: Potential role in immunomodulation and neuroinflammation. *Journal of Neuroimmune Pharmacology, 8*, 608–620. http://dx.doi.org/10.1007/s11481-013-9445-9

Salas-Wright, C. P., Vaughn, M. G., Todic, J., Córdova, D., & Perron, B. E. (2015). Trends in the disapproval and use of marijuana among adolescents and young adults in the United States: 2002–2013. *American Journal of Drug and Alcohol Abuse, 41*, 392–404. http://dx.doi.org/10.3109/00952990.2015.1049493

Schuster, R. M., Gilman, J., & Eden, A. E. (in press). Effects of adolescent cannabis use on brain structure and function: Current findings and recommendations for future research. In K. Sabet & K. Winters (Eds.), *Contemporary health issues on marijuana.* New York: Oxford University Press.

Substance Abuse and Mental Health Services Administration. (2013). *Results from the 2012 National Survey on Drug Use and Health: Summary of national findings.* NSDUH Series H-46, HHS Publication No. (SMA) 13-4795. Rockville, MD: Author.

Volkow, N. D., Baler, R. D., Compton, W. M., & Weiss, S. R. B. (2014). Adverse health effects of marijuana use. *New England Journal of Medicine, 370*, 2219–2227. http://dx.doi.org/10.1056/NEJMra1402309

Volkow, N. D., Wang, G.-J., Telang, F., Fowler, J. S., Alexoff, D., Logan, J., . . . Tomasi, D. (2014). Decreased dopamine brain reactivity in marijuana abusers is associated with negative emotionality and addiction severity. *Proceedings of the National Academy of Sciences, 111*, E3149–E3156. http://dx.doi.org/10.1073/pnas.1411228111

Wen, H., Hockenberry, J. M., & Cummings, J. R. (2015). The effect of medical marijuana laws on adolescent and adult use of marijuana, alcohol, and other substances. *Journal of Health Economics, 42*, 64–80. http://dx.doi.org/10.1016/j.j healeco.2015.03.007

2

International Trends in Cannabis Use

JAMES C. ANTHONY, OMAYMA ALSHAARAWY, AND
CATALINA LOPEZ-QUINTERO

INTRODUCTION

We organized this chapter with an introduction, three main sections, and concluding remarks. The introduction covers several recently reported international trends pertinent to cannabis, which are based upon official statistics submitted by individual countries in response to requests from the United Nations (UN). While covering UN statistics, we address several issues of concept and methods for epidemiological research on cannabis use.

After the introduction, we provide a section of background information intended to be useful to students writing dissertations and other scholars in the field. Readers of this section will gain an appreciation for the work of pioneers, some of whom started thinking about international mental health and behavioral contrasts and trends almost 200 years ago.

Our chapter's second section provides a first approximation of a grand global tour of cannabis smoking estimates and trends, all based on systematic epidemiological surveys of general populations in various countries of the world. We begin with estimates from Canada and other nations of the western hemisphere before a turn toward other regions for which survey-based trend estimates are available.

In the chapter's third main section, we provide an overview of some international trends pertinent to the possibility of a narrowing of the male–female difference in risk of becoming a cannabis user in recent years. This kind of narrowing has been observed in trend estimates for risk of starting to drink alcoholic beverages, as well as for prevalence of drinking alcohol (Cheng, Cantave, & Anthony, 2016). We evaluate whether the same narrowing might be seen in trend estimates for cannabis use, based on multiple repeated surveys of 15- and 16-year-old school-attending teenagers in each of the many countries that participate in the European School Survey Project on Alcohol and Other Drugs (ESPAD), with a comparison to United States estimates from the Monitoring the Future surveys of high school students.

In our concluding remarks for the chapter, we offer some suggestions about future directions in research on cannabis use. We also offer some specifications for future country-level reports of epidemiological survey results, borrowing heavily from prior recommendations made for reports of country-level statistics on mental and behavioral health and including some elements required for meta-analyses and trend analyses of the type attempted in this chapter. Finally, we provide some details on the creation of something akin to an International Cannabis Products Safety Commission, given widespread concern about hazards of cannabis use, about which we now have no truly useful monitoring of international trends.

THE TERM *CANNABIS*

An introductory note on this chapter's use of the term *cannabis* may be in order. Our bibliographic search of the global scientific literature disclosed a clear preference for *marijuana* in the United States literature, with *marihuana* preferred in some of the other western hemisphere countries. Nonetheless, *cannabis* is generally used in the international literature and in articles written by scientists in many other countries of the world. In our view, *cannabis* is the scientific term. As such, we use it to encourage a scientific frame of reference that can be distinguished from the more political or policy-laden frame of reference that historically has been offered by the U.S. Bureau of Narcotics and Dangerous Drugs and by the current Drug Enforcement Administration in the United States.

UN OFFICE ON DRUGS AND CRIME

Before turning to our section on background and historical roots, we should clarify that the United Nations Office on Drugs and Crime has published a series of annual monographs known as the *World Drug Report* (UN; WDR), from which an official statistics view of international cannabis trends can be gained. Each year's WDR typically offers a view of trends of cannabis herb seizures as reported to the agency in recent years, in the form of country-specific maps of recent trends from 2009 through 2010 and in the form of a region-specific graphs from 2003 through 2013. In these maps and estimated trends, some of the evidence shows generally increasing number of metric tons of herbal cannabis products seized, as can be distinguished from other cannabis products in the global market, for which separate estimates could be generated (e.g., resin or oil such as hash oil, synthetic cannabinoid receptor agonists).

Although the information value of these country-specific official seizure reports must be acknowledged as an important element in comprehensive understanding of cannabis epidemiology, there also is a clear element of subjectivity. At the end of the day, the record of cannabis seizures is separately determined by each country and is entirely dependent upon details such as whether the police officer is following a policy of random stops or nonrandom stops of pedestrians or vehicles or something else. Classification of a cannabis seizure as wholesale or as retail remains uncertain (e.g., see Manski et al., 2001). The result is a mosaic of information, each piece of which deserves more careful scrutiny than might be apparent in estimated trends of this type. Fortunately, each WDR now includes a self-critique section with notes to help the reader evaluate of the validity of the statistics.

Table 2.1, based entirely on the WDR, shifts perspective from official reports of trend data on increases and reductions in product seizures in the direction of a perspective on actual consumption or use of cannabis products. As shown in the table, for the past 10 years or so, there seems to have been a relative stability in the prevalence of being a recently active user of cannabis products, both globally and for individual regions of the world, notwithstanding what can be seen in the ups and downs of official seizures.

Consider the first rows of Table 2.1, where *recent use* of cannabis refers to use in the year prior to some specified date, such as the date of a field survey assessment. As shown at the bottom of the table, the global estimate reported in the *WDR 2004* (UN, 2004) suggested that there were as many (or as few) as 146 or 147 million recently active cannabis users at that time worldwide, corresponding with a global prevalence estimate of about 3.7% of adults age 15 to 64 years old. Subsequent WDR values for 2009 (UN, 2009) and 2015 (UN, 2015) provide upper and lower bounds to depict some actual uncertainty in the size of the reported estimates.

An interesting perspective can be gained by looking at whether the global estimate published in 2004 falls outside or inside the global estimates for the later years. Table 2.1 shows that the *WDR 2004* (UN 2004) estimate of 146.3 million recently active users falls well within the lower and upper bounds of estimates presented in *WDR 2009* (UN 2009) and in *WDR 2015* (UN 2015), shown in the later global rows of this chapter's table. This observation helps substantiate the claim that official statistics show us a relatively stable international trend in global cannabis prevalence, as aggregated from each country's official reports to the agency, even though the *WDR 2015* point estimate for the number of active cannabis users worldwide is more than 182 million, which is numerically larger than the *WDR 2004* point estimate of 146 million active users. Despite the fluctuation of these point estimates, when margins of error are taken into account, it is difficult to claim a statistically robust increase in this trend in numbers of users globally.

A similar stability can be seen in Table 2.1 for the Africa estimates and the Asia estimates. In contrast, estimates for the Americas suggest a trend of increasing prevalence, whereas declines are suggested for Europe and Oceania.

VALIDITY OF DATA

Here again we must draw attention to open questions about the validity of these official statistics, as reported to the UN from each country. In some countries,

Table 2.1 YEAR- AND REGION-SPECIFIC ESTIMATES FOR PREVALENCE (%) AND
NUMBER OF RECENTLY ACTIVE CANNABIS USERS (PAST YEAR), 2004, 2009, AND 2015

Region	Year	Estimated Prevalence of Recently Active Cannabis Users		Bound Estimate (in Millions)	
		%	N (in Millions)	Lower	Upper
Oceania	2004	16.4	3.4	N.R.	N.R.
Africa	2004	7.7	34.6	N.R.	N.R.
Americas	2004	6.3	34.9	N.R.	N.R.
North America	2004	10.3	28.5	N.R.	N.R.
South America	2004	2.4	6.5	N.R.	N.R.
Europe	2004	5.3	28.8	N.R.	N.R.
West Europe	2004	6.7	20.4	N.R.	N.R.
East Europe	2004	3.6	8.4	N.R.	N.R.
Asia	2004	1.9	44.7	N.R.	N.R.
Global	2004	3.7	146.3	N.R.	N.R.
Oceania	2009	N.R.	N.R.	2,460	2,570
Africa	2009	N.R.	N.R.	28,850	56,390
Americas[a]	2009	N.R.	N.R.	41,450	42,080
North America	2009	N.R.	N.R.	31,260	31,260
South America	2009	N.R.	N.R.	8,500	8,510
Rest of Americas	2009	N.R.	N.R.	1,690	2,310
Europe[b]	2009	N.R.	N.R.	28,890	29,660
West/Central Europe	2009	N.R.	N.R.	20,810	20,940
East/SE Europe	2009	N.R.	N.R.	8,080	8,720
Asia	2009	N.R.	N.R.	40,930	59,570
Global	2009	N.R.	N.R.	142,580	190,270
Oceania	2015	10.7	2.65	2,220	3,570
Africa	2015	7.5	45.8	20,380	59,120
Americas	2015	8.4	54.2	53,510	55,620
North America	2015	11.6	36.7	36,470	36,870
South America	2015	5.9	16.1	16,010	16,050
Rest of Americas	2015	2.5	1.5	1,030	2,700
Europe	2015	4.3	23.7	22,980	24,380
West/Central Europe	2015	5.7	18.4	18,330	18,460
East/SE Europe	2015	2.3	5.3	4,650	5,920
Asia	2015	1.9	55.5	29,390	89,380
Global	2015	3.9	181.8	128,480	232,070

[a] North and South Americas were listed as subregions in 2004, while other parts of Americas were added for the 2009 and 2015 World Drug Reports.

[b] Subregions of Europe were re-specified after 2004, with new labels as shown here.

NOTE: N.R. = not reported.

SOURCES: United Nations Office of Drugs and Crime (2004, 2009, 2015).

official statistics are based on formal epidemiological field surveys with nationally representative samples, as illustrated in the chapter's next section. In other countries, the statistics are from interviews with small snowball samples, respondent driven samples, or rapid assessment approaches, yielding estimates that are distinguished more by their practicality and cost-efficiency than by metrics of established validity.

At this point in the chapter, it might be useful to clarify that prevalence of being a recently active user often refers to having used the drug within some defined interval of time, often specified to be one year. Prevalence is not at all the same as incidence, by which we mean the appearance of first-time cannabis users in a given population as time passes.

Regrettably, even when it is based upon rigorous epidemiological field research approaches, the prevalence proportion estimated in this fashion is one that hides the relative contribution of (a) the incidence rate for becoming a newly incident cannabis user (for the first time) and (b) the duration of cannabis use once it starts. Why is this situation regrettable? The answer can be traced to an epidemiological principle about prevalence estimates, according to which a prevalence estimate always will vary as a function of (a) incidence rate for a disease or for a behavioral condition such as cannabis use and (b) the duration of the disease or other condition. Consequently, for any region with increasing prevalence of a disease, the rising prevalence might be due to an increase in healthcare access and the benefit of life-saving therapies, which might affect duration in various ways, perhaps shortening the condition via cure or extending its duration via reduced case fatality rates; there may be no contribution whatsoever from an increasing or declining risk of becoming a case of the disease. Or, where health services are deteriorating, and when the life-saving therapies for a disease are withdrawn, there can be a reduction in prevalence of the condition simply because the people affected are not living as long as they once lived (i.e., case fatality rates have increased). Consequently, whenever we see an increasing prevalence of cannabis use in a region (e.g., in the Americas), it might be due to an increasing duration of each cannabis user's smoking history, even when never-users show no increasing risk of starting to use cannabis. Alternately, there might be increasing risk of never-users starting to use cannabis, with no change in duration of use. Of course, other possibilities exist, making it very difficult to make a definitive interpretation of trends in prevalence estimates of cannabis use, except when the two complementary trends are shown (i.e., the incidence rate trend and the trend in duration of use). A recent contribution by Parker and Anthony (2015) may be of interest to chapter readers interested in technical details (e.g., how to derive estimates of duration when estimates of both incidence rates and prevalence proportions are available).

Epidemiological principles such as these should prompt scientists to look more closely at estimates of the risk of becoming a newly incident case of disease (given no prior history of the disease), or in this case, the risk of becoming a newly incident user of cannabis, given no prior or past history of cannabis use. We have no good international trend data on the incidence rates for becoming a cannabis user, but we have some first approximations from the World Mental Health Surveys (WMHS) completed in the early 21st century. The WMHS program asked community participants in multiple countries to state when they had started to use cannabis. By combining these retrospective onset ages with each participant's birth year, it has become possible to visualize the pattern of age-specific increasing incidence or risk of becoming a cannabis user in multiple countries, generally with a low incidence rate before adolescence, increasing rates during the adolescent and young adult years, followed by a return to low incidence values in middle-to-late adulthood, when risk of starting to use cannabis is quite low, if not zero. Estimates of this type have been presented by Degenhardt and our WMHS colleagues, in a series of tables and graphs that convey a clear increase in risk of starting cannabis use, birth cohort by birth cohort, and country by country, for individuals born before 1990 (Degenhardt et al., 2008). The estimates suggest a generalizable period effect; the increased incidence in cannabis use from 1965 through 1990 does not appear to be specific to any cohorts born prior to 1945.

A note about a useful epidemiological estimator of this type may be useful at this point in our introduction. Sometimes erroneously called *lifetime prevalence* by individuals without graduate or postgraduate training in epidemiology, a commonly presented epidemiological estimator actually is a cumulative incidence proportion (CIP) in that it is affected by the incidence rate for a condition but is unaffected by the duration of the condition. The error in using the name *lifetime prevalence* can be seen by noting that this particular estimator is unaffected by the duration of the condition, and, as noted in an earlier paragraph of this introduction, the basic epidemiological principle is that a prevalence estimate is determined by both an incidence rate and a condition's duration. As such, lifetime prevalence as an epidemiological estimator does not meet the standard specifications for a prevalence proportion in epidemiology (e.g., see Streiner et al., 2009).

When we are conducting epidemiological research on nonfatal conditions, such as cannabis smoking, it is clear that the lifetime history of becoming, being, or having become a cannabis user is essentially unaffected by the duration of cannabis use. For the CIP as an estimate, we start with a denominator that consists of all persons in a population or population subgroup (e.g., all persons 12 years old and older, all persons 12–64 years old, all persons 15–70 years old, etc.), none of whom have self-administered cannabis at birth, but some of whom start cannabis self-administration in childhood, in adolescence, or (more typically) in the young to middle adult years. Age by age, working forward from birth, as cannabis use starts, an increasing number of the never-users start to use cannabis and carry this history of cannabis use forward with them, even if they used only one time and then stopped using. In analyses of retrospective cannabis data from cross-sectional surveys, it becomes possible to form an age-specific incidence rate by counting the number of never-users of a given age at the start of a year and by counting up how many of the never-users start to use cannabis by the end of the year. By dividing the number of newly incident users by the number of never-users at the start of the interval, we obtain an initial guess/estimation of the annual incidence rate for that age group. Refinements in the annual incidence rate sometimes can be made using a person-months formulation of the rate. In this refinement, there is a counting up the number of months of each individual's never-use during the year, with a stopping point as soon as an individual starts to use. This count of person-months is then substituted as the denominator for the rate, in place of the count of never-users at the start of the year. An intermediate approximation is to base the denominator on the number of never-users as observed as of the midpoint date of the year.

The concept of a CIP builds from the idea of the annual incidence rate. The difference involves the numerator of the proportion. Whereas the annual incidence rate is based on the count of newly incident cannabis users in a given year or time interval, the cumulative incidence keeps counting people who have tried cannabis, even once, irrespective of whether there is persistence of use. Applying the concept to 12-year-olds observed in the population as of a cross-sectional survey assessment date, the denominator for this proportion is the total number of 12-year-olds, irrespective of their past history of cannabis use, and the numerator for the proportion is based on counting up the number of 12-year-olds who have tried cannabis, even once, by the date of the survey assessment. The result is an age-specific estimate for the CIP for cannabis use as derived from a cross-sectional survey.

Finally, consider the total population of all ages surveyed in research on drug use and health, which often has a lower bound such as age 12 years or age 15 years and sometimes has an upper bound of age 54 years, 64 years, or 65 years. The CIP for that population would be formed with a denominator consisting of all persons of the stated age range, and the numerator would be the count of individuals who had tried cannabis, even once, as of the date of survey assessment. The international trend estimates presented in the next section of this chapter have this form. They are not age-specific CIPs. Rather, they are estimated CIPs for cannabis use (with use on at least one occasion), as experienced by the country's total population in the age range under study, generally with data gathering via standardized retrospective self-report survey questions in a questionnaire or interview.

We conclude this introduction by leaving the chapter reader with a general sense that international trends in prevalence of cannabis use show a general stability, but in some regions of the world, there might well be declining trends in the prevalence of cannabis use. Whether these declining prevalence trends can be traced back to reduced incidence rates for becoming a cannabis user in the first place is uncertain. The declines might be due to reduced duration of cannabis use, once it starts. Indeed, the documented increase in relative delta-9-tetrahydrocannabinol (THC) concentration of cannabis products, with corresponding reductions in cannabidiol compound concentrations, might be provoking early adverse (e.g., dysphoric) responses to first cannabis use. One result might well be a shortened duration of use because some first-time users might decide they never want to try the drug again (United Nations, 2009, 2015).

If so, cannabis prevalence estimates might be dropping due to reduced duration of cannabis use once it has started rather than being attributable to reductions in the incidence of starting to use cannabis in the first place. Moreover, the WDR time series data or trend estimates for the prevalence of being a cannabis user will not resolve this uncertainty. What is needed is a time series or set of trend estimates for incidence rates (i.e., becoming a cannabis user for the first time as time passes). At present, we have no statistically valid or precise estimates for these international trend parameters in cannabis epidemiology, except as will be presented in the next section's CIPs.

Before turning to historical background, it might be useful to note that the UN Office of Drugs and Crime is highly self-critical of the shortcomings in its estimates. Each UN report on this topic acknowledges conceptual and method-ological deficiencies in the official country statistics. These deficiencies stretch from A to Z, with A standing for variations in the source of the evidence, and Z standing for variations in statistical methods for estimation of upper and lower bound confidence intervals (CIs). In terms of variations in the source of the evidence, some of the country reports are based on key informant in-formation with no empirical epidemiological estimates available, whereas other countries produce estimates via well-constructed population surveys. In terms of variations in statistical methods, some country reports provide de-tailed information that can be used to derive margins of errors. Other country reports provide insufficient information to gauge margins of error. It is to the credit of the UN Office on Crime and Drugs that it includes this self-criticism in each of its reports. Quite clearly, the UN officials are aware that countries do not always apply World Health Organization (WHO) guidelines developed and refined as described in the next section of this chapter.

EARLY EVOLUTION OF INTERNATIONAL RESEARCH ON MENTAL HEALTH AND DRUGS ISSUES

Writing this chapter in 2015, as we looked backward and forward with an eye toward epidemiology's evidence about international trends, we found interna-tional comparisons that appear the early-mid 19th century work of William Farr (b. 1807–d. 1883). Farr was the father of vital statistics and an original thinker in our field. Farr, as registrar-general for England and Wales, combined med-ical and sociological ideas with his solid foundation of training in statistics. The results were excellent analyses of birth and death records in England and Wales, based largely on the life table form of survival analysis developed by Edmund Halley of comet fame.

Farr imagined a time when it might be possible to make valid international comparisons and to study trends in his areas of interest, which encompassed social inequalities, suicide death rates, and the well-being and survivorship of the mentally ill (Whitehead, 2000). Farr was a visionary who saw that occupa-tional exposures and social status might influence mortality risks, but his work includes no contemplation of health issues pertinent to the use of psychotropic drugs beyond what was known about alcohol. Nonetheless, Farr realized that valid international comparisons were out of reach due to inconsistencies in the way each country's leaders conceptualized, gathered information, analyzed, and reported their results (Farr, 1885).

Morton Kramer (b. 1914–d. 1998) was Farr's mid-late 20th century successor in the specific area of mental health statistics. Kramer launched the first US National Institute of Mental Health (NIMH) epidemiology and biostatistics research initiatives and led these initiatives for almost 30 years, with detailed planning of a series of NIMH Epidemiologic Catchment Area surveys later described by Eaton and Kessler (1985). Kramer's work demonstrates an abiding interest in cross-national comparisons and trends. We think that Kramer should be acknowledged as the first public health scientist to think through problems that we face when making within-country or cross-national comparisons about trends in the use of psychotropic drugs (Kramer, 1957). Kramer's disciplined approach to these comparisons can be seen in several publications, including recommendations for standardization of mental health indicators used in international contrasts, as conceptualized more than 30 years ago (Kramer, 1969; Kramer & Anthony, 1983).

Other concurrent developments along these lines included monographs and guidelines specific to the study of alcohol and other drugs, authored by WHO-affiliated public health scientists of note. For example, the late Patrick Hughes (b. 1934–d. 2010) was lead author for a WHO report entitled "Core Data for Epidemiological Studies of Nonmedical Drug Use" (Hughes et al., 1980), which built from his community-based participatory outreach and intervention experiences as a public health psychiatrist during heroin epidemic years of the late 1960s and 1970s in US inner city communities of Chicago (Hughes & Crawford, 1972). Lead authors for other contributions to the WHO monograph series of the early 1980s included Irving Rootman and Lloyd D. Johnston, as well Reginald Smart (Rootman & Hughes, 1980; Smart et al., 1980). Readers who wish to study a developmental trace of epidemiology's methods and approaches from those early years through to the present time can turn to a UN publication that includes two interesting overview articles, one by Sloboda and Kozel (2003) and the other by Hickman and colleagues (Hickman et al., 2003), each with complementary coverage of drug use and drug problems research. A bibliographic search of works citing these 2003 contributions shows some forward progress, including new applications of mathematical models intended to overcome some of the uncertainties of field survey data (e.g., Orwa, 2014).

A FIRST APPROXIMATION FOR A GLOBAL GRAND TOUR OF CANNABIS TRENDS

This section presents epidemiological field survey estimates for specific countries of the world, starting with Canada and other nations of the western hemisphere.

The result is somewhat of a different picture than was seen in the UN official statistics for world regions. As one might imagine, considerably more variation can be seen within individual countries of a region. Often, the impression of overall stability of a trend line for a region can be due to a mixture of (a) rising numbers of cannabis users in some countries of the region, (b) declining numbers in other countries of that same region, and (c) some countries with stable estimates.

To be included in this overview, we required a minimum of three country-wide general population survey (GPS) estimates from the country, all with data gathering within a span of time from the mid-1990s through the early years of the present decade, with a focus on the (lifetime) cumulative incidence of using cannabis at least one time in any form and either with an analysis-weighted 95% confidence interval, or some indication of each survey's sample size so that we were able to impute a standard error for each estimate, as explained elsewhere (Vselevoloskaya & Anthony, 2014). Most of the time, the form of cannabis used was herbal cannabis. In most countries, there was a stable age range under study, such as the national population age 12 years and older or those age 15 to 64 years, and a single point estimate has been reported for the entire age range; exceptions are noted.

Appreciating that some chapter readers might wish to be able to characterize each country with a single estimate, along with a 95% CI for use as a margin of error in the estimate, we provide a meta-analytic summary (MAS) estimate. This MAS estimate borrows information from each individual country estimate, year by year, with more weight given to years with larger sample sizes. The MAS estimate has greatest utility in countries with quite a bit of stability in the across-year trends. Nonetheless, as shown with various examples in the following discussion, the MAS estimate can be useful even when the estimates show upward or downward trends.

We are hesitant to endorse cross-country comparison of the MAS estimates at this time because too little is known about the comparability of methods used each country's general population surveys. For example, in the United States, there has been relative stability in the survey methods each year since 2004, and there is a strong tradition of federal government research. In addition, the mode of survey assessment is that of audio-enhanced computerized self-interview, such that the assessment of cannabis and other drug use was known to the participant and recorded via the laptop, but no one else was involved. That is, in the US surveys, there is no need for the probabilistically drawn participant to tell a field staff interviewer whether cannabis has been used. No one is watching while the participant sits at the laptop computer and uses the keyboard to answer the survey questions after seeing each item on the laptop screen and listening to the audio soundtrack via headphones. Even in the highly standardized WMHS research described in the chapter's introduction, some countries have used a paper-and-pencil interview with the interviewer reading the items and marking answers spoken aloud, while computers were used in other countries. Intercountry methods variations of this type almost certainly account for some of the variations in observed estimates, within countries across time, and for any between-country comparisons. Nevertheless, we believe these epidemiological trend estimates can be useful as first approximations.

In Figure 2.1, the estimates for Canada's (lifetime) CIP show a pattern of modest steady decline across recent years. A CIP estimate as large as 45% was seen among those age 15 years and older in 2004. In 2011, the corresponding estimate is at the 38% to 39% level. With information borrowed across of the estimates shown, the meta-analysis summary estimate is 42%, and the MAS 95% confidence interval, CI is [41%, 44%]. Readers who wish to make between-country MAS comparisons should study these MAS 95% CI, which reflect margins of error in the survey estimates as best we could derive them from the survey reports. A rule of thumb is that we should not use a difference or ratio of point estimates to declare that one country's estimate is larger or smaller than another country's point estimate. Rather, for one generally trustworthy approach, it is possible to check whether the 95% CI overlap. When this first approximation shows no CI overlap whatsoever, there is a basis for drawing attention to a possible difference of substantive importance.

In Figure 2.2, the corresponding US CIP estimates for persons age 15 years and older are not appreciably different from those just presented for the other North American residents living in Canada. Applying the rule of thumb about margins of error, the US MAS estimate is 43.2% with 95% CI from 42.3% to 44.0%—that is, with considerable overlap of US and Canada 95% CIs and statistically indistinguishable summary estimates with respect to this epidemiological measure of cannabis experience. As for trends over time, there is an indication of a possible increasing CIP estimate from 2011 to 2012. Here again, non-overlapping 95%

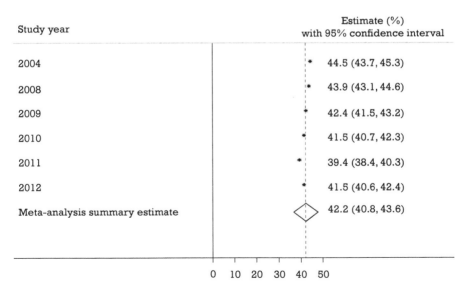

Figure 2.1 Canada: Cumulative occurrence (%) of cannabis use among 15+ year olds.
SOURCE: Data from Health Canada (2012).

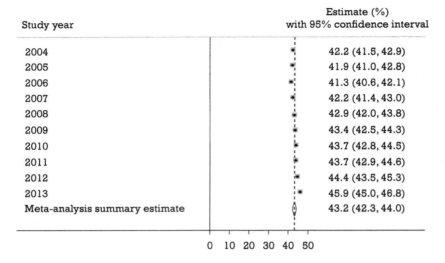

Study year	Estimate (%) with 95% confidence interval
2004	42.2 (41.5, 42.9)
2005	41.9 (41.0, 42.8)
2006	41.3 (40.6, 42.1)
2007	42.2 (41.4, 43.0)
2008	42.9 (42.0, 43.8)
2009	43.4 (42.5, 44.3)
2010	43.7 (42.8, 44.5)
2011	43.7 (42.9, 44.6)
2012	44.4 (43.5, 45.3)
2013	45.9 (45.0, 46.8)
Meta-analysis summary estimate	43.2 (42.3, 44.0)

0 10 20 30 40 50

Figure 2.2 United States: Cumulative occurrence (%) of cannabis use among 15+ year olds. SOURCE: Data from United States (2015).

CI can be seen for CIP estimates in those two successive years. The most recent estimates of annual incidence rates provide a similar indication that risk of becoming a newly incident cannabis use might be increasing in the United States for adolescent subgroups of the population (Lipari et al., 2017).

The US southern border is shared with Mexico's northern border, but as shown in Figure 2.3, unless the survey-based estimates are terrible approximations, the population of Mexico age 12 to 65 years is much less likely than their US

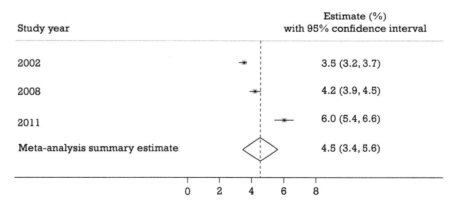

Study year	Estimate (%) with 95% confidence interval
2002	3.5 (3.2, 3.7)
2008	4.2 (3.9, 4.5)
2011	6.0 (5.4, 6.6)
Meta-analysis summary estimate	4.5 (3.4, 5.6)

0   2   4   6   8

Figure 2.3 Mexico. Cumulative occurrence (%) of cannabis use among 12 to 65 year olds.
SOURCE: Villatoro et al. (2012); Instituto Nacional de Psiquiatría Ramón de la Fuente Muñiz; Instituto Nacional de Salud Pública; Secretaría de Salud. Encuesta Nacional de Adicciones (2012).

counterparts to have any experience with cannabis smoking. For the three years depicted in the figure, there appears to be an increasing CIP, from 3.5% in 2002 to 6% in 2011, with no overlap in 95% CI. The MAS estimate is 4%, 95% CI [3.8%, 4.2%].

In the background is a process of migration into and back out of the United States from Mexico, with an underlying theory that migrants might experience cannabis acculturation processes during the intervals of labor visits to the United States. Initial suggestions in support of the theory can be seen in study estimates for Mexico's cannabis CIP from the WMHS of 18- to 65-year-olds in 2001–2002. The Mexico WMHS survey offered cannabis CIP estimates slightly larger than those seen in the Mexico Addiction National Survey and were suggestive of the following pattern: 18% CIP for those who had worked in the United States but were residing in Mexico at that time of the survey, 8.8% CIP for Mexico-residing family members of those who had worked in the United States, and 5.8% for others in Mexico (Borges et al., 2007). Here, the margins of error are indicative of substantively important variations, and the implications stretch toward issues of increasing international tourism and labor migration as might affect cannabis trends in the future. These implications are important not only with respect to the United States and Mexico, but also with respect to other countries experiencing population displacements from countries observed in official statistics to have relatively lower cannabis CIP (e.g., Iraq, Syria) to countries observed to have higher cannabis CIP (e.g., Germany).

Many countries of the western hemisphere are missing in this first approximation of a global tour due to lack of a time series of estimates from general population surveys (GPS). Nonetheless, Costa Rica, midway between Mexico and Colombia of South America, has completed its GPS of 12- to 70-year-olds in 2001, 2006, and 2010, as shown in Figure 2.4. Trend stability is seen between 2006 and 2010, and the MAS estimate for cannabis CIP is 6.7%, with effective 95% CI from 5.5% to 8.0%, more or less robustly above the corresponding estimates for Mexico but well below the CIP estimates for Canada and the United States.

For Colombia, the cannabis CIP estimates are based on three GPSs conducted in 1996 through 2013, with slightly varying denominators (ages 18–60 years until 2008; ages 18–65 in 2013). The GPS cannabis CIP estimates show incrementally increasing trends of population experience with cannabis, each estimate being robustly different from the MAS CIP estimate of 8%, 95% CI [5.2%, 11.4%], and from each other, as gauged by non-overlap of 95% CI (Figure 2.5). Colombia and Costa Rica do not share a border. Nonetheless, the Colombia population's increasing trend is in contrast with Costa Rica's generally stable trend. The most recent estimate for Costa Rica is roughly one half the estimate seen for Colombia in 2013.

Looking southward along the western Pacific coast of South America, the next set of trend estimates is from the Republic of Peru, where GPS from 1998 through 2006 covered 12- to 64-year-olds; in contrast, the 2010 GPS age range was 18 to 65 years. The later estimates are robustly smaller than the earlier estimates, which suggests a declining cannabis CIP trend for Peru over this span of time (Figure

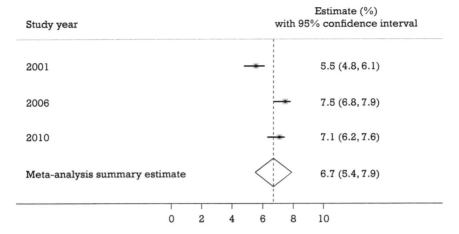

Figure 2.4 Costa Rica. Cumulative occurrence (%) of cannabis among 12 to 70 year old. SOURCE: Data from Instituto sobre Alcoholismo y Farmacodependencia (2001, 2006, 2010).

2.6). Peru's MAS estimate is on a par with the corresponding estimates for Mexico and Costa Rica, at 4.5% (95% CI 3.7%, 5.3%), and is roughly one half the estimate for Colombia, but in this comparison there is an overlap of the 95% CI.

Chile is next in the North–South sequence along the western Pacific coast. Based on successive GPS of 12- to 64-year-olds, Chile's meta-analysis summary estimate for cannabis CIP is 22%, 95% CI [19%, 25%], based on gently increasing

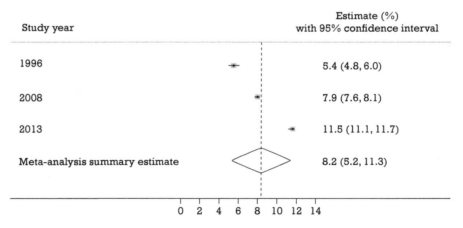

Figure 2.5 Colombia: Cumulative occurrence (%) of cannabis use. The survey in 1996 included individuals 18 to 60 years old, and the 2008 and 2013 surveys included individuals 18 to 65 years old.
SOURCE: Data from Rodríguez Ospina (1997), Ministerio del Interior y de Justicia, Ministerio de la Protección Social, Dirección Nacional de Estupefacientes (2009), and Ministerio de Justicia y del Derecho, Observatorio de Drogas de Colombia, Ministerio de Salud y Protección Social (2013).

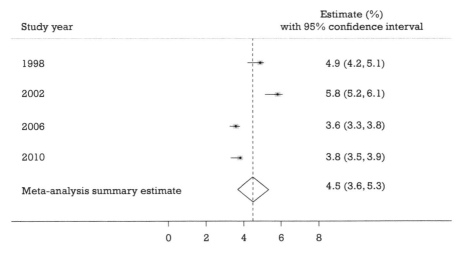

Figure 2.6 Peru: Cumulative occurrence (%) of cannabis use. The surveys between 1998 to 2006 included individuals 12 to 64 years old, and the survey in 2010 included individuals 12 to 65 years old.
SOURCE: Data from Comisión Nacional para el Desarrollo y Vida sin Drogas, DEVIDA. (2002; 2006; 2010).

estimates across the span of years from 1994 through 2012 (Figure 2.7). It is noteworthy that the cannabis CIP estimates for 2010 to 2012 are lower than corresponding estimates for 2006 to 2008, even with margins of error taken into account. But note that the estimate for 2014 is 31.5%, 95% CI [30.9%, 31.8%], signifying a recent larger cannabis CIP estimate than any of the others seen in the western hemisphere south of the United States. It will be interesting to see whether future estimates for Chile show sustained increases in the direction of the estimates for the United States and Canada.

Argentina shares a long border with Chile along the southern extension of the generally traffic-blocking Andean mountain range. Argentina's GPS surveys of 16- to 65-year-olds indicate a very stable trend, with all but one cannabis CIP estimate between 7% and 10% and with overlapping 95% CI (Figure 2.8). The exception, a value greater than 16% in 2006, suggests a possible artifact; the lower 95% CI value of 15.6% for the 2006 estimate is larger than the MAS upper 95% CI of 14.6%. Under these circumstances, given much lower estimates before and after 2006, the possibility of regression upon the mean deserves consideration, and substantive interpretation of the 2006 CIP estimate is difficult from this distance. The Argentina MAS estimate for cannabis CIP is 10.7%, 95% CI [7.1%, 14.1%], not appreciably different from the corresponding estimate for Colombia but about one half the MAS estimate for neighboring Chile.

Uruguay produced GPS estimates for its population 12- to 65-years-old from 2001 through 2014 in a manifestation of a statistically robust increasing trend of cannabis CIP values (Figure 2.9). Uruguay's experience deserves special attention,

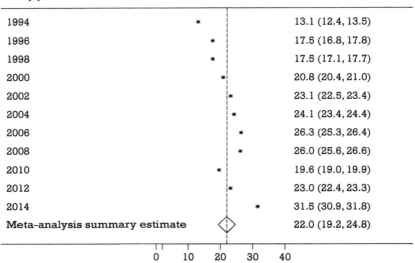

Figure 2.7 Chile: Cumulative occurrence (%) of cannabis use among 12 to 64 year olds.
SOURCE: Data from Ministerio del Interior y Seguridad Pública, Servicio Nacional para la Prevención y Rehabilitación del Consumo de Drogas y Alcohol, and Observatorio Chileno de Drogas (2015).

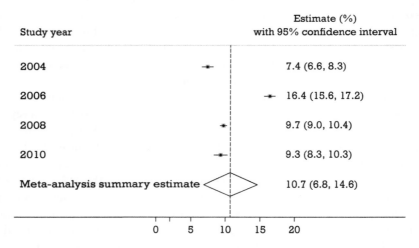

Figure 2.8 Argentina: Cumulative occurrence (%) of cannabis use among 15 to 65 year olds.
SOURCE: Observatorio Argentino de Drogas, Instituto Nacional de Estadística y Censos (2004, 2006, 2008, 2010).

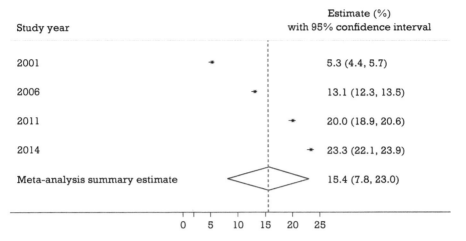

Study year	Estimate (%) with 95% confidence interval
2001	5.3 (4.4, 5.7)
2006	13.1 (12.3, 13.5)
2011	20.0 (18.9, 20.6)
2014	23.3 (22.1, 23.9)
Meta-analysis summary estimate	15.4 (7.8, 23.0)

Figure 2.9 Uruguay: Cumulative occurrence (%) of cannabis use among 15 to 65 year olds.
SOURCE: Data from Junta Nacional de Drogas, Secretaría Nacional de Drogas, and Programa de Naciones Unidas para el Desarrollo (2001). Junta Nacional de Drogas, Secretaría Nacional de Drogas, Observatorio Uruguayo de Drogas, La Oficina de Naciones Unidas Contra las Drogas y el Delito, and La Comisión Interamericana para el Control del Abuso de Drogas (2007), Junta Nacional de Drogas, Secretaría Nacional de Drogas, and Observatorio Uruguayo de Drogas (2011, 2015).

given its recent relaxation of cannabis regulations. Taking differences between successive CIP estimates, we can derive a sense of trends before cannabis policy was relaxed. Differences of 7% to 8% are seen for each of the five-year spans from 2001 to 2006 and from 2006 to 2011, from which a mean annual increasing incidence of 1.5% can be seen. The corresponding value based on the difference of estimates across the three-year span from 2011 and 2014 is close to 1.1% per year. That is, cannabis incidence rates appear to have been accelerating across the decade prior to announcements that Uruguay's cannabis policy would be relaxed. We look forward to comparable estimates from 2016 and beyond, which can be used to make comparisons with the pre-change acceleration observed in Uruguay's trend estimates from the past.

The situation in Uruguay raises several serious problems faced when there is an attempt to evaluate effects of cannabis policy changes. First, it is possible that the societal movement toward policy relaxation is as important or more important than the date of policy change. Second, measurement of cannabis incidence via self-report survey methods can mean that the population is more willing to report its true cannabis experiences when the perceived hazard of being identified as a cannabis user is relaxed. The self-report-measured trend might not be the same as the true trend that one might discover by taking saliva specimens and using bioassay results to quantify cannabis use. Third, the reliance on bioassay generally means that the estimator is a prevalence estimator rather than an incidence estimator, given that affordable saliva tests for cannabinoids detect recent use but not when cannabis use started. Consequently, bioassays make it difficult to tell whether the policy affects persistence of cannabis use among already established users or whether its effect might be seen in a shift of the cannabis incidence rates.

In Figure 2.10, our first approximation of a global tour moves from the western hemisphere across the Atlantic Ocean for a view of an interpretable series survey estimates for Scotland, Ireland, and Northern Ireland and the United Kingdom (exclusive of Scotland and Ireland). Here we see estimates for Scotland, with somewhat of an increase in cannabis CIP from earlier values of 2003–2004, but with relatively stable estimates from 2005 through 2013. The MAS CIP estimate for Scotland is 26%, 95% CI [24%, 29%].

Figure 2.11 shows estimates for Ireland and Northern Ireland across the span from 2002–2003 through 2010–2011, with a statistically robust increasing trend of cannabis CIP estimates toward 25%, 95% CI [24%, 26.5%]. The MAS CIP estimate is 21.5%, 95% CI [17.0%, 26.1%].

In estimates for the United Kingdom (England and Wales, excluding Northern Ireland and Scotland), as shown in Figure 2.12, the GPS of 16- to 59-year-olds from 2001 through 2014 suggest very stable trends in the cannabis CIP estimates, generally hovering around the MAS estimate of 30.2%, with narrow 95% CI of 29.9% to 30.6%.

Turning eastward toward continental Europe, Denmark's 16- to 64-year-old population was surveyed five times between 2000 and 2013, yielding a MAS

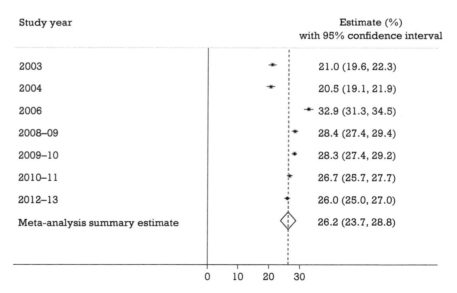

Study year		Estimate (%) with 95% confidence interval
2003		21.0 (19.6, 22.3)
2004		20.5 (19.1, 21.9)
2006		32.9 (31.3, 34.5)
2008–09		28.4 (27.4, 29.4)
2009–10		28.3 (27.4, 29.2)
2010–11		26.7 (25.7, 27.7)
2012–13		26.0 (25.0, 27.0)
Meta-analysis summary estimate		26.2 (23.7, 28.8)

0   10   20   30

Figure 2.10 Scotland: Cumulative occurrence (%) of cannabis use among 16 to 64 year olds.
SOURCE: Data from the Scottish Crime and Justice Surveys.

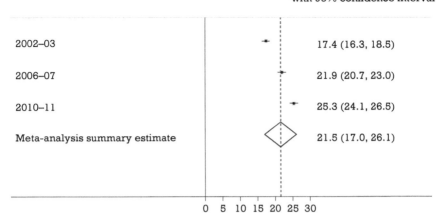

Study year	Estimate (%) with 95% confidence interval
2002–03	17.4 (16.3, 18.5)
2006–07	21.9 (20.7, 23.0)
2010–11	25.3 (24.1, 26.5)
Meta-analysis summary estimate	21.5 (17.0, 26.1)

0 5 10 15 20 25 30

Figure 2.11 Ireland: Cumulative occurrence (%) of cannabis use among 15 to 64 year olds.
SOURCE: Data from the National Advisory Committee on Drugs and Alcohol, Crime and Justice Survey, Drug Use in Ireland and Northern Ireland Surveys.

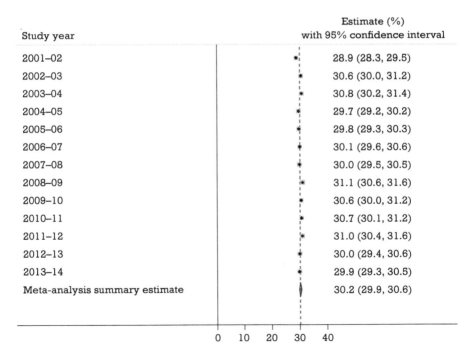

Study year	Estimate (%) with 95% confidence interval
2001–02	28.9 (28.3, 29.5)
2002–03	30.6 (30.0, 31.2)
2003–04	30.8 (30.2, 31.4)
2004–05	29.7 (29.2, 30.2)
2005–06	29.8 (29.3, 30.3)
2006–07	30.1 (29.6, 30.6)
2007–08	30.0 (29.5, 30.5)
2008–09	31.1 (30.6, 31.6)
2009–10	30.6 (30.0, 31.2)
2010–11	30.7 (30.1, 31.2)
2011–12	31.0 (30.4, 31.6)
2012–13	30.0 (29.4, 30.6)
2013–14	29.9 (29.3, 30.5)
Meta-analysis summary estimate	30.2 (29.9, 30.6)

0 10 20 30 40

Figure 2.12 United Kingdom: Cumulative occurrence (%) of cannabis use among 16 to 59 year olds.
SOURCE: Data from the Office for National Statistics, Crime Surveys for England and Wales (previously the British Crime Surveys).

cannabis CIP estimate of 34.8%, 95% CI [32.5%, 37.2%], as shown in Figure 2.13. This value is slightly larger than the just-presented estimates from the British Isles. There is statistically robust fluctuation from one year's survey to the next, but the general trend is stable, with no robust increase or decrease.

Germany's GPS population covers 18- to 64-year-olds and leaves out middle teen years that are encompassed in most of the other GPS seen in this review. It is possible that this different specification for the population coverage helps to account for an MAS cannabis CIP estimate of 23.3%, 95% CI [21.0%, 25.5%], somewhat lower than has been seen in the other countries of the European Union to this point. An increase can be seen from the 2000 GPS estimate to the 2003 GPS estimate, but thereafter, the pattern is one of a fairly stable trend (Figure 2.14).

France conducted GPS of its 15- to 64-year-old population from 1992, but the most recently available estimate is from 2010. As shown in Figure 2.15, across that span of time, there has been a steadily increasing trend in the cannabis CIP estimates, and the most recent estimate, from 2010, is 32.1%, 95% CI [31.5%, 32.7%], on a par with the corresponding 2010 GPS estimates from Denmark and for the United Kingdom (England and Wales). The MAS cannabis CIP estimate for France is 24.2%, 95% CI [18.3%, 30.1%].

Bulgaria is the only other country of Europe for which we have found at least three comparable GPS surveys that produced cannabis CIP estimates during recent years. As shown in Figure 2.16, there was a statistically robust increase in the 2008 CIP estimate (7.3%), relative to the corresponding point estimate of 5.6% from the 2007 GPS, but the trend has been stable from 2008 to 2012. The MAS cannabis

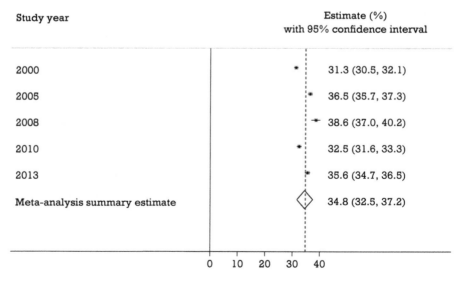

Figure 2.13 Denmark: Cumulative occurrence (%) of cannabis use among 16 to 64 year olds.
SOURCE: Data from the Danish National Institute of Public Health Surveys.

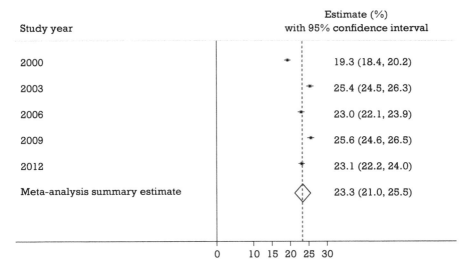

Figure 2.14 Germany: Cumulative occurrence (%) of cannabis use among 18 to 64 year olds.
SOURCE: Data from the Institute for Therapeutic Research, Munich; Federal Ministry of Health and Social Security, Epidemiological Surveys of Substance Abuse.

CIP estimate is 6.3%, 95% CI [5.0%, 7.5%], well below corresponding estimates for the other countries of Europe for which we could find suitable estimates.

Australia is the final country for which we can depict a trend of cannabis CIP estimates based on relatively stable GPS, here with a focus on the population age

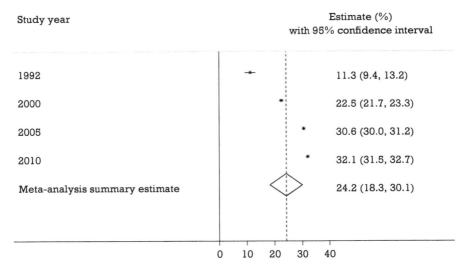

Figure 2.15 France: Cumulative occurrence (%) of cannabis use among 15 to 64 year olds.
SOURCE: Data from the National Institute for Prevention and Health Education, Health Barometer Survey.

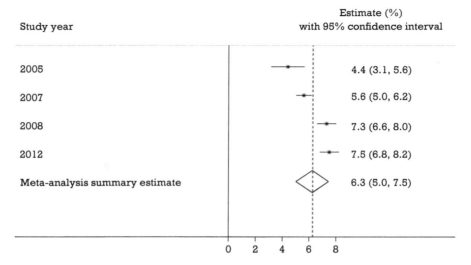

Figure 2.16 Bulgaria: Cumulative occurrence (%) of cannabis use among 15 to 64 year olds.
SOURCE: Data from the National Centre for Addictions, The National Focal Point on Drugs and Drug Addiction.

14 years and older. Figure 2.17 displays relatively stable estimates across the span from 2001 to 2013, except for a statistically robust jump from 33.5% to 35.4% as observed in the comparison of the 2007 GPS estimate and the 2010 GPS estimate. Australia's MAS cannabis CIP estimate is 34.1%, 95% CI [33.2%, 35.0%], not too distant from those seen in several of the countries of Europe but lower than values observed in Canada and the United States. We note that the MAS cannabis CIP estimate for Chile places it in the top rank order of estimates and is greater than 30%. Nevertheless, the estimate for Chile can be differentiated from Australia's MAS estimate, with no overlap of the 95% CI.

A NARROWING OF MALE–FEMALE DIFFERENCES IN CANNABIS INCIDENCE PROPORTIONS?

In our chapter introduction, we drew attention to recently published evidence on a narrowing of male–female differences in the risk of starting to drink alcohol and a female excess seen in some countries when the focus is on risk of starting to drink before mid-adolescence (Cheng et al., 2016). One of the most prominent explanations involves shifts in gender identities and gender-related social roles, as well as greater prominence of women in societal leadership roles, in part traceable to achievement of female parity in finishing secondary school and associated completion of more advanced educational objectives (Cheng & Anthony, 2017).

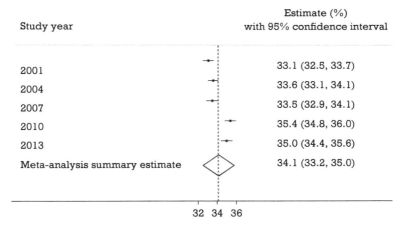

Study year	Estimate (%) with 95% confidence interval
2001	33.1 (32.5, 33.7)
2004	33.6 (33.1, 34.1)
2007	33.5 (32.9, 34.1)
2010	35.4 (34.8, 36.0)
2013	35.0 (34.4, 35.6)
Meta-analysis summary estimate	34.1 (33.2, 35.0)

32 34 36

Figure 2.17 Australia: Cumulative occurrence (%) of cannabis use among 14+ years old.
SOURCE: Data from the (2013) national survey, Australian Institute of Health and Welfare. (2014).

These explanations for a narrowed male–female gap in drinking also might apply to the male–female gap in risk of starting to smoke herbal cannabis before mid-adolescence. Accordingly, we framed a research question about male–female differences in cannabis experience and launched an exploration of these differences for this chapter. These resulting male–female difference estimates are from school surveys completed in multiple countries of Europe from 1999 through 2011, with country-specific results as presented in Figure 2.18 for field survey research completed in 2011. Table 2.2 shows the trends in the form of year-specific MAS estimates of the male–female difference in cannabis CIP.

All of this chapter's evidence about male–female differences in cannabis experience is based on reports from surveys of school-attending 15- to 16-year-olds in each participating country, completed as part of ESPAD. For this chapter, the CIP for cannabis smoking was extracted separately for males and females from each country's ESPAD report. In many instances, the ESPAD surveys were designed to yield nationally representative estimates, and there either was self-weighting or an analysis weight to take into account variation in probabilities of selection for the surveys. Nevertheless, in some countries, the population coverage was based on the most populous metropolitan areas or regions, and there was no attempt to produce a nationally representative sample.

Most ESPAD country reports include the actual number of males and females participating in the surveys, from which an approximate margin of error can be derived, with or without application of a survey design effect based on external sources of information about the degree of school-level clustering of cannabis use within schools (e.g., with a pairwise odds ratio of 1.1 to 1.9). From these extracted country-level statistics, our team differenced the sex-specific CIP and derived approximate 95% CI based on the data available to us. We then

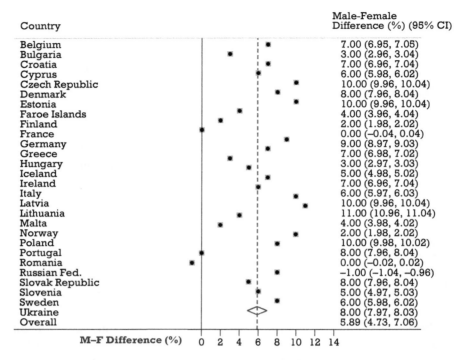

Country	Male-Female Difference (%) (95% CI)
Belgium	7.00 (6.95, 7.05)
Bulgaria	3.00 (2.96, 3.04)
Croatia	7.00 (6.96, 7.04)
Cyprus	6.00 (5.98, 6.02)
Czech Republic	10.00 (9.96, 10.04)
Denmark	8.00 (7.96, 8.04)
Estonia	10.00 (9.96, 10.04)
Faroe Islands	4.00 (3.96, 4.04)
Finland	2.00 (1.98, 2.02)
France	0.00 (−0.04, 0.04)
Germany	9.00 (8.97, 9.03)
Greece	7.00 (6.98, 7.02)
Hungary	3.00 (2.97, 3.03)
Iceland	5.00 (4.98, 5.02)
Ireland	7.00 (6.96, 7.04)
Italy	6.00 (5.97, 6.03)
Latvia	10.00 (9.96, 10.04)
Lithuania	11.00 (10.96, 11.04)
Malta	4.00 (3.98, 4.02)
Norway	2.00 (1.98, 2.02)
Poland	10.00 (9.98, 10.02)
Portugal	8.00 (7.96, 8.04)
Romania	0.00 (−0.02, 0.02)
Russian Fed.	−1.00 (−1.04, −0.96)
Slovak Republic	8.00 (7.96, 8.04)
Slovenia	5.00 (4.97, 5.03)
Sweden	6.00 (5.98, 6.02)
Ukraine	8.00 (7.97, 8.03)
Overall	5.89 (4.73, 7.06)

M–F Difference (%)   0 2 4 6 8 10 12 14

Figure 2.18 Estimated country-specific male–female differences in cumulative incidence proportions for starting to use cannabis by age 15–16 years.
SOURCE: Data from the European Drug Report, 2015.

produced meta-analysis summaries in the form of forest plots for the male–female difference in cannabis CIP estimates observed by mid-adolescence, as well as corresponding MAS CIP estimates for each survey year.

Figure 2.18 discloses that in 2011 there is only survey with a negative sign on the point estimate for the CIP difference as well as both 95% confidence bounds, signifying a statistically robust female excess risk in starting to try cannabis by age 15–16 years; this estimate is from the Russian Federation, for which a survey of Moscow area students was completed. For all of the other countries depicted in Figure 2.18, which are arranged in alphabetical order, the sign on the cannabis CIP point estimate (cumulative to age 15–16 years) is nonnegative, and in all but two instances the sex difference is consistent with a statistically robust male excess risk in starting to smoke cannabis by mid-adolescence. The exceptions are found in France and in Romania, where the traditionally observed male excess was not present in the 2011 survey data.

The largest male excess is seen in Lithuania (estimated CIP = 11%, 95% CI [10.96%, 11.04%]). Norway and Finland have the smallest male excess, with CIP at 2.00% (both 95% CI [1.98%, 2.02%]). The meta-analysis summary estimate based on borrowing information from all of the 2011 surveys is 5.89%, 95% CI [4.73%, 7.06%].

Table 2.2 presents our meta-analysis summary estimates for cannabis CIPs based on years for which comparable survey data could be obtained. No clear trend can be seen in the table's mosaic of meta-analysis summary estimates for male–female differences in the risk of starting to use cannabis; no narrowing of the male–female difference can be claimed. The smallest estimate for the male–female difference is seen in the 1999 survey value of 4.45% (approximate 95% CI [3.15%, 5.75%]). The largest is from 2007 surveys, which produced a point estimate with a male excess of 6.33%, (95% CI [5.09%, 7.58%]). Even without a rigorous approach to the survey design effect (which might have broadened these 95% CI somewhat), none of the year-specific estimates can be said to be different. All have overlapping CIs, as can be seen by observing that the smallest lower bound of the 95% CI is 5.09%, and 5.09% is entrapped within 95% CI for each of the other estimates. The largest upper bound of the 95% CI is 7.58%, which is entrapped within the 95% CI for each of the other estimates.

We conclude that, based on these analyses to date, we have discovered no clear evidence of a narrowing of the male–female difference in risk of starting to use cannabis by mid-adolescence in these European countries. As such, according to

Table 2.2 YEAR-SPECIFIC META-ANALYSIS SUMMARY ESTIMATES FOR THE MALE–FEMALE DIFFERENCE IN CUMULATIVE INCIDENCE PROPORTIONS FOR STARTING TO USE CANNABIS BY AGE 15–16 YEARS

Survey Year	Male–Female Difference in MAS CIP Estimates (Male CIP Minus Female CIP, %)	Approximate Lower 95% Confidence Bound (%)	Approximate Upper 95% Confidence Bound (%)
1995	4.45	3.15	5.75
1999	6.00	4.73	7.27
2003	5.89	4.38	7.40
2007	6.33	5.09	7.58
2011	5.89	4.73	7.06

NOTES: Approximate 95% confidence intervals. Some country-specific reports from the European School Survey Project on Alcohol and Other Drugs state the exact numbers of males and females surveyed; for other countries, an approximation has been made. Issues of survey design effects due to clustering of cannabis experiences within sampled schools have not been addressed fully in construction of these approximate 95% confidence intervals. MAS = meta-analytic summary. CIP = cumulative incidence proportion.

SOURCE: Data from European Drug Report, 2015.

these estimates, the processes governing the observed narrowing of the male–female difference in risk of starting to drink alcohol by mid-adolescence might not be exactly the same as those governing risk of starting to use cannabis.

Notwithstanding limitations on survey data of this type, we can mention that more refined analyses are forthcoming, and the refinements include a constriction of the sample to consistently reporting countries that have provided estimates for all years of these ESPAD surveys. Some degree of variation in population coverage might hide what otherwise could be a narrowing trend when MAS estimates are based on consistently reporting countries. In addition, we are approaching the ESPAD investigators for more information about the numbers of participating males and females, as well as the issue of the survey design effect, in hope that the result will be improved approximations of our 95% CIs. We also hope to incorporate corresponding evidence from the Monitoring the Future surveys as well as the Youth Behavioral Risk Factor Surveys conducted with state-level samples in the United States so that corresponding state-specific CIP differences can be estimated, and overall MAS summary analyses can be derived.

CONCLUSION

Our conclusion is organized in relation to three topics. First, we offer a summary of what we have covered. Second, we offer some specifications for future country-level reports of epidemiological survey results. Finally, we offer some new directions for research on international cannabis trends.

As for chapter coverage, we provided a selection of official statistics reported to the UN from each country with respect to time trends in cannabis product seizures, concurrent with general stability in prevalence of recently active cannabis use globally and in almost all regions of the world. We also provided a section of background information and historical roots that might be studied by graduate students and scholars in the field who wish to reflect upon the pathways that led from 19th and 20th century pioneers and visionaries with early thoughts about international comparisons. For these reflections, we have no data in hand to be confident about observed trends of mental and behavioral health importance during these early years. Our CIPs from GPSs in selected countries disclosed within-region variations that are hidden in the UN statistics on regional trends. Clearly, some countries either are experiencing increased incidence rates for starting to use cannabis, or there is methods turbulence that is affecting the self-report measurements taken in the successive surveys. As such, we regard the available estimates and our meta-analysis summaries and MAS cannabis CIP as first approximations, with somewhat spotty coverage of the people of the world and with no chapter coverage of some regions (e.g., Asia, Africa, and Oceania, exclusive of Australia). Finally, our initial investigation of a narrowing of male–female differences in the risk of starting to use cannabis by mid-adolescence disclosed that the Moscow area of the Russian Federation might be in the vanguard of a female excess risk of cannabis use by mid-adolescence, but the overall trend pattern is one that is consistent with no tangible narrowing of this male–female difference within the European region when considered in aggregate via the MAS cannabis CIP estimates studied year by year. Refinement of this aspect of our chapter coverage is needed and should be addressed in new work on this topic.

As for specifications for future country reports on cannabis use epidemiology, we draw attention to already published recommendations (Kramer & Anthony, 1983), some of which have escaped the attention of cannabis researchers. A crucially important issue to address in any new survey report is the publication of the actual numbers of participants, including important subgroup sample sizes (e.g., number of males, number of females). In addition, we had to construct crude approximations of the 95% CIs because no information about the size of survey design effects was included in the study reports. This deficiency of the reports can be remedied with relative ease, using readily available statistical software and instructions (e.g., see Vselevoloskaya & Anthony, 2014). Without some way of correcting for survey design effects, the 95% CI will remain little more than crude approximations.

Finally, we looked for and found little more than isolated evidence on country-specific trends in the hazards and harmful outcomes now attributed to cannabis use, some of which are thought to be on the rise due to increasing potency of the cannabis products and possibly due to contamination with adulterants or to shifts toward inhalation of vaporized cannabinoids. For these reasons and because there are claims that some forms of cannabis products cause severely disabling conditions to occur de novo (e.g., cannabis-attributable psychoses), we recommend creation and sustained activity of an International Cannabis Products Safety Commission, akin to the Consumer Product Safety Commissions that have been created to protect the public's health and safety from product defects in other realms of commerce. A newly created International Cannabis Products Safety Commission can regularize both passive and active monitoring of claims about adverse cannabis product experiences and can assemble an apparatus to investigate which forms of the cannabis product might be more or less hazardous. To illustrate, it is claimed that the relative balance of various cannabinoids in a cannabis product is a driver of cannabis-attributable psychosis (e.g., with some cannabidiols posited as effect-modulators in the direction of reduced risk). If that is the case, then a newly created International Cannabis Products Safety Commission can create an active international surveillance of new incident cannabis-attributed psychosis cases, with conferencing and diagnostic workup to confirm the phenomenon and with gathering of the implicated cannabis products and pertinent details (e.g., route of administration). These case-associated cannabis products can be compared with samplings of regularly seized cannabis products from the same area (i.e., seized by law enforcement) or with sampling based on controlled buys from both legal and illegal cannabis vendors to nominate constituents of the products that might be accounting for the observed cannabis-associated adversities (e.g., mold or other adulterants; absence of CBD). This type of activity is well known to food safety epidemiologists; the concepts and statistical approaches to food safety data already have been harnessed for new estimates of cannabis-associated harms (e.g., Lopez-Quintero & Anthony, 2015). What is missing is an international organization to systematize international investigations of passive and active surveillance when a claim is made that use of a cannabis product is causing a serious health or other public safety consequence. To date, the approach has been to regulate and essentially to try to ban all cannabis products. Recent trends toward relaxation of cannabis policies and deregulation make it necessary to shift other modes of cannabis product investigation and control. Given the international trafficking in cannabis products, as well as increased cannabis tourism trends, society will need some counterbalancing innovations on the public health and safety side. An International Cannabis Products Safety Commission might represent an especially timely innovation during a time of evolving international trends in use of cannabis products.

ACKNOWLEDGMENTS

The authors wish to acknowledge support from the Michigan State University and the National Institutes of Health (NIH) for preparation of this manuscript. James C. Anthony's work on the article has been supported by an NIH/National Institute on Drug Abuse Senior Scientist and Mentorship Award (K05DA01579), while the NIH/NIDA support of Omayma Alshaarawy and Catalina Lopez-Quintero has been through an institutional research training program award (T32DA021129). In addition, during completion of the article, Alshaarawy received a K99 career development award from the NIH National Center for Complementary and Integrative Health (K99AT009156). Finally, we note that some of the ideas and material covered in this article have appeared in prior articles and chapters, especially with respect to distinctions between the epidemiological parameters of incidence and prevalence and in relation to our proposal for an International Cannabis Products Safety Commission (e.g., Anthony et al. [2016]. Cannabis epidemiology: A selective review. *Current Pharmaceutical Design*, 22, 6340–6352). Necessarily, this article and any of our chapters on the topic of international trends in epidemiological evidence on cannabis use will include similar ideas. Nonetheless, the expression of the ideas will be seen to be different across these contributions, different words are being used to express similar thoughts, and new ideas have been added to this article.

REFERENCES

Anthony, J. C., Lopez-Quintero, C., & Alshaarawy, O. (2016). Cannabis epidemiology: A selective review. *Current Pharmaceutical Design*, 22, 6340–6352. http://dx.doi.org/10.2174/1381612822666160813214023

Australian Institute of Health and Welfare. (2014). *National drug strategy household survey 2013*. Retrieved from http://www.aihw.gov.au/publication-detail/?id=60129549469

Borges, G., Medina-Mora, M. E., Breslau, J., & Aguilar-Gaxiola, S. (2007). The effect of migration to the United States on substance use disorders among returned Mexican migrants and families of migrants. *American Journal of Public Health, 97*, 1847–1851. http://dx.doi.org/10.2105/AJPH.2006.097915

Cheng, H. G., Cantave, M. D., & Anthony, J. C. (2016). Taking the first full drink: Epidemiological evidence on male–female differences in the United States. *Alcoholism: Experimental and Clinical Research, 40*, 816–825. http://dx.doi.org/10.1111/acer.13028

Cheng, H. G., & Anthony, J. C. (2017) A new era for drinking? Epidemiological evidence on adolescent male–female differences in drinking incidence in the United States and Europe. *Social Psychiatry Psychiatric Epidemiology, 2017*, 117–126. http://dx.doi.org/10.1007/s00127-016-1318-0

Chandra, M., Lopez-Quintero, C., Cheng, H., & Anthony, J. C. *Epidemiological evidence on male–female differences in cannabis use in Europe.* Unpublished manuscript.

Degenhardt, L., Chiu, W. T., Sampson, N., Kessler, R. C., Anthony, J. C., Angermeyer, M., . . . Karam, A. (2008). Toward a global view of alcohol, tobacco, cannabis, and cocaine use: findings from the WHO World Mental Health Surveys. *PLoS Medicine 5*(7), e141. http://dx.doi.org/10.1371/journal.pmed.0050141

Eaton, W. W., Kessler, L. G., & NIMH Epidemiologic Catchment Area Program (U.S.). (1985). *Epidemiologic field methods in psychiatry: The NIMH Epidemiologic Catchment Area Program.* Orlando, FL: Academic Press.

European Drug Report. (2015). The European Monitoring Centre for Drugs and Drug addiction, 2015. Retrieved from http://www.emcdda.europa.eu/data/stats2015

Health Canada. (2012). The Canadian Alcohol and Drug Use Monitoring Survey (CADUMS). Retrieved from http://www.hc-sc.gc.ca/hc-ps/drugs-drogues/stat/_2012/summary-sommaire-eng.php

Farr, W. (1885). *Vital statistics: A memorial volume of selections from the reports and writings of William Farr.* London: Offices of the Sanitary Institute.

Hickman, M., Taylor, C., Chatterjee, A., Degenhardt, L., Frischer, M., Hay, G., & Tilling, K. (2003). Estimating drug prevalence: Review of methods with special reference to developing countries. *UN Bulletin of Narcotics, 54*(1–2), 15–32.

Hughes, P. H., & Crawford, G. A. (1972). A contagious disease model for researching and intervening in heroin epidemics. *Archives of General Psychiatry, 27*, 149–155. http://dx.doi.org/10.1001/archpsyc.1972.01750260005001

Instituto Nacional de Psiquiatría Ramón de la Fuente Muñiz; Instituto Nacional de Salud Pública; Secretaría de Salud. Encuesta Nacional de Adicciones. (2011). Reporte de Drogas. Villatoro-Velázquez, J. A., Medina-Mora, M. E., Fleiz-Bautista, C., Téllez-Rojo, M. M., Mendoza-Alvarado, L. R., Romero-Martínez, M., Gutiérrez-Reyes, J. P., Castro-Tinoco, M., Hernández-Ávila, M., Tena-Tamayo, C., Alvear-Sevilla, C. y Guisa-Cruz, V. México, D. F., México:INPRFM; 2012. Retrieved for Figure 3 from www.inprf.gob.mx, last accessed August 2017.

Instituto sobre Alcoholismo y Farmacodependencia. (2001). *Consumo de drogas en Costa Rica: Resultados de la encuesta nacional, 2001* [Consumption of drugs in Costa Rica: Results of the national survey, 2001]. Retrieved from http://www.iafa.go.cr/images/descargables/conocimiento/17.INFORME-ESTUDIO-NACIONAL-2000.pdf

Instituto sobre Alcoholismo y Farmacodependencia. (2006). *Consumo de drogas en Costa Rica: Resultados de la encuesta nacional, 2001* [Consumption of drugs in

Costa Rica:. Results of the national survey, 2006]. Retrieved from http://www.bvs.
sa.cr/tabaquismo/consumo1.pdf

Instituto sobre Alcoholismo y Farmacodependencia. (2010). Consumo de erogas en
Costa Rica: Resultados de la encuesta nacional, 2001 [Consumption of drugs in
Costa Rica: Results of the national survey, 2010]. Retrieved from http://www.bvs.
sa.cr/tabaquismo/cannabis.pdf

Junta Nacional de Drogas, Secretaría Nacional de Drogas, & Programa de Naciones
Unidas para el Desarrollo. (2001). *Tercera encuesta nacional de prevalencia del
consumo de drogas* [Third national household survey on drug use]. Retrieved
from   http://www.infodrogas.gub.uy/html/encuestas/documentos/3ra_encuesta_
prevalencia_drogas_2001-rev6.pdf

Junta Nacional de Drogas, Secretaría Nacional de Drogas, Observatorio Uruguayo
de Drogas, La Oficina de Naciones Unidas Contra las Drogas y el Delito, & La
Comisión Interamericana para el Control del Abuso de Drogas. (2007). Cuarta
encuesta nacional de prevalencia del consumo de drogas [Fourth national household
survey on drug use]. Retrieved from http://www.infodrogas.gub.uy/html/encuestas/
documentos/2007_4ta_encuesta_hogares.pdf

Junta Nacional de Drogas, Secretaría Nacional de Drogas, & Observatorio Uruguayo
de Drogas. (2011). Quinta encuesta nacional de prevalencia del consumo de
drogas [Fifth national household survey on drug use]. Retrieved from http://www.
infodrogas.gub.uy/images/stories/pdf/v_enc_hogares_2011.pdf

Junta Nacional de Drogas, Secretaría Nacional de Drogas, & Observatorio Uruguayo de
Drogas. (2015). Sexta encuesta nacional de prevalencia del consumo de drogas [Sixth
national household survey on drug use]. Retrieved from http://www.infodrogas.gub.
uy/images/stories/pdf/vi_encuesta_hogares_2015.pdf

Kramer, M. (1957). A discussion of the concepts of incidence and prevalence as related
to epidemiologic studies of mental disorders. *American Journal of Public Health and
the Nations Health, 47*(7), 826–840.

Kramer, M. (1969). Cross-national study of diagnosis of the mental disorders: origin
of the problem. *American Journal of Psychiatry, 125*(10S), 1–11. http://dx.doi.org/
10.1176/ajp.125.10S.1

Kramer, M., & Anthony, J. (1983). Review of differences in mental health indicators used
in national publications: recommendations for their standardization. *World health statistics quarterly/Rapport trimestriel de statistiques sanitaires mondiales, 36*, 256–338.

Lipari, R. N., Ahrnsbrak, R. D., Pemberton, M. R., & Porter, J. D. (2017). *Risk and
Protective Factors and Estimates of Substance Use Initiation: Results from the 2016
National Survey on Drug Use and Health*. Rockville, MD: Substance Abuse and
Mental Health Services Administration. 2017. (Last accessed 1 January 2018, https://
www.samhsa.gov/data/sites/default/files/NSDUH-DR-FFR3-2016/NSDUH-DR-
FFR3-2016.htm)

Lopez-Quintero, C., & Anthony, J. C. (2015). Drug use disorders in the polydrug context: New epidemiological evidence from a foodborne outbreak approach. *Annals
of the New York Academy of Sciences, 1349*, 119–126. http://dx.doi.org/10.1111/
nyas.12868

Manski, C. F., Pepper, J. V., & Petrie, C. V. (2001). *Informing America's policy on illegal drugs. What we don't know keeps hurting us*. Washington, DC: National
Academy Press.

Ministerio del Interior y de Justicia, Ministerio de la Protección Social, & Dirección Nacional de Estupefacientes. (2009). *Estudio nacional de consumo de sustancias psicoactivas en Colombia* [National Study of the consumption of psychoactive substances in Colombia]. Retrieved from https://www.unodc.org/documents/colombia/2013/septiembre/Estudio_Nacional_Consumo_2008.pdf

Ministerio de Justicia y del Derecho, Observatorio de Drogas de Colombia, Ministerio de Salud y Protección Social. (2013). *Estudio nacional de consumo de sustancias psicoactivas en Colombia* [National Study on the consumption of psychoactive substances in Colombia]. Retrieved from https://www.unodc.org/documents/colombia/2014/Julio/Estudio_de_Consumo_UNODC.pdf

Ministerio del Interior y Seguridad Pública, Servicio Nacional para la Prevención y Rehabilitación del Consumo de Drogas y Alcohol, & Observatorio Chileno de Drogas. (2015). *Décimo primer estudio nacional de drogas en población general—SENDA, 2014* [Eleventh national study on drugs in the general population—SENDA, 2014]. Retrieved from http://www.senda.gob.cl/media/2015/08/Informe-Ejecutivo-ENPG-2014.pdf

Observatorio Argentino de Drogas, Instituto Nacional de Estadística y Censos. (2004). *Estudio Nacional sobre consumo de sustancias psicoactivas–OAD/INDEC* [National study on the consumption of psychoactive substances–OAD/INDEC]. (Last accessed August 2017: Retrieved from http://scripts.minplan.gob.ar/octopus/archivos.php?file=4310).

Observatorio Argentino de Drogas, Opinión Pública Servicios y Mercados. (2006). *Estudio Nacional sobre consumo de sustancias psicoactivas – OAD/OPSM* [National study on the consumption of psychoactive substances – OAD/OPSM]. (Last accessed August 2017: Retrieved from http://scripts.minplan.gob.ar/octopus/archivos.php?file=4310).

Observatorio Argentino de Drogas, Universidad Nacional de Tres de Febrero. (2008). *Estudio Nacional sobre consumo de sustancias psicoactivas – OAD/UNTREF* [National study on the consumption of psychoactive substances – OAD/UNTREF]. (Last accessed August 2017: Retrieved from http://scripts.minplan.gob.ar/octopus/archivos.php?file=4310).

Observatorio Argentino de Drogas, Universidad Nacional de Tres de Febrero. (2010). *Estudio Nacional sobre consumo de sustancias psicoactivas – OAD/UNTREF* [National study on the consumption of psychoactive substances – OAD/UNTREF]. (Last accessed August 2017: Retrieved from http://scripts.minplan.gob.ar/octopus/archivos.php?file=4310).

Orwa, T. O. (2014). *Modelling the dynamics of alcohol and methamphetamine co-abuse in the Western Cape Province of South Africa* (Unpublished doctoral dissertation). University of Stellenbosch, Stellenbosch, South Africa.

Parker, M. A., & Anthony, J. C. (2015). Epidemiological evidence on extra-medical use of prescription pain relievers: Transitions from newly incident use to dependence among 12-21 yar olds in the United States using meta-analysis, 2002–13. *PeerJ, 3*, e1340. http://dx.doi.org/10.7717/peerj.1340

Rodríguez Ospina, E. (1997) Estudio nacional sobre consumo de sustancias psicoactivas en Colombia—1996 [National study on the consumption of psychoactive substances in Colombia—1996]. Bogotá: Editorial Carrera 7a Ltda.

Rootman, I., & Hughes, P. H. (1980). *Drug-abuse reporting systems*. Geneva: World Health Organization.

Secretaría de Salud, Consejo Nacional Contra las Adicciones, Instituto Nacional de
    Psiquiatría Ramón de la Fuente, & Instituto Nacional de Salud Pública. (2008). *Encuesta*
    nacional de adicciones 2008. Morelos, Mexico: Instituto Nacional de Salud Pública.
Sloboda, Z., & Kozel, N. J. (2003). Understanding drug trends in the United States of
    America: The role of the Community Epidemiology Work Group as part of a com-
    prehensive drug information system. *UN Bulletin on Narcotics, 55*(1–2), 41–51.
Smart, R. G., Wadud, K. A., Varma, V. K., Poshyachinda, V., Navaratnam, V.,
    Mora, M. . . . Hughes, P. H. (1980). *A methodology for student drug-use surveys*.
    Geneva: World Health Organization.
Streiner, D. L., Patten, S. B., Anthony, J. C., & Cairney, J. (2009). Has "lifetime prev-
    alence" reached the end of its life? An examination of the concept. *Psychiatric*
    Research, 18, 221–228. http://dx.doi.org/10.1002/mpr.296
Unidad de Prevención y Rehabilitación de CONTRADROGAS, & Instituto Nacional
    de Estadística e Informática. (1998). *Encuesta nacional de prevención y uso de drogas,*
    1998 [National survey of prevention and drug use, 1998]. Retrieved from http://www.
    unodc.org/documents/peruandecuador/Publicaciones/I_ENCUESTA_1998.pdf
Unidad de Prevención y Rehabilitación de CONTRADROGAS. Comisión Nacional
    para el Desarrollo y Vida sin Drogas, DEVIDA. (2002). *II Encuesta Nacional de*
    Consumo de Drogas de la Población General de Perú, 2002. [Second national survey
    of the consumption of drugs in the general population in Peru, 2002]. (Last accessed
    August 2017: Retrieved for Figure 6 from http://www.unodc.org/documents/
    peruandecuador/Publicaciones/II_ENCUESTA_2002.pdf)
Unidad de Prevención y Rehabilitación de CONTRADROGAS. Comisión Nacional
    para el Desarrollo y Vida sin Drogas, DEVIDA. (2006). *III Encuesta Nacional de*
    Consumo de Drogas de la Población General de Perú, 2006 [Third national survey of
    the consumption of drugs in the general population in Peru, 2006]. (Last accessed
    August 2017: Retrieved for Figure 6 from http://www.devida.gob.pe/uploads/libros/
    III-Encuesta-Nacional-Consumo-Drogas-Poblacion-General-Peru-2006.pdf).
Unidad de Prevención y Rehabilitación de CONTRADROGAS. Comisión Nacional
    para el Desarrollo y Vida sin Drogas, DEVIDA. (2010). *IV Encuesta Nacional de*
    Consumo de Drogas de la Población General de Perú, 2010 [Fourth national survey
    of the consumption of drugs in the general population in Peru, 2006]. (Last accessed
    August 2017: Retrieved for Figure 6 from: http://www.hablafranco.gob.pe/images/
    upload/descarga/20130123143258Informe%20Ejecutivo%20Poblaci%C3%B3n%20
    General%202010%20(2).pdf).
United Nations. Office on Drugs and Crime. (2004). *World drug report 2004*. Vienna:.
    (Last accessed 1 January 2018: http://www.unodc.org/unodc/en/data-and-analysis/
    WDR-2004.html).
United Nations. Office on Drugs and Crime. (2009). *World drug report 2009*. Vienna.
    (Last accessed 1 January 2018: http://www.unodc.org/unodc/en/data-and-analysis/
    WDR-2009.html).
United Nations. Office on Drugs and Crime. (2015). *World drug report 2015*. Vienna.
    (Last accessed 1 January 2018: http://www.unodc.org/wdr2015/).
United States. Substance Abuse and Mental Health Services Administration. Center for
    Behavioral Health Statistics and Quality. Reports and Detailed Tables from the 2015
    National Survey on Drug Use and Health (NSDUH). Rockville, MD: Substance Abuse
    and Mental Health Services Administration. 2016. (Last accessed 1 January 2018:

https://www.samhsa.gov/samhsa-data-outcomes-quality/major-data-collections/
reports-detailed-tables-2015-NSDUH).

Vsevolozhskaya, O. A., Anthony, J. C. (2014). Confidence interval estimation in
R-DAS. *Drug and Alcohol Dependence*, *143*, 95–104. http://dx.doi.org/10.1016/
j.drugalcdep.2014.07.017

Villatoro, J., Medina–Mora M.E., Cravioto, P., Fleiz Bautista, C., Moreno Lopez, M.,
Robles N.O., Bustos Gamiño, M., Fregoso Ito, D. Gutiérrez López, M.L., Buenabad,
N.A., Encuesta Nacional de Adicciones. (2012). México: Capítulo de drogas. Consejo
Nacional Contra las Adicciones - CONADIC, Instituto Nacional de Psiquiatría Ramón
de la Fuente Muñiz, INPRFM, Dirección General de Epidemiología, DGE, Instituto
Nacional Estadística, Geografía e Informática, INEGI; 2003. Retrieved for Figure
3 from HYPERLINK "http://www.inprf.gob.mx" www.inprf.gob.mx, last accessed
August 2017.

Whitehead, M. (2000). William Farr's legacy to the study of inequalities in health.
Bulletin of the World Health Organization, *78*(1), 86–87.

Clinical Characteristics of Cannabis Use Disorder

TAMMY A. CHUNG AND KEN C. WINTERS

INTRODUCTION

This chapter reviews the clinical characteristics of cannabis use disorder (CUD), with consideration of the addictive nature of marijuana, relative to alcohol and tobacco. Prevalence of cannabis use varies by country and across demographic subgroups (e.g., age, gender) within a country. Multiple trajectories of cannabis use have been identified, with most users reporting a peak in cannabis use during young adulthood and a decline in the mid-20s. Changes to diagnostic criteria for a CUD from fourth edition of the *Diagnostic and Statistical Manual of Mental Disorders–Fourth Edition* (DSM–IV; American Psychiatric Association [APA], 1994) to the fifth edition (DSM–5; APA, 2013) have produced little overall change in CUD prevalence, despite the inclusion of cannabis withdrawal and a new craving symptom. Although DSM–5 substance use disorder (SUD) criteria are now applied across substances, there are mixed findings regarding the validity of cannabis withdrawal as a CUD symptom. Cannabis appears to have lower addictive liability compared to alcohol and nicotine. The chapter concludes by outlining future research to improve assessment, diagnosis, and treatment of CUD.

CLINICAL CHARACTERISTICS OF CANNABIS USE DISORDER

Cannabis is one of the most commonly used illicit drugs worldwide (United Nations Office on Drug and Crimes [UNODC], 2014). As cause for concern, time trend data in the United States indicate a gradual increase in the proportion of youth reporting marijuana use in recent years and no signs of less use among adults (Substance Abuse and Mental Health Services Administration [SAMHSA],

2015). The increase in cannabis use in the United States has occurred in parallel with a decrease in perceived risk of harm from marijuana use (Johnston, O'Malley, Miech, Bachman, & Schulenberg, 2014), an increase in the number of states with medical and recreational marijuana laws (Bestrashniy & Winters, 2015), and greater potency of marijuana in recent years (ElSohly, 2014). The increase in cannabis use has occurred despite documentation of cannabis-related health harms (Hall, 2015; Volkow, Baler, Compton, & Weiss, 2014).

In the context of changing legal policy regarding cannabis and increasing potency of cannabis, this chapter reviews the clinical characteristics of CUD, with consideration of its addictive liability relative to commonly used substances such as alcohol and tobacco. This review describes cannabis use prevalence, peak risk of onset and progression of cannabis use, and common trajectories of cannabis use. Next, core features of addiction and diagnostic criteria for CUD according to the fourth and fifth editions of the DSM (APA, 1994, 2013) are discussed. Prevalence of DSM–IV and DSM–5 CUD and CUD symptoms are summarized to identify common and relatively mild, versus more severe, cannabis-related symptoms. The course of CUD and rates of remission and relapse are then described. The chapter concludes with a discussion of future research directions that aim to improve CUD case identification and to increase knowledge regarding CUD etiology and clinical course.

CANNABIS USE PREVALENCE

In 2012, 2.7% to 4.9% of the global population aged 15 to 64 were estimated to have used cannabis (UNODC, 2014). Regions with the highest prevalence of cannabis use include North America, Oceania (New Zealand, Australia), western and central Europe, and parts of Africa (UNODC, 2014). Across countries, cannabis use is generally higher among males compared to females (Australian Institute of Health and Welfare, 2014; Canadian Centre on Substance Abuse and Addiction, 2014; European Monitoring Centre on Drugs and Drug Addiction, 2014; SAMHSA, 2014; ter Bogt et al., 2014). Within the United States, there is some evidence for race/ethnic differences in cannabis use prevalence, such that Black adolescents were less likely to report marijuana use compared to non-Hispanic White adolescents (Keyes et al., 2015). However, in adulthood, Black women, compared to non-Hispanic White women, were more likely to report cannabis use, whereas there was no difference in cannabis use for Black and non-Hispanic White males (Keyes et al., 2015).

The differences in prevalence of cannabis use in terms of subgroups (e.g., gender, race/ethnicity) across countries and within a country may reflect several factors. There is the complexity of characterizing subgroup differences because an individual may belong to multiple subgroups (e.g., gender, race/ethnicity), and subgroup differences in cannabis use may change across development. Also, there are differences in legalization of cannabis use and social norms regarding cannabis use (Anthony, Warner, & Kessler, 1994; Salas-Wright et al., 2015). This issue has received a great deal of focus in the United States where state-level legalization of medical and recreational marijuana varies considerably. Although some studies have found higher rates of cannabis use and cannabis-related problems in states with legalized medical marijuana (Cerda, Wall, Keyes, Galea, & Hasin, 2012; Wall et al., 2011), others have found no difference (Choo et al., 2014; Hasin et al., 2015; Lynne-Landsman, Livingston, & Wagenaar, 2013), or differences across states that may be explained by chance (Ammerman, Ryan, & Adelman, 2015).

Also, mixed findings between countries may be due, for example, to differences in the interval over which change in marijuana use was examined. In the Netherlands, cannabis use among youth increased after enacting more liberal marijuana laws in the mid-1970s (MacCoun & Reuter, 1997) but has since shown a general decline in recent years, consistent with other European nations. Prevalence of cannabis use among youth (ages 15–24) in the Netherlands is higher relative to most European countries but lower compared to the United States (Ammerman et al., 2015).

ONSET AND PROGRESSION OF CANNABIS USE

Initiation of cannabis use commonly occurs in adolescence (ages 15–18), with peak rates of use emerging in late adolescence and young adulthood (Lanza, Vasilenko, Dziak, & Butera, 2015; Wagner & Anthony, 2002; Young et al., 2002). Specifically, past-year cannabis use was reported by 32% of 18- to 25-year-olds in the United States (SAMHSA, 2014); 21% of 20- to 29-year-old Australians (Australian Institute of Health and Welfare, 2014), 20.3% of 15- to 24-year-olds in Canada (Canadian Centre on Substance Abuse and Addiction, 2014), and 14% of 15- to 24-year-olds in Europe (European Monitoring Centre on Drugs and Drug Addiction, 2014).

Most lifetime cannabis users show limited or experimental use (Brook, Zhang, & Brook, 2011; Flory, Lynam, Milich, Leukefeld, & Clayton, 2004); only about 1 in 11 (9%) lifetime users might progress to cannabis dependence (Anthony et al., 1994). Yet, among daily cannabis users, one in two are estimated to be at risk for cannabis dependence (Hall & Pacula, 2003). Also, those with early onset (e.g., initiation prior to ages 15–16) and regular use in adolescence are at greatest risk for later problem use (Coffey, Lynskey, Wolfe, & Patton, 2000; Dennis, Babor, Roebuck, & Donaldson, 2002; Taylor et al., 2017; Winters & Lee, 2008).

The transition from initial use to regular use of a substance, including cannabis, is typically driven by the rewarding effects of use, whereas progression to addiction involves a shift to habit-driven use (Koob & Volkow, 2010). Differences across substances in the probability of transition to dependence may be due to substance-specific physiological effects, which interact with individual differences in drug response and environmental risks (e.g., peer norms regarding drug use, drug availability) associated with progression (Ridenour, Maldonado-Molina, Compton, Spitznagel, & Cottler, 2005). With respect to cannabis, fewer lifetime users of cannabis (9%) progressed to dependence compared to tobacco (67%) and alcohol (23%; Lopez-Quintero et al., 2011). However, the transition to dependence occurred, on average, faster to cannabis, relative to tobacco or alcohol (Lopez-Quintero et al., 2011; Wagner & Anthony, 2002). These results are suggestive of generally lower overall addiction liability (progression to dependence) for cannabis relative to tobacco and alcohol (Anthony et al., 1994), but the faster transition to cannabis dependence also indicates the addictive potential of cannabis among vulnerable individuals.

HETEROGENEITY IN THE COURSE OF CANNABIS USE

The course of cannabis use from adolescence into adulthood varies across individuals. Cannabis use trajectories differ in age at initiation of use, rate of escalation, severity, and chronicity (persistence, desistance; Brook et al., 2011; Ellickson, Martino, & Collins, 2004; Flory et al., 2004; Passarotti, Crane, Hedeker, & Mermelstein, 2015; Schulenberg et al., 2005; Tucker, Ellickson, Orlando, Martino, & Klein, 2005). Trajectory groups representing no to low levels of cannabis use (e.g., experimental use) account for the greatest proportion of community samples followed into adulthood. For those with a history of regular cannabis use, many show an increase in use in mid- to late adolescence, followed by a decline or desistance of use in the mid-20s, which may be associated with young adult role transitions such as becoming a parent and full-time employment (Brook et al., 2011; von Sydow et al., 2001). A minority of regular cannabis users show persistence of high levels of cannabis use into adulthood (Brook et al., 2011). We discuss the course of a CUD in a subsequent section.

CORE FEATURES OF ADDICTION AND DSM CUD DIAGNOSIS

In the two most recent editions of the DSM, DSM–IV (APA, 1994), and DSM–5 (APA, 2013), the dependence syndrome concept (Edwards & Gross, 1976) provided the framework for SUD criteria. Essential clinically descriptive elements of the dependence syndrome, originally described in relation to alcohol use and later extended to other substances, included physical symptoms of tolerance and withdrawal, salience of drug use (e.g., organizing one's day around drug use), narrowing of drug use behavior (e.g., reduced flexibility in timing, dose, and frequency of use), a compulsion to engage in drug use, and recurrence of the syndrome after abstinence (Edwards & Gross, 1976). In addition, the dependence syndrome concept proposed a bi-axial model in which symptoms of dependence formed a separate dimension from negative consequences associated with substance use (e.g., health problems resulting from heavy use; Edwards & Gross, 1976).

Consistent with the dependence syndrome concept, DSM–IV SUD included diagnoses of abuse and dependence, which were defined by non-overlapping criterion sets representing negative social and personal consequences of substance use, and symptoms of dependence. In DSM–IV, a diagnosis of substance dependence precluded a diagnosis of abuse, suggesting that abuse represented a milder form of illness that preceded dependence. Cannabis abuse in DSM–IV required meeting one of four symptoms representing impairment in major role obligations due to use (e.g., working while high on cannabis), hazardous use (e.g., driving when high on cannabis), cannabis-related legal problems, and social problems due to cannabis use (e.g., others expressed concern about cannabis use). DSM–IV cannabis dependence required three of six symptoms, which occurred together within a 12-month period, representing tolerance, using more or longer than intended (larger/longer), difficulties cutting down or stopping use (quit/cut down), much time spent using, reduced activities in favor of cannabis use, and use despite psychological or physical problems caused or exacerbated by use (psychological/physical problems). Importantly, the DSM–IV departed from how withdrawal symptoms were recognized with other substances and did not recognize a cannabis withdrawal syndrome as an indicator of dependence, due to limited data to support its inclusion.

Revisions leading to DSM–5 SUD criteria were based on extensive literature reviews, analyses of population-based and treatment data sets, and expert judgments regarding clinical utility of the diagnostic algorithm (Hasin et al., 2013). A major change in DSM–5 involved combining the separate DSM–IV substance abuse and dependence criteria into a single SUD criterion set, based on research indicating that most of the criteria loaded on a single factor across different substances (e.g., alcohol, cannabis, cocaine; Hasin et al., 2013). Two other substance-wide changes are noteworthy. Since substance-related legal problems generally did not load on the single SUD factor and was a relatively severe symptom, the criterion was removed (Hasin et al., 2013). Further, a new craving criterion was added to DSM–5 based on its importance to addiction as a potential treatment target and its loading on the single SUD factor (Hasin et al., 2013). Whereas improvements in defining SUD with the DSM–5 has been noted (Hasin et al., 2013), the new criteria have been criticized for lack of adjustments when applied to adolescents (Winters, Martin, & Chung, 2011).

A change that was specific to cannabis involved the inclusion of cannabis withdrawal in DSM–5. This decision was based, in part, on empirical work demonstrating the reliable emergence among clinical samples of abstinence effects with discontinuation of cannabis use (Budney, Moore, Vandrey, & Hughes, 2003; Haney, Ward, Comer, Foltin, & Fischman, 1999). These lab-based studies identified a specific time course for cannabis withdrawal in which clinically significant symptoms emerged within one to two days after stopping use, peaked after two to four days, and typically lasted one to three weeks (Budney et al., 2003). Abstinence symptoms also were found to resolve with readministration of cannabis (Budney, Vandrey, Hughes, Moore, & Bahrenburg, 2007). The most commonly reported cannabis withdrawal symptoms included anxiety, decreased appetite, irritability, restlessness, and sleep problems (Budney, Hughes, Moore, & Vandrey, 2004; Milin, Manion, Dare, & Walker, 2008). In samples of adolescent and adult cannabis users, greater severity of cannabis withdrawal predicted worse outcomes (Chung, Martin, Cornelius, & Clark, 2008; Cornelius, Chung, Martin, Wood, & Clark, 2008). Inclusion of cannabis withdrawal in DSM–5 suggests the utility of a common set of SUD criteria across a variety of substances.

DSM–5 defines SUD, including CUD, using a single set of 11 criteria, which includes three of the four DSM–IV abuse criteria (role obligations, hazardous use, social problems), all of the DSM–IV dependence criteria, the addition of the criteria for craving, and the inclusion of a new cannabis withdrawal syndrome. DSM–5 defines cannabis withdrawal as cessation of heavy and prolonged use that leads to at least three symptoms (e.g., irritability, sleep problems, anxiety) that develop within one week of cessation. In DSM–5, mild SUD is indicated by meeting two to three criteria, moderate SUD is met with four to five criteria, and severe SUD is indicated by meeting six or more criteria. For all DSM–5 SUD severity levels, criteria need to cluster within a 12-month period to meet criteria for diagnosis.

PREVALENCE OF DSM–IV CUD

Due to the relatively recent publication of DSM–5, estimates of CUD prevalence focus on DSM–IV SUD. Among survey respondents age 12 and older in the United States, the prevalence of past-year DSM–IV cannabis abuse or dependence was 1.6% in the 2013 National Survey on Drug Use and Health (SAMHSA, 2014). Prevalence of past-year DSM–IV cannabis abuse (1.1%) was higher than cannabis dependence (0.3%) in a US national survey (Stinson, Ruan, Pickering, & Grant, 2006). Similar to CUD prevalence in the United States, in Australia, past-year prevalence of DSM–IV CUD was 1.5% in the 1997 national survey (Swift, Hall, & Teesson, 2001). Only a minority of those with CUD seek treatment (Stinson et al., 2006). In the United States, only 9.8% of individuals with lifetime cannabis abuse and 34.7% with cannabis dependence reported receiving drug treatment (SAMHSA, 2014).

CUD prevalence differs by age, gender, and race/ethnicity. In a US national survey, across age, young adults (ages 18–25) had the highest past-year prevalence of DSM–IV CUD (5.4%), followed by adolescents (ages 12–17; 2.9%), with older adults (ages 26+; 0.8%) having the lowest prevalence (SAMHSA, 2014). The peak in CUD among young adults also was evident in the 2010 Global Burden of Disease study, in which prevalence of DSM–IV cannabis dependence peaked at ages 20 to 24 (Degenhardt et al., 2013). With regard to gender, CUD is more prevalent in males than females (Degenhardt et al., 2013), and young adult males are more likely to have CUD compared to women and older men (Compton, Grant, Colliver, Glantz, & Stinson, 2004).

In the United States, Native American ethnicity is associated with greater odds of CUD, whereas self-identification as Black, Asian, or Hispanic decreased the odds of CUD (Stinson et al., 2006). Differences in CUD prevalence that are associated with demographic characteristics need to be interpreted with some caution, since these differences may reflect individual differences in CUD risk or measurement error (see the following discussion), or a combination of both.

DSM–IV VERSUS DSM–5 CUD

Research suggests relatively small differences in CUD prevalence using DSM–IV versus DSM–5 criteria. In an Australian national sample, lifetime DSM–IV CUD was 6.2% and declined to 5.4% when using DSM–5 (Mewton, Slade, & Teesson, 2013). The decrease when using DSM–5 was due mainly to individuals who only endorsed hazardous use, a criterion that results in a DSM–IV cannabis abuse diagnosis but not the DSM–5 CUD (Mewton et al., 2013). Analyses of a US national sample also indicated a slight decrease in CUD using the DSM–5 compared to the DSM–IV (Agrawal et al., 2014). However, other work using an Australian sample of young adult twins and siblings, suggested a small increase in lifetime DSM–5 CUD compared to the DSM–IV (Kubarych et al., 2014). Overall, the shift from the DSM–IV to the DSM–5 appears to involve a relatively small difference in CUD prevalence.

DSM-BASED CANNABIS SYMPTOMS

As shown in Table 3.1, the most commonly reported cannabis symptoms typically represent difficulties controlling use (larger/longer, quit/cut down), tolerance, and hazardous use. However, there is considerable variation in the rank order prevalence of DSM-based cannabis symptoms based on sample characteristics. Differences in symptom prevalence across age (i.e., differences in symptom endorsement by age of respondent), gender, and countries can indicate factors that foster or constrain the occurrence of specific symptoms and how symptoms may manifest differently in subgroups.

Adolescent and adult cannabis users show some differences in the symptoms most likely to be endorsed. In a US national survey, among individuals who started using marijuana in the past year, adolescents (age 12–17) were twice as likely to report symptoms of DSM–IV cannabis dependence compared to adults (age 18+), specifically, the symptoms of quit/cut down and tolerance, even when controlling for differences in CUD severity (Chen & Anthony, 2003). Other research indicates that among adolescent cannabis users, larger/longer was a commonly reported symptom, suggesting the early emergence of impaired control over cannabis use among young users (Dennis et al., 2002; Hartman et al., 2008). Differences between adolescent and adult cannabis users in symptom endorsement, however, suggest that the symptoms as they are queried in surveys may have a different meaning for adolescents compared to adults, especially when symptoms are endorsed at relatively low levels of use among youth (Chen &

Table 3.1 PREVALENCE OF *DIAGNOSTIC AND STATISTICAL MANUAL OF MENTAL DISORDERS*-BASED CANNABIS SYMPTOMS ACROSS STUDIES

	Wu et al. (2009) US Treatment Sample	Beseler (2010) NESARC	Mewton et al. (2013) Australia	Kubarych et al. (2014) Australia Males	Kubarych et al. (2014) Australia Females	Delforterie et al. (2015) Netherlands Males	Delforterie (2015) Netherlands Females	Nocon et al. (2006) Germany
	Past Year	Lifetime	Lifetime	Lifetime	Lifetime	Lifetime	Lifetime	Lifetime
Role Obligations	–	8.4	2.4	13.9	4.1	9.1	8.7	–
Hazardous Use	–	33.7	4.6	17.8	5.4	13.4	7.1	–
Legal Problems	–	5.9	0.2	4.6	0.3	2.2	0.8	–
Social Problems	–	16.0	2.2	10.8	4.6	9.5	10.2	–
Tolerance	34.1	10.0	3.2	16.6	9.0	15.1	11.8	14.5
Withdrawal	16.7	3.2	2.7	15.4	8.2	13.8	10.2	16.8
Larger/Longer	31.8	7.9	4.7	21.1	8.7	12.9	11.0	13.5
Quit/Cut Down	39.9	33.3	0.9	25.5	10.9	4.7	3.9	3.7
Much Time	32.2	11.5	1.7	13.1	4.6	7.3	7.9	9.8
Reduced Activities	21.9	5.5	1.1	9.6	4.1	4.7	1.6	7.3
Physical/ Psychological Problems	21.5	10.6	2.0	8.1	3.8	5.2	5.5	12.9
Craving	–	–	2.5	18.5	9.3	–	–	–

NOTES: NESARC = National Epidemiologic Survey of Alcohol and Related Conditions. Larger/Longer = use more or longer than intended. Quit/Cut Down = repeated failed attempts to quit or cut down on substance use.

Anthony, 2003). For example, adolescents' report of using more or longer than intended at early stages of use may reflect factors such as impulsivity or peer encouragement of use, rather than a compulsive pattern of use (Chung & Martin, 2005).

Gender differences in CUD symptom endorsement have been observed in some studies (Agrawal & Lynskey, 2007; Martin, Chung, Kirisci, & Langenbucher, 2006; Piontek, Kraus, Legleye, & Buhringer, 2011) but not others (Compton, Saha, Conway, & Grant, 2009; Gizer et al., 2013; Wu et al., 2009). Some research suggests that certain cannabis abuse symptoms reflect greater severity in females, whereas some cannabis dependence criteria indicate greater severity in males. For example, in a US national survey, hazardous use and cannabis-related legal problems were associated with greater severity in women compared to men (Agrawal & Lynskey, 2007); this gender difference also was observed in a sample of treated adolescents (Martin et al., 2006). Gender differences in report of cannabis abuse symptoms may reflect female social roles, which could reduce the likelihood of experiencing legal problems and hazardous use (Agrawal & Lynskey, 2007). Gender differences also suggest that some symptoms may be more salient for one gender, highlighting the importance of refining criteria to reduce possible gender bias in identification of CUD (Agrawal & Lynskey, 2007).

Cross-national comparisons most consistently indicate differences in the prevalence of cannabis-related legal problems and withdrawal. In a study that compared the United States and the Netherlands, cannabis users in the United States were more likely to report cannabis-related legal problems, a finding that was interpreted as possibly reflecting more tolerant attitudes toward cannabis use in the Netherlands (Delforterie et al., 2015). Research that compared cannabis users in the United States, Mexico, and Colombia found that users in Colombia, relative to the United States, were more likely to report cannabis-related legal problems (Fiestas et al., 2010). The greater rate of cannabis-related legal problems in Colombia was discussed as possibly reflecting greater concurrent alcohol and cannabis use in that country, which increased risk for legal involvement (Fiestas et al., 2010). Cross-national differences in the prevalence of cannabis-related legal problems, which appear to be dependent on local laws and patterns of polydrug use, support the exclusion of this symptom from DSM–5.

The rank order prevalence of cannabis withdrawal varies widely across studies (see Table 3.1). Cannabis withdrawal is one of the least prevalent, possibly more severe, symptoms in survey research conducted in the United States (Agrawal & Lynskey, 2007; Gillespie, Neale, Prescott, Aggen, & Kendler, 2007; Wu et al., 2009) and a French study of adolescents (Piontek et al., 2011). In contrast, cannabis withdrawal was reported with relatively high prevalence, possibly reflecting a more mild symptom, in a US Native American sample (Gizer et al., 2013), an Australian sample (Swift et al., 2001), and a young German sample (Nocon, Wittchen, Pfister, Zimmermann, & Lieb, 2006). Across all studies, differences in the assessment of cannabis withdrawal (e.g., type and number of symptoms used to determine presence of cannabis withdrawal, time frame for recall: lifetime or past year); and differences across samples in typical delta-9-tetrahydrocannabinol (THC) content, dosing, and route of administration may explain differences in prevalence of cannabis withdrawal across studies and subgroups within a population (Nocon et al., 2006). Research is needed to determine whether the use of standardized criteria to assess cannabis withdrawal in DSM–5 results in greater consistency in its rank order prevalence across studies.

In sum, differences in the rank order prevalence of DSM-based cannabis symptoms have been identified across countries and in specific subpopulations (e.g., age, gender). Differences in symptom prevalence and performance (e.g., differential item functioning) across subgroups may reflect differences in regional or cultural norms (e.g., social acceptability of cannabis use) and laws regarding cannabis use, mode of administration and potency of cannabis consumed, and individual differences in cannabis effects. Since some cannabis symptoms appear to function differently across subgroups, differences in CUD prevalence and risk factors for CUD need to be interpreted with caution (Delforterie et al., 2015).

COURSE OF CUD

Whereas the average age of CUD onset was found in a US sample to be 18.6 years (Farmer et al., 2015), the pathway to a CUD has been studied. The peak risk for the presence of CUD symptoms typically occurs within one to three years after initiation of cannabis use (Anthony et al., 1994), although among those that progress to dependence, onset of dependence typically occurs within 10 years of first use (Rosenberg & Anthony, 2001; Stinson et al., 2006). Risk factors for the transition from cannabis use to problematic use include early onset of cannabis use (e.g., prior to age 15–16), use of other substances (e.g., alcohol, tobacco), co-occurring psychopathology (e.g., conduct problems), peer substance use, and report of stressful life events (Chen, O'Brien, & Anthony, 2005; Coffey et al., 2000; Perkonigg et al., 2008; Prince van Leeuwen et al., 2014; Winters & Lee, 2008). Many of these risk factors (e.g., co-occurring psychopathology) also predict escalation of use for other substances (Lopez-Quintero et al., 2011). A risk factor specific to CUD progression involves initial and typical positive subjective response to cannabis use (e.g., pleasurable rush or buzz), which appears to be heritable (Agrawal, Madden, Bucholz, Heath, & Lynskey, 2014; Zeiger et al., 2010).

One study (Rosenberg & Anthony, 2001), which examined the sequential emergence of DSM-based cannabis symptoms, found that within one year of initiating cannabis use, more than one fourth of users reported hazardous use and psychological/physical symptoms associated with use. Among those with cannabis dependence, the first symptom to emerge was often larger/longer, a symptom of impaired control over use that was less commonly reported among those with no CUD or cannabis abuse only. The early emergence of larger/longer among those with cannabis dependence suggests that this symptom may serve as an early marker of risk for dependence. Among noncases, the most common cannabis symptom to emerge early, in 44% of this group, was quit/cut down. Of note, quit/cut down was never the first symptom to be reported by those with cannabis dependence. In this study, cannabis withdrawal emerged relatively late, as a more severe symptom of dependence (Rosenberg & Anthony, 2001). Further research is needed to characterize the sequential development of DSM–5 CUD symptoms, which can guide efforts to identify individuals with early problem use who could benefit from early intervention.

REMISSION AND RECOVERY FROM CUD

Relative to other substances (e.g., alcohol), cannabis has the highest rate of cessation of use (Anthony et al., 1994; Calabria et al., 2010), suggesting its possible lower addiction liability. Also, legalization, availability, and community norms may also influence cannabis's relative cessation rates compared to other substances. Among those with a lifetime CUD, most show remission of symptoms (Calabria et al., 2010; Farmer et al., 2015; Lopez-Quintero et al., 2011). In a US regional sample, 81.8% with a lifetime CUD recovered by age 30 (Farmer et al., 2015). A longitudinal community study of German youth found that among those with DSM–IV cannabis abuse, half (56.6%) improved over a one-year follow-up, 41.3% retained an abuse diagnosis, and 2.2% developed cannabis dependence (von Sydow et al., 2001). Among those with cannabis dependence, 19.0% remained dependent, but most showed full remission (44.2% with no disorder; 20.6% with abuse or partial remission) over a one-year follow-up (von Sydow et al., 2001); 82% of those with cannabis dependence at baseline showed remission over 10-year follow-up (Perkonigg et al., 2008). In a US national sample, median time to remission after onset of cannabis dependence was six years, with more than one third retaining a dependence diagnosis 10 years later (Lopez-Quintero et al., 2011). Although the majority of individuals with CUD show remission, a subgroup, particularly those with a cannabis dependence diagnosis, show a chronic course.

The period of highest risk for relapse to CUD occurs in the first year after remission (Florez-Salamanca et al., 2013). Longer duration of remission has been shown to be inversely related to risk for relapse over follow-up in a US national survey (Florez-Salamanca et al., 2013). Over a three-year follow-up in a US national sample, among individuals with CUD in remission at baseline, the CUD recurrence rate was 6.6% (Florez-Salamanca et al., 2013), which is lower than the rate observed in treatment samples (Witkiewitz & Marlatt, 2004) and may reflect the lower average severity of CUD in a population-based sample. Predictors of CUD recurrence are similar to predictors of progression and include, for example, other substance use and co-occurring psychopathology (Florez-Salamanca et al., 2013; Moore & Budney, 2003). The chronic nature of cannabis dependence among a subgroup of users suggests the importance of continuing care to maintain recovery (Scott, Dennis, Laudet, Funk, & Simeone, 2011).

RESEARCH AND TREATMENT GAPS

Basic questions regarding the impact of cannabis-related legislation on rates of use and cannabis-related health harms remain to be addressed. Given legalization of medical marijuana in several US states, as well as legal recreational use allowed in a few states, information is needed on rates of misuse of medical marijuana, including diversion of medical marijuana (Hopfer, 2014), and the impact of medical marijuana use on treatment for other substance use. Research also is needed on development of addiction to cannabis among medical marijuana users. In addition, little is known regarding the course of DSM–5 CUD, which included two new symptoms, cannabis withdrawal and craving. In particular, there are mixed findings regarding whether cannabis withdrawal is fairly prevalent or relatively rare. Another continuing issue involves whether substance-specific criteria and thresholds should be used (Budney, 2006), since the salience of certain SUD symptoms differs by substance. An important area for future research is the need to bring diagnostic systems into closer alignment with contemporary theories of the neurobiology of addiction (Koob, 2006). In this regard, Research Domain Criteria has been proposed as a framework to classify and characterize mental disorders based on neurobiological and behavioral measures and cross-cutting dimensional domains (e.g., cognitive systems, positive and negative valence systems) that underlie various forms of psychopathology (Cuthbert, 2014). Research that applies the Research Domain Criteria framework to addictive behaviors, such as CUD, is needed (Litten et al., 2015).

CONCLUSION

Core features of addiction as reflected by DSM criteria apply to cannabis, although certain SUD symptoms are less salient to cannabis relative to other substances. There is a need to bring diagnostic systems into closer alignment with neurobiological processes underlying addictive behavior (Litten et al., 2015). Cannabis activates brain reward circuitry common to addictive substances (Koob & Volkow, 2010) but generally has lower addiction liability compared to alcohol and tobacco (Anthony et al., 1994). There is variability in the prevalence of cannabis symptoms across countries and subgroups (e.g., age, gender); this variability may reflect differential impact of risk factors, environmental and cultural differences, and possible measurement error. The course of CUD is variable, with remission typically occurring with lower levels of severity and a subgroup of individuals at risk for chronic CUD. Divergent views on the legalization of marijuana for medical and recreational purposes (Loflin & Earleywine, 2015; Wright, 2015) provide compelling arguments for further research on the clinical features and course of CUD to inform public policy regarding cannabis.

REFERENCES

Agrawal, A., & Lynskey, M. T. (2007). Does gender contribute to heterogeneity in criteria for cannabis abuse and dependence? Results from the national epidemiological survey on alcohol and related conditions. *Drug and Alcohol Dependence, 88,* 300–307. http://dx.doi.org/10.1016/j.drugalcdep.2006.10.003

Agrawal, A., Lynskey, M. T., Bucholz, K. K., Kapoor, M., Almasy, L., Dick, D. M., . . . Bierut, L. J. (2014). DSM–5 cannabis use disorder: A phenotypic and genomic perspective. *Drug and Alcohol Dependence, 134,* 362–369. http://dx.doi.org/10.1016/j.drugalcdep.2013.11.008

Agrawal, A., Madden, P. A., Bucholz, K. K., Heath, A. C., & Lynskey, M. T. (2014). Initial reactions to tobacco and cannabis smoking: A twin study. *Addiction, 109,* 663–671. http://dx.doi.org/10.1111/add.12449

American Psychiatric Association. (1994). *Diagnostic and statistical manual of mental disorders* (4th ed.). Washington, DC: Author.

American Psychiatric Association. (2013). *Diagnostic and statistical manual of mental disorders* (5th ed.). Washington, DC: Author.

Ammerman, S., Ryan, S., & Adelman, W. P. (2015). The impact of marijuana policies on youth: Clinical, research, and legal update. *Pediatrics, 135,* e769–e785. http://dx.doi.org/10.1542/peds.2014-4147

Anthony, J. C., Warner, L. A., & Kessler, R. C. (1994). Comparative epidemiology of dependence on tobacco, alcohol, controlled substances, and inhalants. *Experimental and Clinical Psychopharmacology, 2,* 264–268. http://dx.doi.org/10.1037/1064-1297.2.3.244

Australian Institute of Health and Welfare. (2014). *National Drug Strategy Household Survey detailed report: 2013.* Drug statistics series no. 28. Cat. no. PHE 183. Canberra, AU: Author.

Beseler, C. L., & Hasin, D. S. (2010). Cannabis dimensionality: dependence, abuse and consumption. *Addictive Behaviors, 35*(11), 961–969.

Bestrashniy, J., & Winters, K. C. (2015). Variability in medical marijuana laws in the United States. *Psychology of Addictive Behaviors, 29,* 639–642. http://dx.doi.org/10.1037/adb0000111

Brook, J. S., Zhang, C., & Brook, D. W. (2011). Antisocial behavior at age 37: Developmental trajectories of marijuana use extending from adolescence to adulthood. *American Journal on Addictions, 20,* 509–515. http://dx.doi.org/10.1111/j.1521-0391.2011.00179.x

Budney, A. J. (2006). Are specific dependence criteria necessary for different substances: How can research on cannabis inform this issue? *Addiction, 101*(Suppl 1), 125–133. http://dx.doi.org/10.1111/j.1360-0443.2006.01582.x

Budney, A. J., Hughes, J. R., Moore, B. A., & Vandrey, R. (2004). Review of the validity and significance of cannabis withdrawal syndrome. *American Journal of Psychiatry, 161,* 1967–1977. http://dx.doi.org/10.1176/appi.ajp.161.11.1967

Budney, A. J., Moore, B. A., Vandrey, R. G., & Hughes, J. R. (2003). The time course and significance of cannabis withdrawal. *Journal of Abnormal Psychology, 112*, 393–402. http://dx.doi.org/10.1037/0021-843X.112.3.393

Budney, A. J., Vandrey, R. G., Hughes, J. R., Moore, B. A., & Bahrenburg, B. (2007). Oral delta-9-tetrahydrocannabinol suppresses cannabis withdrawal symptoms. *Drug and Alcohol Dependence, 86*, 22–29. http://dx.doi.org/10.1016/j.drugalcdep.2006.04.014

Calabria, B., Degenhardt, L., Briegleb, C., Vos, T., Hall, W., Lynskey, M., . . . McLaren, J. (2010). Systematic review of prospective studies investigating "remission" from amphetamine, cannabis, cocaine or opioid dependence. *Addictive Behaviors, 35*, 741–749. http://dx.doi.org/10.1016/j.addbeh.2010.03.019

Canadian Centre on Substance Abuse and Addiction. (2014). *Canadian drug summary.* Retrieved from http://www.ccsa.ca/Eng/topics/Marijuana/Pages/default.aspx

Cerda, M., Wall, M., Keyes, K. M., Galea, S., & Hasin, D. (2012). Medical marijuana laws in 50 states: Investigating the relationship between state legalization of medical marijuana and marijuana use, abuse and dependence. *Drug and Alcohol Dependence, 120*, 22–27. http://dx.doi.org/10.1016/j.drugalcdep.2011.06.011

Chen, C. Y., & Anthony, J. C. (2003). Possible age-associated bias in reporting of clinical features of drug dependence: Epidemiological evidence on adolescent-onset marijuana use. *Addiction, 98*, 71–82.

Chen, C. Y., O'Brien, M. S., & Anthony, J. C. (2005). Who becomes cannabis dependent soon after onset of use? Epidemiological evidence from the United States: 2000–2001. *Drug and Alcohol Dependence, 79*, 11–22. http://dx.doi.org/10.1016/j.drugalcdep.2004.11.014

Choo, E. K., Benz, M., Zaller, N., Warren, O., Rising, K. L., & McConnell, K. J. (2014). The impact of state medical marijuana legislation on adolescent marijuana use. *Journal of Adolescent Health, 55*, 160–166. http://dx.doi.org/10.1016/j.jadohealth.2014.02.018

Chung, T., & Martin, C. S. (2005). What were they thinking? Adolescents' interpretations of DSM–IV alcohol dependence symptom queries and implications for diagnostic validity. *Drug and Alcohol Dependence, 80*, 191–200. http://dx.doi.org/10.1016/j.drugalcdep.2005.03.023

Chung, T., Martin, C. S., Cornelius, J. R., & Clark, D. B. (2008). Cannabis withdrawal predicts severity of cannabis involvement at 1-year follow-up among treated adolescents. *Addiction, 103*, 787–799. http://dx.doi.org/10.1111/j.1360-0443.2008.02158.x

Coffey, C., Lynskey, M., Wolfe, R., & Patton, G. C. (2000). Initiation and progression of cannabis use in a population-based Australian adolescent longitudinal study. *Addiction, 95*, 1679–1690.

Compton, W. M., Grant, B. F., Colliver, J. D., Glantz, M. D., & Stinson, F. S. (2004). Prevalence of marijuana use disorders in the United States: 1991–1992 and 2001–2002. *JAMA, 291*, 2114–2121. http://dx.doi.org/10.1001/jama.291.17.2114

Compton, W. M., Saha, T. D., Conway, K. P., & Grant, B. F. (2009). The role of cannabis use within a dimensional approach to cannabis use disorders. *Drug and Alcohol Dependence, 100*, 221–227. http://dx.doi.org/10.1016/j.drugalcdep.2008.10.009

Cornelius, J. R., Chung, T., Martin, C., Wood, D. S., & Clark, D. B. (2008). Cannabis withdrawal is common among treatment-seeking adolescents with cannabis dependence and major depression, and is associated with rapid relapse to dependence. *Addictive behaviors, 33*, 1500–1505. http://dx.doi.org/10.1016/j.addbeh.2008.02.001

Cuthbert, B. N. (2014). The RDoC framework: Facilitating transition from ICD/DSM to dimensional approaches that integrate neuroscience and psychopathology. *World Psychiatry, 13*, 28–35. http://dx.doi.org/10.1002/wps.20087

Degenhardt, L., Ferrari, A. J., Calabria, B., Hall, W. D., Norman, R. E., McGrath, J., . . . Vos, T. (2013). The global epidemiology and contribution of cannabis use and dependence to the global burden of disease: Results from the GBD 2010 study. *PloS One, 8*, e76635. http://dx.doi.org/10.1371/journal.pone.0076635

Delforterie, M., Creemers, H., Agrawal, A., Lynskey, M., Jak, S., van der Ende, J., . . . Huizink, A. (2015). Functioning of cannabis abuse and dependence criteria across two different countries: The United States and The Netherlands. *Substance Use & Misuse, 50*, 242–250. http://dx.doi.org/10.3109/10826084.2014.952445

Dennis, M., Babor, T. F., Roebuck, M. C., & Donaldson, J. (2002). Changing the focus: The case for recognizing and treating cannabis use disorders. *Addiction, 97*(Suppl 1), 4–15. http://dx.doi.org/10.1046/j.1360-0443.97.s01.10.x

Edwards, G., & Gross, M. M. (1976). Alcohol dependence: provisional description of a clinical syndrome. *British Medical Journal, 1*, 1058–1061.

Ellickson, P. L., Martino, S. C., & Collins, R. L. (2004). Marijuana use from adolescence to young adulthood: Multiple developmental trajectories and their associated outcomes. *Health Psychology, 23*, 299–307. http://dx.doi.org/10.1037/0278-6133.23.3.299

ElSohly, M. (2014). *Potency monitoring program quarterly report no.123—Reporting period: 09/16/2013–12/15/2013*. Oxford, MS: University of Mississippi, National Center for Natural Products Research.

European Monitoring Centre on Drugs and Drug Addiction. (2014). *European Drug Report 2014: Trends and developments*. Retrieved from http://www.emcdda.europa.eu/publications/edr/trends-developments/2014 Retrieved 03-24-15

Farmer, R. F., Kosty, D. B., Seeley, J. R., Duncan, S. C., Lynskey, M. T., Rohde, P., . . . Lewinsohn, P. M. (2015). Natural course of cannabis use disorders. *Psychological Medicine, 45*, 63–72. http://dx.doi.org/10.1017/S003329171400107X

Fiestas, F., Radovanovic, M., Martins, S. S., Medina-Mora, M. E., Posada-Villa, J., & Anthony, J. C. (2010). Cross-national differences in clinically significant cannabis problems: Wpidemiologic evidence from "cannabis-only" smokers in the United States, Mexico, and Colombia. *BMC Public Health, 10*, 152. http://dx.doi.org/10.1186/1471-2458-10-152

Florez-Salamanca, L., Secades-Villa, R., Budney, A. J., Garcia-Rodriguez, O., Wang, S., & Blanco, C. (2013). Probability and predictors of cannabis use disorders relapse: Results of the National Epidemiologic Survey on Alcohol and Related Conditions (NESARC). *Drug and Alcohol Dependence, 132*, 127–133. http://dx.doi.org/10.1016/j.drugalcdep.2013.01.013

Flory, K., Lynam, D., Milich, R., Leukefeld, C., & Clayton, R. (2004). Early adolescent through young adult alcohol and marijuana use trajectories: Early predictors, young adult outcomes, and predictive utility. *Development and Psychopathology, 16*, 193–213.

Gillespie, N. A., Neale, M. C., Prescott, C. A., Aggen, S. H., & Kendler, K. S. (2007). Factor and item-response analysis DSM–IV criteria for abuse of and dependence on cannabis, cocaine, hallucinogens, sedatives, stimulants and opioids. *Addiction, 102*, 920–930. http://dx.doi.org/10.1111/j.1360-0443.2007.01804.x

Gizer, I. R., Gilder, D. A., Lau, P., Wang, T., Wilhelmsen, K. C., & Ehlers, C. L. (2013). Contributions of ethnicity to differential item functioning of cannabis abuse and dependence symptoms. *Journal of Studies on Alcohol and Drugs, 74*, 320–328.

Hall, W. (2015). What has research over the past two decades revealed about the adverse health effects of recreational cannabis use? *Addiction, 110*, 19–35. http://dx.doi.org/10.1111/add.12703

Hall, W., & Pacula, R. L. (2003). *Cannabis use and dependence: Public health and public policy.* Cambridge, UK: Cambridge University Press.

Haney, M., Ward, A. S., Comer, S. D., Foltin, R. W., & Fischman, M. W. (1999). Abstinence symptoms following smoked marijuana in humans. *Psychopharmacology, 141*, 395–404.

Hartman, C. A., Gelhorn, H., Crowley, T. J., Sakai, J. T., Stallings, M., Young, S. E., . . . Hopfer, C. J. (2008). Item response theory analysis of DSM–IV cannabis abuse and dependence criteria in adolescents. *Journal of the American Academy of Child and Adolescent Psychiatry, 47*, 165–173. http://dx.doi.org/10.1097/chi.0b013e31815cd9f2

Hasin, D. S., O'Brien, C. P., Auriacombe, M., Borges, G., Bucholz, K., Budney, A., . . . Grant, B. F. (2013). DSM–5 criteria for substance use disorders: Recommendations and rationale. *American Journal of Psychiatry, 170*, 834–851. http://dx.doi.org/10.1176/appi.ajp.2013.12060782

Hasin, D. S., Wall, M., Keyes, K. M., Cerdá, M., Schulenberg, J., O'Malley, P. M., . . . Feng, T. (2015). Medical marijuana laws and adolescent marijuana use in the USA from 1991 to 2014: Results from annual, repeated cross-sectional surveys. *The Lancet: Psychiatry, 2*, 601–68. http://dx.doi.org/10.1016/S2215-0366(15)00217-5

Hopfer, C. (2014). Implications of marijuana legalization for adolescent substance use. *Substance abuse, 35*, 331–335. http://dx.doi.org/10.1080/08897077.2014.943386

Johnston, L. D., O'Malley, P. M., Miech, R. A., Bachman, J. G., & Schulenberg, J. E. (2014). *Monitoring the Future national results on drug use: 1975-2013: Overview, Key Findings on Adolescent Drug Use.* Ann. Arbor: Institute for Social Research, The University of. Michigan. Institute for Social Research.

Keyes, K. M., Vo, T., Wall, M. M., Caetano, R., Suglia, S. F., Martins, S. S., . . . Hasin, D. (2015). Racial/ethnic differences in use of alcohol, tobacco, and marijuana: is there a cross-over from adolescence to adulthood? *Social Science in Medicine, 124*, 132–141. http://dx.doi.org/10.1016/j.socscimed.2014.11.035

Koob, G. F. (2006). The neurobiology of addiction: a neuroadaptational view relevant for diagnosis. *Addiction, 101*(Suppl 1), 23–30. http://dx.doi.org/10.1111/j.1360-0443.2006.01586.x

Koob, G. F., & Volkow, N. D. (2010). Neurocircuitry of addiction. *Neuropsychopharmacology, 35*, 217–238. http://dx.doi.org/10.1038/npp.2009.110

Kubarych, T. S., Kendler, K. S., Aggen, S. H., Estabrook, R., Edwards, A. C., Clark, S. L., . . . Gillespie, N. A. (2014). Comparing factor, class, and mixture models of cannabis initiation and DSM cannabis use disorder criteria, including craving, in the Brisbane longitudinal twin study. *Twin Research and Human Genetics, 17*, 89–98. http://dx.doi.org/10.1017/thg.2014.9

Lanza, S. T., Vasilenko, S. A., Dziak, J. J., & Butera, N. M. (2015). Trends Among US high school seniors in recent marijuana use and associations with other substances: 1976–2013. *Journal of Adolescent Health, 57*, 198–204. http://dx.doi.org/10.1016/j.jadohealth.2015.04.006

Litten, R. Z., Ryan, M. L., Falk, D. E., Reilly, M., Fertig, J. B., & Koob, G. F. (2015). Heterogeneity of alcohol use disorder: Understanding mechanisms to advance personalized treatment. *Alcoholism: Clinical and Experimental Research*, 39, 579–584. http://dx.doi.org/10.1111/acer.12669

Loflin, M., & Earleywine, M. (2015). The case for medical marijuana: An issue of relief. *Drug and Alcohol Dependence*, 149, 293–297. http://dx.doi.org/10.1016/j.drugalcdep.2015.01.006

Lopez-Quintero, C., Perez de los Cobos, J., Hasin, D. S., Okuda, M., Wang, S., Grant, B. F., & Blanco, C. (2011). Probability and predictors of transition from first use to dependence on nicotine, alcohol, cannabis, and cocaine: Results of the National Epidemiologic Survey on Alcohol and Related Conditions (NESARC). *Drug and Alcohol Dependence*, 115, 120–130. http://dx.doi.org/10.1016/j.drugalcdep.2010.11.004

Lynne-Landsman, S. D., Livingston, M. D., & Wagenaar, A. C. (2013). Effects of state medical marijuana laws on adolescent marijuana use. *American Journal of Public Health*, 103, 1500–1506. http://dx.doi.org/10.2105/AJPH.2012.301117

MacCoun, R., & Reuter, P. (1997). Interpreting Dutch cannabis policy: Reasoning by analogy in the legalization debate. *Science*, 278(5335), 47–52.

Martin, C. S., Chung, T., Kirisci, L., & Langenbucher, J. W. (2006). Item response theory analysis of diagnostic criteria for alcohol and cannabis use disorders in adolescents: implications for DSM-V. *Journal of Abnormal Psychology*, 115, 807–814. http://dx.doi.org/10.1037/0021-843X.115.4.807

Mewton, L., Slade, T., & Teesson, M. (2013). An evaluation of the proposed DSM-5 cannabis use disorder criteria using Australian national survey data. *Journal of Studies on Alcohol and Drugs*, 74, 614–621. http://dx.doi.org/10.15288/jsad.2013.74.614

Milin, R., Manion, I., Dare, G., & Walker, S. (2008). Prospective assessment of cannabis withdrawal in adolescents with cannabis dependence: A pilot study. *Journal of the American Academy of Child and Adolescent Psychiatry*, 47, 174–178. http://dx.doi.org/10.1097/chi.0b013e31815cdd73

Moore, B. A., & Budney, A. J. (2003). Relapse in outpatient treatment for marijuana dependence. *Journal of Substance Abuse Treatment*, 25, 85–89.

Nocon, A., Wittchen, H. U., Pfister, H., Zimmermann, P., & Lieb, R. (2006). Dependence symptoms in young cannabis users? A prospective epidemiological study. *Journal of Psychiatric Research*, 40, 394–403. http://dx.doi.org/10.1016/j.jpsychires.2005.07.011

Passarotti, A. M., Crane, N. A., Hedeker, D., & Mermelstein, R. J. (2015). Longitudinal trajectories of marijuana use from adolescence to young adulthood. *Addictive behaviors*, 45, 301–308. http://dx.doi.org/10.1016/j.addbeh.2015.02.008

Perkonigg, A., Goodwin, R. D., Fiedler, A., Behrendt, S., Beesdo, K., Lieb, R., & Wittchen, H. U. (2008). The natural course of cannabis use, abuse and dependence during the first decades of life. *Addiction*, 103, 439–449; discussion 450–431. http://dx.doi.org/10.1111/j.1360-0443.2007.02064.x

Piontek, D., Kraus, L., Legleye, S., & Buhringer, G. (2011). The validity of DSM-IV cannabis abuse and dependence criteria in adolescents and the value of additional cannabis use indicators. *Addiction*, 106, 1137–1145. http://dx.doi.org/10.1111/j.1360-0443.2010.03359.x

Prince van Leeuwen, A., Creemers, H. E., Verhulst, F. C., Vollebergh, W. A., Ormel, J., van Oort, F., & Huizink, A. C. (2014). Legal substance use and the development of a

DSM–IV cannabis use disorder during adolescence: The TRAILS study. *Addiction, 109*, 303–311. http://dx.doi.org/10.1111/add.12346

Ridenour, T. A., Maldonado-Molina, M., Compton, W. M., Spitznagel, E. L., & Cottler, L. B. (2005). Factors associated with the transition from abuse to dependence among substance abusers: Implications for a measure of addictive liability. *Drug and Alcohol Dependence, 80*, 1–14. http://dx.doi.org/10.1016/j.drugalcdep.2005.02.005

Rosenberg, M. F., & Anthony, J. C. (2001). Early clinical manifestations of cannabis dependence in a community sample. *Drug and Alcohol Dependence, 64*, 123–131.

Salas-Wright, C. P., Vaughn, M. G., Todic, J., Córdova, D., & Perron, B. E. (2015). Trends in the disapproval and use of marijuana among adolescents and young adults in the United States: 2002–2013. *American Journal of Drug and Alcohol Abuse, 41*, 392–404. http://dx.doi.org/10.3109/00952990.2015.1049493

Schulenberg, J., Merline, A., Johnston, L., O'Malley, P., Bachman, J., & Laetz, V. (2005). Trajectories of marijuana use during the transition to adulthood: The big picture based on national panel data. *Journal of Drug Issues, 35*, 255–279. http://dx.doi.org/10.1177/002204260503500203

Scott, C. K., Dennis, M. L., Laudet, A., Funk, R. R., & Simeone, R. S. (2011). Surviving drug addiction: The effect of treatment and abstinence on mortality. *American Journal of Public Health, 101*, 737–744. http://dx.doi.org/10.2105/AJPH.2010.197038

Stinson, F. S., Ruan, W. J., Pickering, R., & Grant, B. F. (2006). Cannabis use disorders in the USA: Prevalence, correlates and co-morbidity. *Psychological Medicine, 36*, 1447–1460. http://dx.doi.org/10.1017/S0033291706008361

Substance Abuse and Mental Health Services Administration. (2014). *Results from the 2013 National Survey on Drug Use and Health: Summary of national findings*, NSDUH Series H-48, HHS Publication No. (SMA) 14-4863. Rockville, MD: Author.

Substance Abuse and Mental Health Services Administration. (2015). *Behavioral health barometer: United States, 2014*. HHS Publication No. SMA-15-4895. Rockville, MD: Author.

Swift, W., Hall, W., & Teesson, M. (2001). Characteristics of DSM–IV and ICD-10 cannabis dependence among Australian adults: Results from the National Survey of Mental Health and Wellbeing. *Drug and Alcohol Dependence, 63*, 147–153. http://dx.doi.org/10.1016/S0376-8716(00)00197-6

Taylor, M., Collin, S. M., Munafò, M. R., MacLeod, J., Hickman, M., & Heron, J. (2017). Patterns of cannabis use during adolescence and their association with harmful substance use behaviour: Findings from a UK birth cohort. *Journal of Epidemiology and Community Health, 71*, 764–770.

ter Bogt, T. F., de Looze, M., Molcho, M., Godeau, E., Hublet, A., Kokkevi, A., . . . Pickett, W. (2014). Do societal wealth, family affluence and gender account for trends in adolescent cannabis use? A 30 country cross-national study. *Addiction, 109*, 273–283. http://dx.doi.org/10.1111/add.12373

Tucker, J., Ellickson, P., Orlando, M., Martino, S., & Klein, D. (2005). Substance use trajectories from early adolescence to emerging adulthood: A comparison of smoking, binge drinking, and marijuana use. *Journal of Drug Issues, 35*, 307–331. http://dx.doi.org/10.1177/002204260503500205

United Nations Office on Drugs and Crime. (2014). *World drug report 2014*. United Nations publication, Sales No. E.14.XI.7. New York: Author.

Volkow, N. D., Baler, R. D., Compton, W. M., & Weiss, S. R. (2014). Adverse health effects of marijuana use. *New England Journal of Medicine, 370*, 2219–2227. http://dx.doi.org/10.1056/NEJMra1402309

von Sydow, K., Lieb, R., Pfister, H., Hofler, M., Sonntag, H., & Wittchen, H. U. (2001). The natural course of cannabis use, abuse and dependence over four years: A longitudinal community study of adolescents and young adults. *Drug and Alcohol Dependence, 64,* 347–361.

Wagner, F. A., & Anthony, J. C. (2002). From first drug use to drug dependence: Developmental periods of risk for dependence upon marijuana, cocaine, and alcohol. *Neuropsychopharmacology, 26,* 479–488. http://dx.doi.org/10.1016/S0893-133X(01)00367-0

Wall, M. M., Poh, E., Cerda, M., Keyes, K. M., Galea, S., & Hasin, D. S. (2011). Adolescent marijuana use from 2002 to 2008: Higher in states with medical marijuana laws, cause still unclear. *Annals of Epidemiology, 21,* 714–716. http://dx.doi.org/10.1016/j.annepidem.2011.06.001

Winters, K. C., & Lee, C. Y. (2008). Likelihood of developing an alcohol and cannabis use disorder during youth: Association with recent use and age. *Drug and Alcohol Dependence, 92,* 239–247. http://dx.doi.org/10.1016/j.drugalcdep.2007.08.005

Winters, K. C., Martin, C. S., & Chung, T. (2011). Commentary on O'Brien: Substance use disorders in DSM-5 when applied to adolescents. *Addiction, 106,* 882–884. http://dx.doi.org/10.1111/j.1360-0443.2010.03334.x

Witkiewitz, K., & Marlatt, G. A. (2004). Relapse prevention for alcohol and drug problems: That was Zen, this is Tao. *American Psychologist, 59,* 224–235. http://dx.doi.org/10.1037/0003-066X.59.4.224

Wright, J. (2015). Legalizing marijuana for medical purposes will increase risk of long-term, deleterious consequences for adolescents. *Drug and Alcohol Dependence, 149,* 298–303. http://dx.doi.org/10.1016/j.drugalcdep.2015.01.005

Wu, L. T., Pan, J. J., Blazer, D. G., Tai, B., Stitzer, M. L., Brooner, R. K., . . . Blaine, J. D. (2009). An item response theory modeling of alcohol and marijuana dependences: A National Drug Abuse Treatment Clinical Trials Network study. *Journal of Studies on Alcohol and Drugs, 70,* 414–425. http://dx.doi.org/10.15288/jsad.2009.70.414

Young, S. E., Corley, R. P., Stallings, M. C., Rhee, S. H., Crowley, T. J., & Hewitt, J. K. (2002). Substance use, abuse and dependence in adolescence: Prevalence, symptom profiles and correlates. *Drug and Alcohol Dependence, 68,* 309–322. http://dx.doi.org/10.1016/S0376-8716(02)00225-9

Zeiger, J. S., Haberstick, B. C., Corley, R. P., Ehringer, M. A., Crowley, T. J., Hewitt, J. K., . . . Rhee, S. H. (2010). Subjective effects to marijuana associated with marijuana use in community and clinical subjects. *Drug and Alcohol Dependence, 109,* 161–166. http://dx.doi.org/10.1016/j.drugalcdep.2009.12.026

4

Effects of Adolescent Cannabis Use on Brain Structure and Function

Current Findings and Recommendations

for Future Research

RANDI MELISSA SCHUSTER, JODI GILMAN, AND A. EDEN EVINS

INTRODUCTION

Cannabis is the most commonly used illicit substance among adolescents in the United States and is one of the only substances with steadily increasing prevalence estimates. In fact, cannabis is now used at higher rates than tobacco (Johnston et al., 2012), and the gap between alcohol and marijuana use among middle and high school students has closed considerably in the past decade (Substance Abuse and Mental Health Services Administration [SAMHSA], 2014). Recent estimates suggest that over half of 18 to 25 year olds have tried cannabis (SAMHSA, 2014), with rates of experimental use increasing with age (e.g., 30.1% of 9th graders, 48.6% of 12th graders; Kann et al., 2014). Nearly one fourth (23.4%) of high school students report use at least one or more times per month (Kann et al., 2014).

Rising prevalence of use in recent years has mirrored an overall decrease in perceived harm of cannabis use (Johnston et al., 2012, 2013) as well as a steady increase in social and legal permissiveness for recreational and medicinal use (Cohen, 2010; Elikkottil, Gupta, & Gupta, 2009; Jarvis et al., 2008; O'Connell & Bou-Matar, 2007). Further, the potency of cannabis available for purchase in the United States has steadily increased such that some versions (e.g., sinsemilla, skunk) contain up to 25-fold higher concentrations of delta-9-tetrahydrocannabinol (THC) than varieties available in previous decades (Burgdorf, Kilmer, & Pacula, 2011; ElSohly, 2014).

The more prevalent usage of a more potent drug in an era of increasing social acceptance of use is a significant public health concern if such use causes
harm. The lifetime risk for cannabis dependence is 17% (one in six) when use
is initiated during teenage years (Anthony, 2006), approximately 9% when use
is initiated in adulthood (Lopez-Quintero et al., 2011), and 25% to 50% in those
who use daily (Hall, 2009; Hall & Degenhardt, 2009); yet it should be noted
that some of these studies involve data that are more than two decades old, and
updating is warranted as rates may have changed with the shifting pattern of use
over time. The rate of transition from non-problematic to problematic cannabis
use may occur more rapidly with cannabis than nicotine or alcohol use (Lopez-
Quintero et al., 2011), although fewer lifetime users of cannabis (9%) progress to
dependence compared to tobacco (67%) and alcohol (23%; Lopez-Quintero et al.,
2011). Also of note, there are sex differences in trajectories of use. Males are more
likely than females to use cannabis and initiate use at an earlier age (Gfroerer
& Epstein, 1999; Pope et al., 2003; SAMHSA, 2014). Females develop tolerance
more rapidly than males (Cocchetto, Owens, Perez-Reyes, DiGuiseppi, & Miller,
1981; Narimatsu, Watanabe, Yamamoto, & Yoshimura, 1991), experience greater
sensitivity to the subjective effects of cannabis intoxication (Cooper & Haney,
2009, 2014), and enter treatment for cannabis use disorders earlier, after fewer
years of use, and less cumulative exposure (Ehlers et al., 2010; Hernandez-Avila,
Rounsaville, & Kranzler, 2004; Khan et al., 2013).

In addition to adolescent cannabis use being associated with reduced education, employment, income, and relationship and life satisfaction (Brook,
Lee, Finch, Seltzer, & Brook, 2013; Fergusson & Boden, 2008), specific brain
and neurocognitive sequelae of adolescent cannabis use has become an area of
increased interest. This chapter will attempt to synthesize what we know about
cannabis's relationship to neurocognitive abnormalities among individuals who
are undergoing ongoing neurodevelopment, delineate what remains unknown
(and why), and outline what scientific steps are needed to gain a better understanding of the relationship between early cannabis exposure and cognitive
health.

THE DEVELOPING CENTRAL NERVOUS SYSTEM

Adolescence is a period of profound and dynamic changes throughout the brain.
Changes to micro- and macrostructure are occurring, particularly in the prefrontal cortex, limbic system, and white matter association fibers, accompanied
by neurochemical alterations (Bava & Tapert, 2010; Huttenlocher & Dabholkar,
1997; Sowell et al., 1999). Although the overall size of the brain does not change
substantially beyond early childhood (Pfefferbaum et al., 1994), longitudinal
morphometric studies reveal global cortical development through middle adolescence (Giedd et al., 1999; Gogtay et al., 2004) with pruning of superfluous
synaptic connections and reductions in glial cells (Huttenlocher & Dabholkar,
1997; Paus, Keshavan, & Giedd, 2008; Tamnes et al., 2010). The development of

cortical grey matter follows an inverted parabolic trajectory, with a peak in density at age 12 to 14 years followed by synaptic pruning that results in a steady decline in neuronal density across the remainder of adolescence (Giedd et al., 1999; Gogtay et al., 2004). Changes in brain volumetry tend to progress in the rostral to caudal direction with attenuations in cortical thickness occurring earlier in the striatum and sensorimotor cortices and later in higher-order association areas such as the prefrontal cortex (Gogtay et al., 2004; Sowell et al., 1999). White matter is also developing in adolescence, undergoing a more protracted and linear increase in volume well into young adulthood (Durston et al., 2001; Giedd et al., 1999), with little regional variation except for exaggerated axonal growth in fronto-parietal lobules (Huttenlocher, 1990; Nagel et al., 2006). The adolescent brain also undergoes dramatic alterations involving multiple neurotransmitter systems. From adolescence into adulthood, there is an increase in dopaminergic projections to the prefrontal cortex (Lambe, Krimer, & Goldman-Rakic, 2000; Tunbridge et al., 2007), increased synthesis and turnover of dopamine (Andersen, Dumont, & Teicher, 1997; Teicher et al., 1993), and increased input to GABAergic inhibitory interneurons in the prefrontal cortex (Lewis, 1997; Spear, 2000).

In terms of sex differences, total brain volume peaks later in males (i.e., 14–15 years of age) compared to females (i.e., 10–11 years of age; Lenroot et al., 2007). Similarly, cortical and subcortical grey matter volumes peak approximately one to two years later in males than females (Lenroot et al., 2007). The overall net volume change and rate of change in both grey and white matter volume are greater in males than females (Giedd et al., 1999). There are also sex differences in the endocannabinoid system. Males exhibit greater type 1 cannabinoid receptor (CB1) density in certain brain regions as well as greater desensitization after THC exposure of CB1 receptors in the prefrontal cortex, hippocampus, striatum, amygdala, and midbrain structures central to higher-order cognitive processing (Burston, Wiley, Craig, Selley, & Sim-Selley, 2010; Rubino et al., 2008).

HEIGHTENED VULNERABILITY TO CANNABIS DURING ADOLESCENCE

Overview

Increased brain plasticity during adolescence allows for more refined higher-order cognitive processing than in earlier developmental epochs but also may render adolescents more vulnerable than adults to effects of psychoactive compounds on these developmental processes. THC is one psychoactive compound in cannabis that binds to endogenous cannabinoid receptors (CB1), which are primarily found on presynaptic central and peripheral neurons and are largely inhibitory in their modulation of synaptic signaling (Freund, Katona, & Piomelli, 2003; Howlett et al., 2002; Viveros, Llorente, Moreno, & Marco, 2005). CB1 receptors are among the most abundant G-protein (i.e., specialized proteins with the ability to bind with guanosine triphosphate and guanosine diphosphate) coupled receptors in the central nervous system (CNS), and they are most densely located in the hippocampus (memory), amygdala (emotion), basal ganglia (movement coordination), and prefrontal cortex (executive functions; Mackie, 2005; Piomelli, 2003), making frontal-limbic neurocircuitry structure and function a prime target of study of the CNS effects of THC (Martin-Santos et al., 2010).

Vulnerability to Neurobiological Structural Abnormalities during Adolescence

Because the endocannabinoid system plays a central role in overall CNS neuromaturation (Mechoulam & Parker, 2013; Viveros et al., 2012) and undergoes substantial development during adolescence (e.g., dramatic pruning of receptor density levels in subcortical and frontal regions; Heng, Beverley, Steiner, & Tseng, 2011; Rodriguez de Fonseca, Ramos, Bonnin, & Fernandez-Ruiz, 1993), exposure to exogenous cannabinoids during this period may influence brain development (Bava & Tapert, 2010; Lubman, Cheetham, & Yucel, 2015). Animal models have demonstrated heightened vulnerability to neurobiological alterations with early exposure to cannabinoids. Chronic exposure to THC in adolescent rats is associated with blunted serotonergic activity in the brainstem (Bambico, Nguyen, Katz, & Gobbi, 2010). Human studies with adults indicate an association of chronic use of cannabis and disrupted dopaminergic activity in the midbrain (Pistis et al., 2004). Exposure to a CB1 receptor agonist (WIN) in early and mid-adolescence, but not in late adolescence, downregulates prefrontal cortex GABAergic transmission with subsequent disinhibition of the prefrontal cortex in adulthood (Cass et al., 2014). Cannabinoid administration may disrupt normal pruning, perhaps through altered functioning of astrocytes, which are macroglial cells in the CNS that, among many other functions, are involved in establishing the micro-architecture of the brain parenchyma as well as synaptogenesis and synaptic maintenance (Bindukumar et al., 2008; Stevens et al., 2007).

Cannabis users show region-specific alterations in cortical thickness, including decreased volume of the insula and frontal cortices and increased volume in temporal, parietal, and paracentral regions (Ashtari et al., 2011; Churchwell, Lopez-Larson, & Yurgelun-Todd, 2010; Filbey et al., 2014; Lopez-Larson et al., 2011). These neuroanatomical alterations may persist for extended periods following cannabis discontinuation (Jacobus et al., 2012) and are inversely correlated with age of cannabis initiation (Lopez-Larson et al., 2011; Wilson et al., 2000), consistent with that reported for other substances, such as alcohol (De Bellis et al., 2000, 2008). Adolescent cannabis exposure has also been associated with compromised white matter integrity (Arnone et al., 2008; Ashtari et al., 2009; Bava et al., 2009; Delisi et al., 2006; Gruber, Silveri, Dahlgren, & Yurgelun-Todd, 2011), including microstructural abnormalities in the splenium of the corpus callosum and the fornix (Gruber, Dahlgren, Sagar, Gonenc, & Lukas, 2014; Rigucci et al., 2016; Zalesky et al., 2012), which is consistent with the role of the endocannabinoid system in developmental synapse formation (Gaffuri, Ladarre, & Lenkei, 2012).

While most studies of adult cannabis users report reduced or no difference in brain volume compared to nonusers, a study of adolescents (Medina et al., 2007) reported hippocampal volume enlargement in users compared with nonusing control subjects. Exposure-dependent nucleus accumbens enlargement, increased gray matter density, and shape abnormalities were reported among recreational adolescent cannabis users compared to matched control nonusers, adjusting for potential confounds (e.g., age, sex, alcohol and cigarette use; Gilman et al., 2014). Adolescents who use cannabis have demonstrated reduced interhemispheric resting state functional connectivity as well as increased connectivity of the middle frontal gyrus and right hemisphere compared to nonusers (Houck, Bryan, & Feldstein Ewing, 2013; Orr et al., 2013), and a pattern of negative functional connectivity of the nucleus accumbens and the medial prefrontal cortex (Lichenstein et al., 2017). Some studies employing magnetic resonance spectroscopy have found metabolic alterations including lower levels of glutamate, GABA, *N-acetyl-asparate*, creatine, and myo-inositol in subcortical grey matter (Silveri, Jensen, Rosso, Sneider, & Yurgelun-Todd, 2011), lower NAA/tCr ratios in the prefrontal cortex (Sung et al., 2013), and reduced myo-inositol levels in white matter (Silveri et al., 2011) in cannabis users compared with nonusers. Although some studies have suggested that these neurobiological abnormalities may not be unique to cannabis use (Becker, Wagner, Gouzoulis-Mayfrank, Spuentrup, & Daumann, 2010; Jacobus et al., 2009; Jacobus, Squeglia, Bava, & Tapert, 2013), others have provided preliminary evidence speaking to the specificity of these effects (Gilman et al., 2014) and argue for the possibility of sensitive biomarkers for cannabis's effect on brain structure and function during vulnerable neuromaturational periods. Further research is clearly needed to replicate the findings and further understand the structure-function relationships as well as dose and age of onset effects. These studies are cross sectional in design, and ideal studies would have assessments prior to onset of cannabis use, during cannabis use, and ideally, after extended abstinence from cannabis use.

There is preliminary evidence that sex plays a role in the effect of cannabis exposure in adolescence on brain morphometry. Female chronic cannabis users had larger amygdala volumes (Jarvis et al., 2008; McQueeny et al., 2011; Medina, Nagel, & Tapert, 2010) and prefrontal cortices (Medina et al., 2009; Medina et al., 2010) than nonusing control subjects, whereas male cannabis users had comparable amygdala volumes (McQueeny et al., 2011) and smaller prefrontal cortices (Medina et al., 2009; Medina et al., 2010) than nonusers; however, these studies did not present specific a priori hypotheses for gender effects, and the sample sizes were small (range: 16 to 35 cannabis users) and disproportionately male, requiring need for replication across larger studies that are balanced for gender. If replicated, such morphometric differences may have important implications on cognition, as larger prefrontal cortical volume has been associated with poorer executive functioning among adolescent cannabis users, whereas the opposite pattern is observed among control subjects (Medina et al., 2009; Medina et al., 2010). Additionally, amount of cannabis use in males has been related to psychomotor processing (Lisdahl & Price, 2012) and decision-making (Crane, Schuster, Fusar-Poli, & Gonzalez, 2013), and to memory (Crane et al., 2013) and visuospatial processing in females (Pope, Jacobs, Mialet, Yurgelun-Todd, & Gruber, 1997), although the moderating effect of gender on cannabis use and neurocognition is not universally reported (Solowij et al., 2011; Tait, Mackinnon, & Christensen, 2011). Together, findings suggest that cannabis use may lead to or result from sex-specific aspects of brain structure and cognition, especially in regions involved in higher-order cognitive processing.

Vulnerability to Neurocognitive Functioning Abnormalities during Adolescence

In addition to heightened vulnerability to effects on brain structure with initiation of cannabis use in adolescence, evidence is accumulating that adolescent-initiated cannabis use is associated with greater risk for neurocognitive difficulties. Rats exposed to chronic doses of THC in early but not late adolescence showed impairments into adulthood in learning (Harte & Dow-Edwards, 2010; Jager & Ramsey, 2008; Schneider & Koch, 2003, 2007) and working memory (O'Shea, Singh, McGregor, & Mallet, 2004; Rubino et al., 2009). Additionally, rats exposed to chronic, heavy THC during adolescence and tested in adulthood long after exposure had stopped exhibiting impaired spatial working memory, marker protein alterations indicating altered hippocampal neuroplasticity, and altered dendritic morphology in the dentate gyrus (Rubino et al., 2009). Similarly, pretreatment with repeated intraperitoneal injections of THC or cannabinoid agonists such as CP 55,940 resulted in greater lasting object recognition memory and working memory decrements as well as hippocampal alterations in adolescent rats compared to adult rats even after extended washout periods (O'Shea et al., 2004; Quinn et al., 2008).

Human studies also indicate that adolescence is a vulnerable developmental window during which cannabis appears to have the greatest impact on neurocognitive functioning. Controlling for multiple potential confounds, those who initiate cannabis use before 18 years show greater impairments compared to those with later onset in terms of visual attention (Ehrenreich et al., 1999), visual search efficiency (Huestegge, Radach, Kunert, & Heller, 2002), verbal fluency (Gruber, Dahlgren, Sagar, Gonenc, & Killgore, 2012; Gruber, Sagar, Dahlgren, Racine, & Lukas, 2012; Pope et al., 2003), episodic memory (Gruber, Dahlgren, et al., 2012; Pope et al., 2003; Solowij et al., 2011), and executive functioning (Fontes et al., 2011; Gruber, Sagar, et al., 2012; Solowij et al., 2011) as well as declines in intellectual functioning (Meier et al., 2012; Pope, Gruber, Hudson, Huestis, & Yurgelun-Todd, 2002). For example, initiation before age 16 was predictive of impaired reaction times on a visual scanning task, above and beyond the effects of current age, THC plasma levels and cumulative lifetime cannabis exposure as compared to later onset users who were not different from control subjects (Ehrenreich et al., 1999). Solowij et al. (2011) reported that earlier age of initiation of cannabis use was associated with poorer learning and retention and retrieval of novel verbal information, controlling for the frequency and amount of cannabis exposure. The neural correlates of the effects of early cannabis use on neurocognitive performance are beginning to be elucidated. For example, those with earlier onset chronic cannabis use made more errors on a behavioral inhibition task and showed more focal activation of the middle anterior cingulate cortex than later onset chronic users (Gruber, Dahlgren, et al., 2012). A summary of this literature is provided in the following discussion, and an overview is offered in Table 4.1.

GLOBAL INTELLECTUAL AND NEUROCOGNITIVE FUNCTIONING

The relationship between cannabis use and global neurocognitive functioning is only a topic of recent inquiry. Hooper, Woolley, and De Bellis (2014) reported that adolescents with cannabis use disorders did not differ from psychiatric and healthy control subjects in intellectual functioning, but their academic achievement scores were significantly below healthy control subjects and comparable to psychiatric control subjects, respectively. Younger age of onset of regular and maximum daily use were correlated with lower achievement scores as well

Table 4.1 SUMMARY OF LITERATURE ON THE EXTENT TO WHICH THERE IS A RESIDUAL IMPACT OF MARIJUANA USE ON ADOLESCENT NEUROCOGNITIVE FUNCTIONING

Neurocognitive Domain	Studies	Agreement among Studies	Finding
Intelligence and Global Neurocognitive Functioning	Very Few	No consensus	Unknown
Memory	Many	High consensus	Detrimental
Processing Speed and Attention	Few	Consensus	Detrimental
Working Memory	Few	No consensus	Unknown
Inhibitory Control	Very Few	No consensus	Unknown
Decision-Making	Few	Consensus	Detrimental
Set-Shifting	Very Few	No consensus	Unknown
Abstract Reasoning	Very Few	No consensus	Unknown
Language	Very Few	No consensus	Unknown

NOTES: ≥10 studies was classified as "many"; 5–9 studies was classified as "few"; <5 studies was classified as "very few."

as moderately correlated with composite estimates of overall neurocognitive functioning (Hooper et al., 2014). Similarly, in a longitudinal study of 1,037 individuals followed from birth to age 38, individuals who initiated cannabis earlier in adolescence showed the greatest decline in intellectual functioning in adulthood (i.e., a decline of on average 8 points) even in the context of sustained abstinence and after matching for the number of cannabis dependence symptoms (Meier et al., 2012). A longitudinal study of two twin samples found that those who subsequently used marijuana, relative to nonusers, experienced significantly greater cognitive decline from late childhood (9–12 years old) to late adolescence (18–20 years old) in measures of verbal ability (vocabulary) and general knowledge (information), but not for performance subtests (Jackson et al., 2016). However, the co-twin control analysis revealed a different pattern of results. This analysis holds constant the potentially confounding influences of genetics and shared environment. Twin pairs that were discordant for marijuana use did not reveal significant differences in IQ change between MZ or DZ siblings for Vocabulary, Similarities, Information, Block Design, or Picture Arrangement subtests, suggesting that familial confounds were responsible for the association between adolescent marijuana use and decline in IQ scores (Jackson et al., 2016). Binge alcohol drinkers who also used cannabis exhibited subtly poorer global neurocognitive functioning than binge drinkers who did not use cannabis at an 18-month follow-up and were no different than binge drinkers at three-year follow-up (Jacobus et al., 2013). Although preliminary and not without exceptions, these data suggest that cannabis use may be associated with poorer global functioning, particularly among those with earlier onset of use, but this association may also be accounted for by common psychiatric and substance use comorbidities.

Memory

Memory is a multifaceted set of faculties involving one's ability to encode, consolidate, and retrieve newly learned information. The relationship between cannabis use and indices of memory is robustly documented (Dougherty et al., 2013). Generally speaking, adolescent regular users who have maintained between 12 hr and 23 days of cannabis abstinence show poorer immediate recall (Becker, Collins, & Luciana, 2014; Gonzalez et al., 2012; Hanson et al., 2010; Harvey, Sellman, Porter, & Frampton, 2007; Solowij et al., 2011), delayed recall (Becker et al., 2014; Gonzalez et al., 2012; Harvey et al., 2007; Solowij et al., 2011), and recognition discriminability (Solowij et al., 2011) of novel verbal information presented in both unstructured and contextualized formats (Fried, Watkinson, & Gray, 2005; Medina et al., 2007; Schwartz, Gruenewald, Klitzner, & Fedio, 1989) relative to nonusers or non-regular cannabis users. The degree of learning and memory impairments among cannabis users has been associated with the duration, quantity, and age of onset of cannabis use (Solowij et al., 2011) and concomitant use of other substances (Schuster, Crane, Mermelstein, &

Gonzalez, 2015) and is not often correctly recognized by individuals (McClure, Lydiard, Goddard, & Gray, 2015). Although some studies suggest that cannabis users perform worse than nonusers on memory tasks even after six months of supervised abstinence (Schwartz et al., 1989), more recent investigations report that deficits normalize in two weeks (Hanson et al., 2010) to three months (Fried et al., 2005). However, other studies do not find links between cannabis use and compromised memory functioning ((Hooper et al., 2014) whereas others find that cognitive deficits are contingent on common comorbidities (Jacobsen, Pugh, Constable, Westerveld, & Mencl, 2007) or how memory is probed. For example, cannabis may confer risk for poor verbal list learning but not other aspects of memory such as associative learning (Harvey et al., 2007; Jager, Block, Luijten, & Ramsey, 2010; Schweinsburg et al., 2010) and visuo-spatial memory (Mahmood, Jacobus, Bava, Scarlett, & Tapert, 2010; Medina et al., 2007).

Neuroimaging protocols have found unique brain-based patterns during memory tasks among cannabis users even in the absence of group differences in cognitive task performance. For example, Medina et al. (2007) reported an abnormal correlation between hippocampal volume and verbal memory performance among cannabis users compared to control subjects with heavy cannabis users with long-term abstinence (mean of approximately seven months) having smaller bilateral hippocampi than healthy control subjects despite no differences on verbal list learning (Medina et al., 2007). In another study, control subjects but not cannabis users demonstrated a positive relationship between hippocampal volume and verbal memory; cannabis users had an inverse correlation between right hippocampal volume and total cannabis exposure (Ashtari et al., 2011). There has even been some research to suggest that cannabis may actually yield some neuroprotective, anti-inflammatory properties that may buffer against the effect of common confounding conditions such as heavy alcohol use (Hampson, Grimaldi, Axelrod, & Wink, 1998). For example, abstinent cannabis users performed comparably to binge drinkers and control subjects on a verbal encoding task, but binge drinkers who also used cannabis showed functional activity that resembled nonusers (i.e., decreased blood oxygenation level dependent response in the dorsal frontal and parietal cortices and increased activation in inferior frontal regions relative to binge drinkers alone). These data together indicate that cannabis use is associated with impaired memory performance at least acutely, and neuroanatomical and functional effects in regions critical to learning and memory, but the extent, significance, duration, and moderators of these effects need further investigation due to inconsistencies in the literature.

Processing Speed and Attention

Several studies have reported that processing speed and attention are impaired in adolescent cannabis users compared to nonusing control subjects after one month of sustained abstinence (Hanson et al., 2010; Medina et al., 2007). The degree of attentional compromise is dose dependently associated with amount of lifetime cannabis use, adjusting for potential confounds such as alcohol use and depressive symptoms (Medina et al., 2007). In an eight-year longitudinal study of polysubstance users and control subjects from adolescence into young adulthood, amount of cannabis use was inversely associated with attention performance (heavier use associated with lower performance, and vice versa) above and beyond the effects of recent use, baseline cognitive functioning, age, and practice effects (Tapert, Granholm, Leedy, & Brown, 2002). However, other studies have reported no effect of cannabis use on processing speed and attention (Hooper et al., 2014; Pope et al., 1997). For instance, cannabis use was not associated with attention among nonpsychotic patients; however, psychotic patients with a cannabis use disorder performed worse on attention measures than psychotic patients without problematic cannabis use, and this relationship was associated with reduced surface area of the right caudal anterior cingulate cortex (Epstein & Kumra, 2014). To further complicate the picture, some have found that cannabis users' processing speed and attention performance were significantly better than nonusers. Yet, these studies employ simple psychomotor paradigms (Becker et al., 2014) and require very little lifetime cannabis use for study inclusion (Piechatzek et al., 2009), which may limit the generalizability of these findings.

Executive Functioning

Executive functioning is an umbrella term that describes a set of cognitive processes that help an individual engage in effortful, goal-directed behavior. Although executive functioning is comprised of multiple skills, the ones most frequently investigated and hence covered in this review include working memory, inhibitory control, and decision-making. The relationship of cannabis use to executive functioning during adolescence is a central topic of scientific inquiry given that these processes are coordinated in large part (but not exclusively so) by the frontal lobes which are undergoing ongoing maturation into young adulthood.

WORKING MEMORY
The literature describing working memory task performance differences between cannabis users and nonusers is complex and at times contradictory. This may be due to differences in task complexity, as abstinent regular cannabis users perform comparably to control subjects on simple paradigms but show impairments on more challenging working memory tasks (Hanson et al., 2010), with the degree of impairment related to frequency of cannabis use (Harvey et al., 2007). Additionally, there have been inconsistent reports of duration of effects of cannabis use following abstinence. Whereas some studies report differences in working memory between users and nonusers 28 days following cannabis

cessation (Jacobsen, Mencl, Westerveld, & Pugh, 2004), others have found that deficits do not persist this long (Hanson et al., 2010; Padula, Schweinsburg, & Tapert, 2007; Schweinsburg, Brown, & Tapert, 2008; Schweinsburg et al., 2010). Some investigations have documented comparable performances by 12 to 36 hr of abstinence (Becker et al., 2014).

Despite inconsistent evidence suggesting impaired working memory performance with cannabis use, many studies document unique patterns of brain activity while performing tasks heavily mediated by working memory functioning (Cabeza & Nyberg, 2000; Wager & Smith, 2003). For example, cannabis users compared to nonusers have increased task related activity in the right basal ganglia, precuneus, postcentral gyrus, and bilateral parietal lobes (Padula et al., 2007) and decreased activity in the dorsolateral prefrontal cortex and occipital and temporal lobes (Schweinsburg et al., 2008). Patterns of activation may, however, differ when considering pertinent task and participant characteristics. Cannabis using adolescent boys showed exaggerated hyperactivation in the prefrontal cortex during the initial phases of a verbal working memory task when encoding was most likely at its peak (Jager et al., 2010). Further, discrepant patterns may emerge when considering common co-occurring conditions. Drinkers with co-morbid problematic cannabis use showed more activation in the dorsolateral prefrontal cortex and more deactivation in the anterior cingulate, right inferior frontal cortex, and superior temporal region during a spatial working memory task compared to healthy control subjects; however, compared to adolescents who only consumed alcohol but in equivalent doses, drinkers with cannabis use disorders showed more medial frontal deactivation and less right inferior frontal and bilateral temporal activation (Schweinsburg et al., 2005). Finally, adolescents with recent (two to seven days) and extended (27 to 60 days) abstinence had similar performances on a simple working memory task, yet recently abstinent cannabis users showed greater activity in the medial and left superior prefrontal cortices and bilateral insula whereas users with more extended abstinence showed greater activity in the right precentral gyrus (Schweinsburg et al., 2010). Together, these data show that even in the absence of behavioral differences, unique neural activation patterns during working memory tasks emerge in the context of cannabis use. Recruitment of ancillary brain regions may suggest that it is more effortful for cannabis users to achieve adequate task performance, particularly during task components that require the most cognitive control and in the early stages of abstinence.

INHIBITORY CONTROL

Few studies have reported behavioral differences between cannabis users and nonusers on measures of inhibition and psychomotor control during adolescence (Abdullaev, Posner, Nunnally, & Dishion, 2010; Harvey et al., 2007; Tapert et al., 2007). For example, among a sample of young adults with attention deficient hyperactivity disorder, there was no main effect of cannabis use or interaction between cannabis use and a diagnosis of attention deficient hyperactivity disorder on a timed measure of verbal response inhibition; however, individuals who initiated cannabis prior to the age of 16 exhibited worse inhibitory control than those who initiated later (Tamm et al., 2013). Importantly, inclusion into the cannabis using group in this study only required monthly use in the past year, and results may therefore not apply to more persistent chronic cannabis users. However, even in studies with relatively low cannabis use thresholds for inclusion, cannabis users may still show distinct patterns of activation during inhibition tasks. Tapert et al. (2007) did not find behavioral differences on a computerized response inhibition task between control subjects and 28-day abstinent cannabis users with just a minimum of 60 lifetime cannabis use occasions, but cannabis users showed increased blood oxygenation level dependent response in right dorsolateral prefrontal cortex, bilateral medial frontal, bilateral inferior and superior parietal lobules, and right occipital gyri.

DECISION-MAKING

Decision-making is a multifactorial construct that involves how one appraises a given situation and adjusts his or her behavior according to given environmental contingencies. Factors such as problem-solving, risk-taking, impulsivity, and reward valuations all contribute to decision-making capacity. A burgeoning area of research has been devoted to understanding cannabis's association with adolescent decision-making, in part given the heavy reliance of decision-making on frontal lobe processing and the potential real-world functional consequences that may be associated with impairments in this domain.

Although research is still in its nascent stage, preliminary evidence suggests that cannabis use may be associated with diminished decision-making abilities (Dougherty et al., 2013). Cannabis users have been shown to perform worse than alcohol users and healthy control subjects, and the degree of impairment may be independent of recency of use but associated with other indices of cannabis use severity including age of first use and cumulative exposure (Solowij et al., 2012). For example, cannabis users show more impulsive, less efficient, and less accurate responding than nonusers on problem-solving tasks (Becker et al., 2014; Lane, Cherek, Tcheremissine, Steinberg, & Sharon, 2007; see review by Lorenzetti et al., 2016). A growing number of studies have also documented small but positive effects between cannabis use and risk-taking (Hanson, Thayer, & Tapert, 2014). For example, regular adolescent cannabis users with 12 days of abstinence showed a preference for frequent gains despite infrequent but large losses whereas their nonusing counterparts took a more conservative approach and tended to choose smaller gains with smaller losses (Becker et al., 2014). They also report greater propensity for risk-taking in specific domains, such as ethical, health/safety, and social risk-taking (Gilman et al., 2014). Although all studies do not consistently demonstrate group differences on behavioral decision-making tasks (e.g., Hooper et al., 2014; Medina et al., 2007), cannabis dependent adolescents in remission may exhibit distinct patterns of neural activation compared to psychiatric and healthy control subjects, including hyperactivation in the left superior parietal lobule, left lateral occipital cortex, and bilateral precuneus when making risky decisions and hypoactivation when processing rewards in the left orbito-frontal cortex (De Bellis et al., 2013).

Further, decision-making may be an important moderator of cannabis severity and cannabis-associated problems. Data from overlapping samples found that there were no group differences in decision-making between two-day abstinent cannabis users and nonusers, but decision-making impairments were associated with *Diagnostic and Statistical Manual of Mental Disorders* (fourth edition; American Psychiatric Association, 1993) symptoms of cannabis dependence and amount of cannabis used was related to problems from use among those with poorer decision-making capacity (Gonzalez et al., 2012). These effects may be contingent on gender (Crane et al., 2013) and may have important implications for real-world, functional outcomes (e.g., sexual risk-taking; Schuster, Crane, Mermelstein, & Gonzalez, 2012).

OTHER LESS COMMONLY STUDIED DOMAINS OF EXECUTIVE FUNCTIONING
As previously discussed, executive functioning is a heterogeneous construct, yet all dimensions in relation to cannabis use have not yet been extensively studied. Small but growing bodies of research include effortful word retrieval, set-shifting, and abstract reasoning. There is some evidence that cannabis users with varied abstinence intervals exhibit poor planning and self-monitoring (Cuzen, Koopowitz, Ferrett, Stein, & Yurgelun-Todd, 2015), more repetition errors during a phonemic fluency paradigm (Tapert et al., 2007), and worse set shifting and sequencing errors (Medina et al., 2007; Tapert et al., 2007) compared to nonusing control subjects. However, these differences are not universally found (Fried et al., 2005; Harvey et al., 2007), and some even indicate that cannabis users may show an advantage in some cognitive domains (e.g., phonemic fluency; Becker et al., 2014).

METHODOLOGICAL LIMITATIONS

Cannabis's neurocognitive profile during adolescence is, at best, tenuous and this is likely due to extensive methodological variability in the current literature. We will, therefore, briefly discuss what we view to be the most prominent areas of heterogeneity and discuss why these preclude a firm understanding of this topic at this time.

What Constitutes an Adolescent?

Significant variability in age inclusion criteria might contribute to discrepant findings because of rapid neurodevelopment occurring during in adolescence. Indeed, the World Health Organization and the American Psychological Association recommend 21 as the demarcation for adolescence, yet research has suggested that the age of biological maturation occurs well into the third decade of life (Giedd et al., 1999). It is therefore not surprising that there is a broad age range across studies that aim to focus on effects during adolescence. For this chapter, we excluded studies that examined people beyond the age of 24, given the stabilization in neuromaturation and psychosocial transitions that begin to occur during this time; yet, interested readers can also examine manuscripts that include a broader age range (e.g., Anderson, Rizzo, Block, Pearlson, & O'Leary, 2010; Becker et al., 2010; Clark, Roiser, Robbins, & Sahakian, 2009; Grant, Chamberlain, Schreiber, & Odlaug, 2012; Gruber, Sagar, et al., 2012; Indlekofer et al., 2009; Piechatzek et al., 2009; Pope & Yurgelun-Todd, 1996; Tamm et al., 2013). Moving forward, it will be important to analyze effects of cannabis use across more similar ages to better control for effects of physical, emotional, cognitive, and social development that vary considerably within a relatively narrow age range of adolescence.

What Threshold of Cannabis Exposure Is Necessary to Qualify as a Cannabis User?

Studies vary in cannabis exposure requirements for inclusion. Whereas some studies require only occasional use, others include regular cannabis use (with variability in how *regular use* is operationalized) or cannabis dependence, which requires insight about and reporting of negative functional consequences of cannabis use by definition. Clearly, these are discrepant groups in terms of severity of use and likely risk for adverse consequences. Although results are generally combined across studies when consequences from cannabis use are discussed, it remains unclear whether findings generalize across groups of cannabis users. As it is unlikely that minimal exposure confers comparable neurocognitive consequences (if any at all) to more significant use, it will be critical to determine exposure thresholds after which individuals are at risk for adverse consequences. Dose/frequency/duration exposure guidelines are needed for definition of recreational, regular, and problematic use in future studies. Further, future studies should consider factors that influence exposure such as methods of use (e.g., inhaled vs. edible) and potencies (e.g., different THC/CBD ratios, variations of THC concentration within cannabis; particularly at issue is current THC concentrations are much higher than what was). Of particular importance is that current THC concentrations of readily available cannabis are considerably much higher than what was available in the recent past. Indeed, no studies to date have specifically examined the impact of high THC concentrations (e.g., as seen in butane hash oils, waxes, or concentrates) on neurocognitive functioning, which is needed given that today's marijuana smoker does not resemble the smoker of the 1960s in terms of potency of the drug used and the variable methods of administration.

Are Some at Higher Risk for Adverse CNS Effects
of Cannabis Use Than Others?

We have discussed research that supports the view that that early age of onset confers greater use of adverse consequences of cannabis use. Future research should delineate whether exposure thresholds are absolute—such that anyone who uses beyond a certain point will likely experience problematic outcomes—or, more likely, that exposure thresholds denote susceptibility to neurocognitive compromise but that demographic, genetic, psychological, and sociological factors moderate these effects. That is, perhaps many individuals can use cannabis on a regular basis without adverse effects, but those with specific phenotypes/genotypes who surpass a certain exposure threshold are likely to experience functional difficulties. If this is the case, it will be critical as a field to conduct longitudinal studies to detail not only exposure thresholds but high-risk populations so that prevention and intervention efforts can be developed in a more targeted and efficient manner. Gender in particular appears to be an important variable in explaining behavioral patterns of cannabis use as well patterns of neurodevelopment. Data have begun to indicate that the distinct patterns of cannabis use in the context of unique neurodevelopmental trajectories may result in sex-based differences in the neurobehavioral disturbances from adolescent cannabis. There is some evidence in animal studies that acute THC administration may result in more impaired learning in female than male adolescent rats (Cha, Jones, Kuhn, Wilson, & Swartzwelder, 2007; Mateos et al., 2011), yet sex differences in the acute effects of cannabis on human neurocognitive functioning have not yet been documented (Makela et al., 2006; McDonald, Schleifer, Richards, & de Wit, 2003; Rogers, Wakeley, Robson, Bhagwagar, & Makela, 2007; Roser et al., 2009). This is clearly an important area of research to pursue.

How Long Do Cannabis Users Need to Be Drug-Free
to Examine Residual Effects?

At this juncture, there is significant variability in the length of abstinence intervals across investigations. This makes it difficult to determine the chronicity of neurocognitive recovery following cessation of cannabis use. That is, it is currently difficult to determine the rate at which neurocognitive functions improve and at what point in time cannabis users perform comparably to nonusers. One aim of future investigations should be to assess cannabis users at multiple intervals (e.g., 24 hr, 72 hr, one week, two weeks, four weeks, eight weeks), particularly in the one to two months following termination of use, to examine within-person variability over time and therefore more precisely determine the course of symptom resolution.

As a cautionary note, we strongly recommend that researchers fully consider how to minimize or avoid the effects of repeated assessments with this type of study design. The phenomenon of practice effects is well known (Grund et al., 2013; Hinton-Bayre, 2010; Machulda et al., 2013), and data show that repeated exposure to testing materials may result in learning and therefore interfere with the target process in question. Therefore, multiple safeguards should be put in place to limit biased findings. For examples, multiple comparisons should be accounted for in statistical models. Additionally, researchers may consider including a practice assessment prior to the collection of baseline data to minimize the effects of task novelty and initial learning. Finally, to the extent that it is possible, it is advisable to employ measures with multiple versions or that have been developed with repeated measurement in mind.

To Whom Do We Compare Cannabis Users?

The control groups to which cannabis users have been compared vary dramatically, including groups such as healthy individuals, noncannabis substance users, nonsubstance using psychiatric patients, and cannabis users with and without co-occurring alcohol and/or other drug use. Comparisons with all such groups are critical; however, it is important to remember that the interpretation and implications of group differences (or lack thereof) varies depending on the comparison group selected. Therefore, future work should continue to employ heterogeneous control groups, yet our dialogue about the findings that emerge should be reflective of this intentional approach.

Is All Cannabis the Same?

The potency of cannabis has increased in recent decades, and the concentrations of the various psychoactive constituents can vary dramatically. Future studies will need to systematically account for cannabis composition when examining the effect of cannabis on brain structure and function and neurocognition. For example, it is possible that individuals who use more potent cannabis may experience more significant neurocognitive declines, and this can be quantified with urine toxicology testing. In contrast, accounting for such potentially important variables as THC to cannabidiol ratio may present a larger methodological challenge as cannabidiol dose is not easily measured. Although some research has supported the use of saliva to measure cannabidiol levels (Concheiro, Lee, Lendoiro, & Huestis, 2013), the window of detection is narrow (approximately 6 hr). Novel methods to measure cannabidiol levels are needed, given evidence for neuroprotective, anti-oxidative and anti-apoptotic effects (Hampson et al., 1998, 2000; Iuvone et al., 2004).

What Indices of Neurocognitive Task Performance Should Be Examined?

Domains of neurocognition are complex and involve multiple component processes. For example, memory is not a unitary construct but instead involves one's ability to encode, consolidate, and retrieve newly learned information. As a field, we should strive to identify the specific processes impacted by cannabis rather than generalizing results across an entire domain. A more nuanced and sophisticated discussion surrounding the specific processes impacted by cannabis will allow for a more precise estimate of cannabis's neurobiological substrates, will permit the development of intervention strategies tailored to a specific neuropsychological profile, and will facilitate an understanding of how and when cannabis may impede function.

What Is the Functional Significance of Aberrant Brain Structure and Function during Neurocognitive Tasks?

Several studies have documented abnormal patterns of brain structure and function during task performance in the context of normal behavioral performance (Halsband & Lange, 2006; Cabeza & Nyberg, 2000; Wager & Smith, 2003). Some have suggested a functional compensation hypothesis; that is, a compensatory neural effort is needed to achieve normal behavioral performance. However, this has not been tested directly, the functional significance of these brain-based differences is unknown, and it is an open question to what extent cannabis use promotes or impairs a possible compensatory phenomenon.

Can Causation Be Inferred from Correlational Data?

Most studies to date are cross-sectional in nature such that associations are correlational: performance among a group of cannabis users are compared to performance of a control group. Causality cannot be determined using this research methodology. Indeed, in cases where cannabis is associated with poor neurocognitive functioning, four possible scenarios are plausible. First, it is possible that prolonged adolescent cannabis exposure causes neurotoxic effects due to disruption to ongoing neurodevelopmental processes, with adverse brain structural, functional, and/or neurocognitive outcomes. Second, brain structural, functional, and/or neurocognitive differences may reflect a pre-existing risk for cannabis use. Third, another variable that is not systematically accounted for in the extant literature is responsible for differences in brain structural, functional, and/or neurocognitive differences between groups. Finally, some combination of the aforementioned scenarios is responsible for the differences observed in cross-sectional studies. Longitudinal studies that examine brain and behavior characteristics prior to first cannabis use, during use, and following extended abstinence are needed. Additionally, designs that involve random assignment and experimental manipulation (e.g., THC administration) will be crucial in understanding the directionality of effects between cannabis and neurocognitive functioning.

AREAS FOR FUTURE SCIENTIFIC INQUIRY AND SUMMARY

After considering the data available and the methodological variability in the current literature, we recommend that the following areas be priorities for future cannabis research:

1. Because protracted neurodevelopment occurs during adolescence with substantial interindividual variability in these processes, future studies are needed with large samples across a broad developmental window. This will be critical to determine whether relationships vary according to current age and age of first use. Reliance solely on convenience samples or averaging across ages during such a dynamic developmental period may obscure findings.
2. Delineate common terminology for various patterns of use (e.g., regular use, recreational use). Related to this, ways to measure THC exposure based on different methods of consumption are also needed. This line of work will ultimately lead to a better understanding of exposure thresholds (i.e., in terms of cumulative amount, frequency, and consistency of use) for brain structural, functional, and/or neurocognitive compromise.
3. It will be important to understand the clinical significance of brain differences between cannabis users and nonusers. That is, do these differences reflect a pre-existing phenotype for risk for use or rather a consequence from cannabis exposure? Further, does delineating these unique brain signatures yield predictive value for important functional outcomes such as risk for problematic use, use of other substances, mental health, and achievement of life goals (e.g., academics, relationships, occupational pursuits)?
4. Inclusion of potential moderators of effects on brain structural, functional, and/or neurocognitive outcomes will be essential. For example, although recruitment of homogenous cannabis using groups that are free of other potential confounds may be an important first step in isolating the effects of cannabis, future studies should examine subgroups that may be uniquely susceptible to cannabis's effects (e.g., by genotype, mental health diagnosis, or co-occurring other substance use). Further, effort should be devoted toward understanding how neurobiological effects may differ based on the chemical composition of the cannabis used.
5. Longitudinal studies will be essential for understanding temporal precedence and thus causality between cannabis use and neurobiological outcomes.

In summary, although there is much to learn and methodological issues remain, converging evidence supports the view that cannabis affects multiple cognitive systems including attentional processing, several aspects of memory, and higher-order executive functioning. These adverse effects on neurocognition persist beyond acute intoxication, and the extent to which they resolve with abstinence and what other factors, such as dose, duration, or age of initiation of use, may influence the degree to which cognitive effects resolve and over what time course is not yet known. Earlier age of onset of regular cannabis use is associated with worse neurocognitive outcomes. Finally, even when cannabis users achieve normative levels of performance on neurocognitive and behavioral tasks, there are brain-based signatures indicating that cannabis users may have to work harder to achieve comparable performance.

Our ability to fully understand how cannabis is associated with brain structural, functional, and/or neurocognitive outcomes in adolescence is complex and could take years to fully delineate given all the factors to consider. However, this issue has been thrust upon the scientific community by voters, clearly reflecting an issue of significant political priority. To potentially avoid mistakes made during initial tobacco legislation, objectively investigating the impact of cannabis on youth is a scientific priority to inform both intervention efforts and policy decisions.

ACKNOWLEDGMENTS

This publication was made possible by the National Institute on Drug Abuse (NIDA; 1K23DA042946-01, PI: Schuster; 1K01DA034093-01A1, PI: Gilman; K24 DA030443, PI: Evins) and by the Norman E. Zinberg Fellowship in Addiction Psychiatry and Livingston Fellowship from Harvard Medical School and the Louis V. Gerstner III Research Scholar Award through Massachusetts General Hospital (Schuster). Its contents are solely the responsibility of the authors and do not necessarily represent the official views of NIDA or the National Institutes of Health. The authors declare no conflicts of interest.

REFERENCES

Abdullaev, Y., Posner, M. I., Nunnally, R., & Dishion, T. J. (2010). Functional MRI evidence for inefficient attentional control in adolescent chronic cannabis abuse. *Behavioural Brain Research*, *215*, 45–57. http://dx.doi.org/10.1016/j.bbr.2010.06.023

American Psychiatric Association. (1994). *Diagnostic and statistical manual of mental disorders* (4th ed.). Washington, DC: Author.

Andersen, S. L., Dumont, N. L., & Teicher, M. H. (1997). Developmental differences in dopamine synthesis inhibition by (+/–)-7-OH-DPAT. *Naunyn-Schmiedeberg's Archives of Pharmacology*, *356*, 173–181.

Anderson, B. M., Rizzo, M., Block, R. I., Pearlson, G. D., & O'Leary, D. S. (2010). Sex, drugs, and cognition: effects of marijuana. *Journal of Psychoactive Drugs, 42*, 413–424. http://dx.doi.org/10.1080/02791072.2010.10400704

Anthony, J. C. (2006). The epidemiology of cannabis dependence. In R. A. & S. Roffman (Eds.), *Cannabis dependence: Its Nature, Consequences and Treatment* (pp 58–105). Cambridge, UK: Cambridge University Press.

Arnone, D., Barrick, T. R., Chengappa, S., Mackay, C. E., Clark, C. A., & Abou-Saleh, M. T. (2008). Corpus callosum damage in heavy marijuana use: preliminary evidence from diffusion tensor tractography and tract-based spatial statistics. *Neuroimage, 41*, 1067–1074. http://dx.doi.org/10.1016/j.neuroimage.2008.02.064

Ashtari, M., Avants, B., Cyckowski, L., Cervellione, K. L., Roofeh, D., Cook, P., . . . Kumra, S. (2011). Medial temporal structures and memory functions in adolescents with heavy cannabis use. *Journal of Psychiatric Reseach, 45*, 1055–1066. http://dx.doi. org/10.1016/j.jpsychires.2011.01.004

Ashtari, M., Cervellione, K., Cottone, J., Ardekani, B. A., Sevy, S., & Kumra, S. (2009). Diffusion abnormalities in adolescents and young adults with a history of heavy cannabis use. *Journal of Psychiatric Reseach, 43*, 189–204. http://dx.doi.org/10.1016/j.jpsychires.2008.12.002

Bambico, F. R., Nguyen, N. T., Katz, N., & Gobbi, G. (2010). Chronic exposure to cannabinoids during adolescence but not during adulthood impairs emotional behaviour and monoaminergic neurotransmission. *Neurobiology of Diseases, 37*, 641–655. http://dx.doi.org/10.1016/j.nbd.2009.11.020

Bava, S., Frank, L. R., McQueeny, T., Schweinsburg, B. C., Schweinsburg, A. D., & Tapert, S. F. (2009). Altered white matter microstructure in adolescent substance users. *Psychiatry Research, 173*, 228–237. http://dx.doi.org/10.1016/j.pscychresns.2009.04.005

Bava, S., & Tapert, S. F. (2010). Adolescent brain development and the risk for alcohol and other drug problems. *Neuropsychology Review, 20*, 398–413. http://dx.doi.org/10.1007/s11065-010-9146-6

Becker, B., Wagner, D., Gouzoulis-Mayfrank, E., Spuentrup, E., & Daumann, J. (2010). Altered parahippocampal functioning in cannabis users is related to the frequency of use. *Psychopharmacology, 209*, 361–374. http://dx.doi.org/10.1007/s00213-010-1805-z

Becker, M. P., Collins, P. F., & Luciana, M. (2014). Neurocognition in college-aged daily marijuana users. *Journal of Clinical and Experimental Neuropsychology, 36*, 379–398. http://dx.doi.org/10.1080/13803395.2014.893996

Bindukumar, B., Mahajan, S. D., Reynolds, J. L., Hu, Z., Sykes, D. E., Aalinkeel, R., & Schwartz, S. A. (2008). Genomic and proteomic analysis of the effects of cannabinoids on normal human astrocytes. *Brain Research, 1191*, 1–11. http://dx.doi.org/10.1016/j.brainres.2007.10.062

Brook, J. S., Lee, J. Y., Finch, S. J., Seltzer, N., & Brook, D. W. (2013). Adult work commitment, financial stability, and social environment as related to trajectories of marijuana use beginning in adolescence. *Substance Abuse, 34*, 298–305. http://dx.doi.org/10.1080/08897077.2013.775092

Burgdorf, J. R., Kilmer, B., & Pacula, R. L. (2011). Heterogeneity in the composition of marijuana seized in California. *Drug and Alcohol Dependence, 117*, 59–61. http://dx.doi.org/10.1016/j.drugalcdep.2010.11.031

Burston, J. J., Wiley, J. L., Craig, A. A., Selley, D. E., & Sim-Selley, L. J. (2010). Regional enhancement of cannabinoid CB₁ receptor desensitization in female adolescent rats following repeated Delta-tetrahydrocannabinol exposure. *British Journal of Pharmacology*, *161*, 103–112. http://dx.doi.org/10.1111/j.1476-5381.2010.00870.x

Cabeza, R., & Nyberg, L. (2000). Neural bases of learning and memory: functional neuroimaging evidence. *Current Opinion in Neurology*, *13*, 415–421.

Cass, D. K., Flores-Barrera, E., Thomases, D. R., Vital, W. F., Caballero, A., & Tseng, K. Y. (2014). CB1 cannabinoid receptor stimulation during adolescence impairs the maturation of GABA function in the adult rat prefrontal cortex. *Molecular Psychiatry*, *19*, 536–543. http://dx.doi.org/10.1038/mp.2014.14

Cha, Y. M., Jones, K. H., Kuhn, C. M., Wilson, W. A., & Swartzwelder, H. S. (2007). Sex differences in the effects of delta9-tetrahydrocannabinol on spatial learning in adolescent and adult rats. *Behavioural Pharmacology*, *18*, 563–569. http://dx.doi.org/10.1097/FBP.0b013e3282ee7b7e

Churchwell, J. C., Lopez-Larson, M., & Yurgelun-Todd, D. A. (2010). Altered frontal cortical volume and decision making in adolescent cannabis users. *Frontiers in Psychology*, *1*, 225. http://dx.doi.org/10.3389/fpsyg.2010.00225

Clark, L., Roiser, J. P., Robbins, T. W., & Sahakian, B. J. (2009). Disrupted "reflection" impulsivity in cannabis users but not current or former ecstasy users. *Journal of Psychopharmacology*, *23*, 14–22. http://dx.doi.org/10.1177/0269881108089587

Cocchetto, D. M., Owens, S. M., Perez-Reyes, M., DiGuiseppi, S., & Miller, L. L. (1981). Relationship between plasma delta-9-tetrahydrocannabinol concentration and pharmacologic effects in man. *Psychopharmacology)*, *75*, 158–164.

Cohen, P. J. (2010). Medical marijuana 2010: It's time to fix the regulatory vacuum. *Journal of Law, Medicine, & Ethics*, *38*, 654–666. http://dx.doi.org/10.1111/j.1748-720X.2010.00519.x

Concheiro, M., Lee, D., Lendoiro, E., & Huestis, M. A. (2013). Simultaneous quantification of delta(9)-tetrahydrocannabinol, 11-nor-9-carboxy-tetrahydrocannabinol, cannabidiol and cannabinol in oral fluid by microflow-liquid chromatography-high resolution mass spectrometry. *Journal of Chromatography A*, *1297*, 123–130. http://dx.doi.org/10.1016/j.chroma.2013.04.071

Cooper, Z. D., & Haney, M. (2009). Comparison of subjective, pharmacokinetic, and physiological effects of marijuana smoked as joints and blunts. *Drug and Alcohol Dependence*, *103*, 107–113. http://dx.doi.org/10.1016/j.drugalcdep.2009.01.023

Cooper, Z. D., & Haney, M. (2014). Investigation of sex-dependent effects of cannabis in daily cannabis smokers. *Drug and Alcohol Dependence*, *136*, 85–91. http://dx.doi.org/10.1016/j.drugalcdep.2013.12.013

Crane, N. A., Schuster, R. M., Fusar-Poli, P., & Gonzalez, R. (2013). Effects of cannabis on neurocognitive functioning: recent advances, neurodevelopmental influences, and sex differences. *Neuropsychology Review*, *23*, 117–137. http://dx.doi.org/10.1007/s11065-012-9222-1

Cuzen, N. L., Koopowitz, S. M., Ferrett, H. L., Stein, D. J., & Yurgelun-Todd, D. (2015). Methamphetamine and cannabis abuse in adolescence: A quasi-experimental study on specific and long-term neurocognitive effects. *BMJ Open*, *5*(1), e005833. http://dx.doi.org/10.1136/bmjopen-2014-005833

De Bellis, M. D., Clark, D. B., Beers, S. R., Soloff, P. H., Boring, A. M., Hall, J., . . . Keshavan, M. S. (2000). Hippocampal volume in adolescent-onset alcohol use disorders. *American Journal of Psychiatry*, *157*, 737–744.

De Bellis, M. D., Van Voorhees, E., Hooper, S. R., Gibler, N., Nelson, L., Hege, S. G., . . . MacFall, J. (2008). Diffusion tensor measures of the corpus callosum in adolescents with adolescent onset alcohol use disorders. *Alcoholism: Clinical and Experimental Research*, *32*, 395–404. http://dx.doi.org/10.1111/j.1530-0277.2007.00603.x

De Bellis, M. D., Wang, L., Bergman, S. R., Yaxley, R. H., Hooper, S. R., & Huettel, S. A. (2013). Neural mechanisms of risky decision-making and reward response in adolescent onset cannabis use disorder. *Drug and Alcohol Dependence*, *133*, 134–145. http://dx.doi.org/10.1016/j.drugalcdep.2013.05.020

Delisi, L. E., Bertisch, H. C., Szulc, K. U., Majcher, M., Brown, K., Bappal, A., & Ardekani, B. A. (2006). A preliminary DTI study showing no brain structural change associated with adolescent cannabis use. *Harm Reduction Journal*, *3*, 17. http://dx.doi.org/10.1186/1477-7517-3-17

Dougherty, D. M., Mathias, C. W., Dawes, M. A., Furr, R. M., Charles, N. E., Liguori, A., . . . Acheson, A. (2013). Impulsivity, attention, memory, and decision-making among adolescent marijuana users. *Psychopharmacology*, *226*, 307–319. http://dx.doi.org/10.1007/s00213-012-2908-5

Durston, S., Hulshoff Pol, H. E., Casey, B. J., Giedd, J. N., Buitelaar, J. K., & van Engeland, H. (2001). Anatomical MRI of the developing human brain: What have we learned? *Journal of the American Academy of Child and Aodlescent Psychiatry*, *40*, 1012–1020. http://dx.doi.org/10.1097/00004583-200109000-00009

Ehlers, C. L., Gizer, I. R., Vieten, C., Gilder, D. A., Stouffer, G. M., Lau, P., & Wilhelmsen, K. C. (2010). Cannabis dependence in the San Francisco Family Study: age of onset of use, DSM-IV symptoms, withdrawal, and heritability. *Addictive Behaviors*, *35*, 102–110. http://dx.doi.org/10.1016/j.addbeh.2009.09.009

Ehrenreich, H., Rinn, T., Kunert, H. J., Moeller, M. R., Poser, W., Schilling, L., . . . Hoehe, M. R. (1999). Specific attentional dysfunction in adults following early start of cannabis use. *Psychopharmacology*, *142*, 295–301.

Elikkottil, J., Gupta, P., & Gupta, K. (2009). The analgesic potential of cannabinoids. *Journal of Opiod Management*, *5*, 341–357.

ElSohly, M. A. (2014). *Potency Monitoring Program Quarterly Report Number 124. Reporting period: 12/16/2013-03/15/2014*. Bethesda, MD: National Institute on Drug Abuse.

Epstein, K. A., & Kumra, S. (2014). Executive attention impairment in adolescents with schizophrenia who have used cannabis. *Schizophrenia Research*, *157*, 48–54. http://dx.doi.org/10.1016/j.schres.2014.04.035

Fergusson, D. M., & Boden, J. M. (2008). Cannabis use and later life outcomes. *Addiction*, *103*, 969–976; discussion 977–968. http://dx.doi.org/10.1111/j.1360-0443.2008.02221.x

Filbey, F. M., Aslan, S., Calhoun, V. D., Spence, J. S., Damaraju, E., Caprihan, A., & Segall, J. (2014). Long-term effects of marijuana use on the brain. *Proceedings of the National Academy of Sciences*, *111*, 16913–16918.

Fontes, M. A., Bolla, K. I., Cunha, P. J., Almeida, P. P., Jungerman, F., Laranjeira, R. R., . . . Lacerda, A. L. (2011). Cannabis use before age 15 and subsequent executive functioning. *British Journal of Psychiatry*, *198*, 442–447. http://dx.doi.org/10.1192/bjp.bp.110.077479

Freund, T. F., Katona, I., & Piomelli, D. (2003). Role of endogenous cannabinoids in synaptic signaling. *Physiological Reviews*, *83*, 1017–1066. http://dx.doi.org/10.1152/physrev.00004.2003

Fried, P. A., Watkinson, B., & Gray, R. (2005). Neurocognitive consequences of marihuana--a comparison with pre-drug performance. *Neurotoxicology and Teratology, 27*, 231–239. http://dx.doi.org/10.1016/j.ntt.2004.11.003

Gaffuri, A. L., Ladarre, D., & Lenkei, Z. (2012). Type-1 cannabinoid receptor signaling in neuronal development. *Pharmacology, 90*, 19–39. http://dx.doi.org/10.1159/000339075

Gfroerer, J. C., & Epstein, J. F. (1999). Marijuana initiates and their impact on future drug abuse treatment need. *Drug and Alcohol Dependence, 54*, 229–237.

Giedd, J. N., Blumenthal, J., Jeffries, N. O., Castellanos, F. X., Liu, H., Zijdenbos, A., . . . Rapoport, J. L. (1999). Brain development during childhood and adolescence: A longitudinal MRI study. *Nature Neuroscience, 2*, 861–863. http://dx.doi.org/10.1038/13158

Gilman, J. M., Kuster, J. K., Lee, S., Lee, M. J., Kim, B. W., Makris, N., . . . Breiter, H. C. (2014). Cannabis use is quantitatively associated with nucleus accumbens and amygdala abnormalities in young adult recreational users. *Journal of Neuroscience, 34*, 5529–5538. http://dx.doi.org/10.1523/JNEUROSCI.4745-13.2014

Gogtay, N., Giedd, J. N., Lusk, L., Hayashi, K. M., Greenstein, D., Vaituzis, A. C., . . . Thompson, P. M. (2004). Dynamic mapping of human cortical development during childhood through early adulthood. *Proceedings of the National Academy of Sciences, 101*, 8174–8179. http://dx.doi.org/10.1073/pnas.0402680101

Gonzalez, R., Schuster, R. M., Mermelstein, R. J., Vassileva, J., Martin, E. M., & Diviak, K. R. (2012). Performance of young adult cannabis users on neurocognitive measures of impulsive behavior and their relationship to symptoms of cannabis use disorders. *Journal of Clinical and Experimental Neuropsychology, 34*, 962–976. http://dx.doi.org/10.1080/13803395.2012.703642

Grant, J. E., Chamberlain, S. R., Schreiber, L., & Odlaug, B. L. (2012). Neuropsychological deficits associated with cannabis use in young adults. *Drug and Alcohol Dependence, 121*, 159–162. http://dx.doi.org/10.1016/j.drugalcdep.2011.08.015

Gruber, S. A., Dahlgren, M. K., Sagar, K. A., Gonenc, A., & Killgore, W. D. (2012). Age of onset of marijuana use impacts inhibitory processing. *Neuroscience Letters, 511*, 89–94. http://dx.doi.org/10.1016/j.neulet.2012.01.039

Gruber, S. A., Dahlgren, M. K., Sagar, K. A., Gonenc, A., & Lukas, S. E. (2014). Worth the wait: Effects of age of onset of marijuana use on white matter and impulsivity. *Psychopharmacology, 231*, 1455–1465. http://dx.doi.org/10.1007/s00213-013-3326-z

Gruber, S. A., Sagar, K. A., Dahlgren, M. K., Racine, M., & Lukas, S. E. (2012). Age of onset of marijuana use and executive function. *Psychology of Addictive Behaviors, 26*, 496–506. http://dx.doi.org/10.1037/a0026269

Gruber, S. A., Silveri, M. M., Dahlgren, M. K., & Yurgelun-Todd, D. (2011). Why so impulsive? White matter alterations are associated with impulsivity in chronic marijuana smokers. *Experimental and Clinical Psychopharmacology, 19*, 231–242. http://dx.doi.org/10.1037/a0023034

Grund, B., Wright, E. J., Brew, B. J., Price, R. W., Roediger, M. P., Bain, M. P., . . . Group, I. S. S. (2013). Improved neurocognitive test performance in both arms of the SMART study: impact of practice effect. *Journal of NeuroVirology, 19*, 383–392. http://dx.doi.org/10.1007/s13365-013-0190-x

Hall, W. (2009). The adverse health effects of cannabis use: what are they, and what are their implications for policy? *International Journal of Drug Policy, 20*, 458–466. http://dx.doi.org/10.1016/j.drugpo.2009.02.013

Hall, W., & Degenhardt, L. (2009). Adverse health effects of non-medical cannabis use. *Lancet, 374,* 1383–1391. http://dx.doi.org/10.1016/S0140-6736(09)61037-0

Halsband, U., & Lange, R. K. (2006). Motor learning in man: a review of functional and clinical studies. *Journal of Physiology, 99,* 414–424. http://dx.doi.org/10.1016/j.jphysparis.2006.03.007

Hampson, A. J., Grimaldi, M., Axelrod, J., & Wink, D. (1998). Cannabidiol and (-) Delta9-tetrahydrocannabinol are neuroprotective antioxidants. *Proceedings of the National Academy of Sciences, 95,* 8268–8273.

Hampson, A. J., Grimaldi, M., Lolic, M., Wink, D., Rosenthal, R., & Axelrod, J. (2000). Neuroprotective antioxidants from marijuana. *Annals of the New York Academy of Sciences, 899,* 274–282.

Hanson, K. L., Thayer, R. E., & Tapert, S. F. (2014). Adolescent marijuana users have elevated risk-taking on the balloon analog risk task. *Journal of Psychopharmacology, 28,* 1080–1087. http://dx.doi.org/10.1177/0269881114550352

Hanson, K. L., Winward, J. L., Schweinsburg, A. D., Medina, K. L., Brown, S. A., & Tapert, S. F. (2010). Longitudinal study of cognition among adolescent marijuana users over three weeks of abstinence. *Addictive Behaviors, 35,* 970–976. http://dx.doi.org/10.1016/j.addbeh.2010.06.012

Harte, L. C., & Dow-Edwards, D. (2010). Sexually dimorphic alterations in locomotion and reversal learning after adolescent tetrahydrocannabinol exposure in the rat. *Neurotoxicology and Teratology, 32,* 515–524. http://dx.doi.org/10.1016/j.ntt.2010.05.001

Harvey, M. A., Sellman, J. D., Porter, R. J., & Frampton, C. M. (2007). The relationship between non-acute adolescent cannabis use and cognition. *Drug and Alcohol Review, 26,* 309–319. http://dx.doi.org/10.1080/09595230701247772

Heng, L., Beverley, J. A., Steiner, H., & Tseng, K. Y. (2011). Differential developmental trajectories for CB1 cannabinoid receptor expression in limbic/associative and sensorimotor cortical areas. *Synapse, 65,* 278–286. http://dx.doi.org/10.1002/syn.20844

Hernandez-Avila, C. A., Rounsaville, B. J., & Kranzler, H. R. (2004). Opioid-, cannabis- and alcohol-dependent women show more rapid progression to substance abuse treatment. *Drug and Alcohol Dependence, 74,* 265–272. http://dx.doi.org/10.1016/j.drugalcdep.2004.02.001

Hinton-Bayre, A. D. (2010). Deriving reliable change statistics from test-retest normative data: comparison of models and mathematical expressions. *Archives of Clinical Neuropsychology, 25,* 244–256. http://dx.doi.org/10.1093/arclin/acq008

Hooper, S. R., Woolley, D., & De Bellis, M. D. (2014). Intellectual, neurocognitive, and academic achievement in abstinent adolescents with cannabis use disorder. *Psychopharmacology, 231,* 1467–1477. http://dx.doi.org/10.1007/s00213-014-3463-z

Houck, J. M., Bryan, A. D., & Feldstein Ewing, S. W. (2013). Functional connectivity and cannabis use in high-risk adolescents. *American Journal of Drug and Alcohol Abuse, 39,* 414–423. http://dx.doi.org/10.3109/00952990.2013.837914

Howlett, A. C., Barth, F., Bonner, T. I., Cabral, G., Casellas, P., Devane, W. A., . . . Pertwee, R. G. (2002). International Union of Pharmacology. XXVII. Classification of cannabinoid receptors. *Pharmacological Reviews, 54,* 161–202.

Huestegge, L., Radach, R., Kunert, H. J., & Heller, D. (2002). Visual search in long-term cannabis users with early age of onset. *Progress in Brain Research, 140*, 377–394. http://dx.doi.org/10.1016/S0079-6123(02)40064-7

Huttenlocher, P. R. (1990). Morphometric study of human cerebral cortex development. *Neuropsychologia, 28*, 517–527.

Huttenlocher, P. R., & Dabholkar, A. S. (1997). Regional differences in synaptogenesis in human cerebral cortex. *Journal of Comparative Neurology, 387*, 167–178.

Indlekofer, F., Piechatzek, M., Daamen, M., Glasmacher, C., Lieb, R., Pfister, H., . . . Schutz, C. G. (2009). Reduced memory and attention performance in a population-based sample of young adults with a moderate lifetime use of cannabis, ecstasy and alcohol. *Journal Psychopharmacology, 23*, 495–509. http://dx.doi.org/10.1177/0269881108091076

Iuvone, T., Esposito, G., Esposito, R., Santamaria, R., Di Rosa, M., & Izzo, A. A. (2004). Neuroprotective effect of cannabidiol, a non-psychoactive component from Cannabis sativa, on beta-amyloid-induced toxicity in PC12 cells. *Journal of Neurochemistry, 89*, 134–141. http://dx.doi.org/10.1111/j.1471-4159.2003.02327.x

Jackson, N. J., Isen, J. D., Khoddam, R., Irons, D., Tuvblad, C., Iacono, W. G., . . . Baker, L. A. (2016). Impact of adolescent marijuana use on intelligence: Results from two longitudinal twin studies. *Proceedings of the National Academy of Sciences, 113*, E500–E508.

Jacobsen, L. K., Mencl, W. E., Westerveld, M., & Pugh, K. R. (2004). Impact of cannabis use on brain function in adolescents. *Annals of the New York Academy of Sciences, 1021*, 384–390. http://dx.doi.org/10.1196/annals.1308.053

Jacobsen, L. K., Pugh, K. R., Constable, R. T., Westerveld, M., & Mencl, W. E. (2007). Functional correlates of verbal memory deficits emerging during nicotine withdrawal in abstinent adolescent cannabis users. *Biological Psychiatry, 61*, 31–40. http://dx.doi.org/10.1016/j.biopsych.2006.02.014

Jacobus, J., Goldenberg, D., Wierenga, C. E., Tolentino, N. J., Liu, T. T., & Tapert, S. F. (2012). Altered cerebral blood flow and neurocognitive correlates in adolescent cannabis users. *Psychopharmacology, 222*, 675–684. http://dx.doi.org/10.1007/s00213-012-2674-4

Jacobus, J., McQueeny, T., Bava, S., Schweinsburg, B. C., Frank, L. R., Yang, T. T., & Tapert, S. F. (2009). White matter integrity in adolescents with histories of marijuana use and binge drinking. *Neurotoxicology and Teratology, 31*, 349–355. http://dx.doi.org/10.1016/j.ntt.2009.07.006

Jacobus, J., Squeglia, L. M., Bava, S., & Tapert, S. F. (2013). White matter characterization of adolescent binge drinking with and without co-occurring marijuana use: a 3-year investigation. *Psychiatry Research, 214*, 374–381. http://dx.doi.org/10.1016/j.pscychresns.2013.07.014

Jager, G., Block, R. I., Luijten, M., & Ramsey, N. F. (2010). Cannabis use and memory brain function in adolescent boys: A cross-sectional multicenter functional magnetic resonance imaging study. *Journal of the American Academy of Child and Adolescent Psychiatry, 49*(6), 561–572. http://dx.doi.org/10.1016/j.jaac.2010.02.001

Jager, G., & Ramsey, N. F. (2008). Long-term consequences of adolescent cannabis exposure on the development of cognition, brain structure and function: an overview of animal and human research. *Current Drug Abuse Reviews, 1*, 114–123.

Jarvis, K., DelBello, M. P., Mills, N., Elman, I., Strakowski, S. M., & Adler, C. M. (2008). Neuroanatomic comparison of bipolar adolescents with and without cannabis use disorders. *Journal of Child and Adolescent Psychopharmacology, 18*, 557–563. http://dx.doi.org/10.1089/cap.2008.033

Johnston, L. D., O'Malley, P.M., Bachman, J.G., & Schulenberg, J.E. (2012). *Monitoring the Future national results on adolescent drug use: Overview of key findings, 2011.* Ann Arbor: Institute for Social Research, University of Michigan.

Johnston, L. D., O'Malley, P. M., Bachman, J.G., & Schulenberg, J. E. (2013). *Monitoring the Future national results on drug use: 2012 Overview, key findings on adolescent drug use.* Ann Arbor: Institute for Social Research, University of Michigan.

Kann, L. K., Shanklin, S. L., Flint, K. H., Hawkins, J., Harris, W. A., Lowry, R., . . . Zaza, S. (2014). *Youth Risk Behavior Surveillance—United States, 2013.* Rockville, MD: ICF International.

Khan, S. S., Secades-Villa, R., Okuda, M., Wang, S., Perez-Fuentes, G., Kerridge, B. T., & Blanco, C. (2013). Gender differences in cannabis use disorders: results from the National Epidemiologic Survey of Alcohol and Related Conditions. *Drug and Alcohol Dependence, 130,* 101–108. http://dx.doi.org/10.1016/j.drugalcdep.2012.10.015

Lambe, E. K., Krimer, L. S., & Goldman-Rakic, P. S. (2000). Differential postnatal development of catecholamine and serotonin inputs to identified neurons in prefrontal cortex of rhesus monkey. *Journal of Neuroscience, 20,* 8780–8787.

Lane, S. D., Cherek, D. R., Tcheremissine, O. V., Steinberg, J. L., & Sharon, J. L. (2007). Response perseveration and adaptation in heavy marijuana-smoking adolescents. *Addictive Behaviors, 32,* 977–990. http://dx.doi.org/10.1016/j.addbeh.2006.07.007

Lenroot, R. K., Gogtay, N., Greenstein, D. K., Wells, E. M., Wallace, G. L., Clasen, L. S., . . . Giedd, J. N. (2007). Sexual dimorphism of brain developmental trajectories during childhood and adolescence. *Neuroimage, 36,* 1065–1073. http://dx.doi.org/10.1016/j.neuroimage.2007.03.053

Lewis, D. A. (1997). Development of the prefrontal cortex during adolescence: Insights into vulnerable neural circuits in schizophrenia. *Neuropsychopharmacology, 16,* 385–398. http://dx.doi.org/10.1016/S0893-133X(96)00277-1

Lichenstein, S. D., Musselman, S., Shaw, D. S., Sitnick, S., & Forbes, E. E. (2017). Nucleus accumbens functional connectivity at age 20 is associated with trajectory of adolescent cannabis use and predicts psychosocial functioning in young adulthood. *Addiction, 112,* 1893–2080. http://dx.doi.org/10.1111/add.13882

Lisdahl, K. M., & Price, J. S. (2012). Increased marijuana use and gender predict poorer cognitive functioning in adolescents and emerging adults. *Journal of the International Neuropsychological Society, 18,* 678–688. http://dx.doi.org/10.1017/S1355617712000276

Lopez-Larson, M. P., Bogorodzki, P., Rogowska, J., McGlade, E., King, J. B., Terry, J., & Yurgelun-Todd, D. (2011). Altered prefrontal and insular cortical thickness in adolescent marijuana users. *Behavioural Brain Research, 220,* 164–172. http://dx.doi.org/10.1016/j.bbr.2011.02.001

Lopez-Quintero, C., Perez de los Cobos, J., Hasin, D. S., Okuda, M., Wang, S., Grant, B. F., & Blanco, C. (2011). Probability and predictors of transition from first use to dependence on nicotine, alcohol, cannabis, and cocaine: results of the National Epidemiologic Survey on Alcohol and Related Conditions (NESARC). *Drug and Alcohol Dependence, 115,* 120–130. http://dx.doi.org/10.1016/j.drugalcdep.2010.11.004

Lorenzetti, V., Alonso-Lana, S., Youssef, G. J., Verdejo-Garcia, A., Suo, C., Cousijn, J., . . . Solowij, N. (2016). Adolescent cannabis use: What is the evidence for functional brain alteration? *Current Pharmaceutical Design, 22,* 6353–6365. http://dx.doi.org/10.2174/1381612822666160805155922

Lubman, D. I., Cheetham, A., & Yucel, M. (2015). Cannabis and adolescent brain development. *Pharmacology and Therapeutics*, *148*, 1–16. http://dx.doi.org/10.1016/j.pharmthera.2014.11.009

Machulda, M. M., Pankratz, V. S., Christianson, T. J., Ivnik, R. J., Mielke, M. M., Roberts, R. O., . . . Petersen, R. C. (2013). Practice effects and longitudinal cognitive change in normal aging vs. incident mild cognitive impairment and dementia in the Mayo Clinic Study of Aging. *Clinical Neuropsychologist*, *27*, 1247–1264. http://dx.doi.org/10.1080/13854046.2013.836567

Mackie, K. (2005). Distribution of cannabinoid receptors in the central and peripheral nervous system. *Handbook of Experimental Pharmacology*, *168*, 299–325.

Mahmood, O. M., Jacobus, J., Bava, S., Scarlett, A., & Tapert, S. F. (2010). Learning and memory performances in adolescent users of alcohol and marijuana: Interactive effects. *Journal of Studies on Alcohol and Drugs*, *71*, 885–894. http://dx.doi.org/10.15288/jsad.2010.71.885

Makela, P., Wakeley, J., Gijsman, H., Robson, P. J., Bhagwagar, Z., & Rogers, R. D. (2006). Low doses of delta-9 tetrahydrocannabinol (THC) have divergent effects on short-term spatial memory in young, healthy adults. *Neuropsychopharmacology*, *31*, 462–470. http://dx.doi.org/10.1038/sj.npp.1300871

Martin-Santos, R., Fagundo, A. B., Crippa, J. A., Atakan, Z., Bhattacharyya, S., Allen, P., . . . McGuire, P. (2010). Neuroimaging in cannabis use: a systematic review of the literature. *Psychological Medicine*, *40*, 383–398. http://dx.doi.org/10.1017/S0033291709990729

Mateos, B., Borcel, E., Loriga, R., Luesu, W., Bini, V., Llorente, R., . . . Viveros, M. P. (2011). Adolescent exposure to nicotine and/or the cannabinoid agonist CP 55,940 induces gender-dependent long-lasting memory impairments and changes in brain nicotinic and CB(1) cannabinoid receptors. *Journal of Psychopharmacology*, *25*, 1676–1690. http://dx.doi.org/10.1177/0269881110370503

McClure, E. A., Lydiard, J. B., Goddard, S. D., & Gray, K. M. (2015). Objective and subjective memory ratings in cannabis-dependent adolescents. *American Journal of Addiction*, *24*, 47–52. http://dx.doi.org/10.1111/ajad.12171

McDonald, J., Schleifer, L., Richards, J. B., & de Wit, H. (2003). Effects of THC on behavioral measures of impulsivity in humans. *Neuropsychopharmacology*, *28*, 1356–1365. http://dx.doi.org/10.1038/sj.npp.1300176

McQueeny, T., Padula, C. B., Price, J., Medina, K. L., Logan, P., & Tapert, S. F. (2011). Gender effects on amygdala morphometry in adolescent marijuana users. *Behavioural Brain Research*, *224*, 128–134. http://dx.doi.org/10.1016/j.bbr.2011.05.031

Mechoulam, R., & Parker, L. A. (2013). The endocannabinoid system and the brain. *Annual Review of Psychology*, *64*, 21–47. http://dx.doi.org/10.1146/annurev-psych-113011-143739

Medina, K. L., Hanson, K. L., Schweinsburg, A. D., Cohen-Zion, M., Nagel, B. J., & Tapert, S. F. (2007). Neuropsychological functioning in adolescent marijuana users: Subtle deficits detectable after a month of abstinence. *Journal of the International Neuropsychological Society*, *13*, 807–820. http://dx.doi.org/10.1017/S1355617707071032

Medina, K. L., McQueeny, T., Nagel, B. J., Hanson, K. L., Yang, T. T., & Tapert, S. F. (2009). Prefrontal cortex morphometry in abstinent adolescent marijuana users: Subtle gender effects. *Addiction Biology*, *14*, 457–468. http://dx.doi.org/10.1111/j.1369-1600.2009.00166.x

Medina, K. L., Nagel, B. J., & Tapert, S. F. (2010). Abnormal cerebellar morphometry in abstinent adolescent marijuana users. *Psychiatry Research*, *182*, 152–159. http://dx.doi.org/10.1016/j.pscychresns.2009.12.004

Meier, M. H., Caspi, A., Ambler, A., Harrington, H., Houts, R., Keefe, R. S., . . . Moffitt, T. E. (2012). Persistent cannabis users show neuropsychological decline from childhood to midlife. *Proceedings of the National Academy of Sciences*, *109*, e2657–e2664. http://dx.doi.org/10.1073/pnas.1206820109

Nagel, B. J., Medina, K. L., Yoshii, J., Schweinsburg, A. D., Moadab, I., & Tapert, S. F. (2006). Age-related changes in prefrontal white matter volume across adolescence. *Neuroreport*, *17*, 1427–1431. http://dx.doi.org/10.1097/01.wnr.0000233099.97784.45

Narimatsu, S., Watanabe, K., Yamamoto, I., & Yoshimura, H. (1991). Sex difference in the oxidative metabolism of delta 9-tetrahydrocannabinol in the rat. *Biochemical Pharmacology*, *41*, 1187–1194.

O'Connell, T. J., & Bou-Matar, C. B. (2007). Long term marijuana users seeking medical cannabis in California (2001-2007): Demographics, social characteristics, patterns of cannabis and other drug use of 4117 applicants. *Harm Reduction Jorunal*, *4*, 16. http://dx.doi.org/10.1186/1477-7517-4-16

Orr, C., Morioka, R., Behan, B., Datwani, S., Doucet, M., Ivanovic, J., . . . Garavan, H. (2013). Altered resting-state connectivity in adolescent cannabis users. *American Journal of Drug and Alcohol Abuse*, *39*, 372–381. http://dx.doi.org/10.3109/00952990.2013.848213

O'Shea, M., Singh, M. E., McGregor, I. S., & Mallet, P. E. (2004). Chronic cannabinoid exposure produces lasting memory impairment and increased anxiety in adolescent but not adult rats. *Journal of Psychopharmacology*, *18*, 502–508. http://dx.doi.org/10.1177/0269881104047277

Padula, C. B., Schweinsburg, A. D., & Tapert, S. F. (2007). Spatial working memory performance and fMRI activation interaction in abstinent adolescent marijuana users. *Psychology of Addictive Behaviors*, *21*, 478–487. http://dx.doi.org/10.1037/0893-164X.21.4.478

Paus, T., Keshavan, M., & Giedd, J. N. (2008). Why do many psychiatric disorders emerge during adolescence? *Nature Reviews Neuroscience*, *9*, 947–957. http://dx.doi.org/10.1038/nrn2513

Pfefferbaum, A., Mathalon, D. H., Sullivan, E. V., Rawles, J. M., Zipursky, R. B., & Lim, K. O. (1994). A quantitative magnetic resonance imaging study of changes in brain morphology from infancy to late adulthood. *Archives of Neurology*, *51*, 874–887.

Piechatzek, M., Indlekofer, F., Daamen, M., Glasmacher, C., Lieb, R., Pfister, H., . . . Schutz, C. G. (2009). Is moderate substance use associated with altered executive functioning in a population-based sample of young adults? *Human Psychopharmacology*, *24*, 650–665. http://dx.doi.org/10.1002/hup.1069

Piomelli, D. (2003). The molecular logic of endocannabinoid signalling. *Nature Reviews Neuroscience*, *4*, 873–884. http://dx.doi.org/10.1038/nrn1247

Pistis, M., Perra, S., Pillolla, G., Melis, M., Muntoni, A. L., & Gessa, G. L. (2004). Adolescent exposure to cannabinoids induces long-lasting changes in the response to drugs of abuse of rat midbrain dopamine neurons. *Biological Psychiatry*, *56*, 86–94. http://dx.doi.org/10.1016/j.biopsych.2004.05.006

Pope, H. G., Jr., Gruber, A. J., Hudson, J. I., Cohane, G., Huestis, M. A., & Yurgelun-Todd, D. (2003). Early-onset cannabis use and cognitive deficits: What is the nature of the association? *Drug and Alcohol Dependence*, *69*, 303–310.

Pope, H. G., Jr., Gruber, A. J., Hudson, J. I., Huestis, M. A., & Yurgelun-Todd, D. (2002). Cognitive measures in long-term cannabis users. *Journal of Clinical Pharmacology*, *42*(Suppl 1), 41–47.

Pope, H. G., Jr., Jacobs, A., Mialet, J. P., Yurgelun-Todd, D., & Gruber, S. (1997). Evidence for a sex-specific residual effect of cannabis on visuospatial memory. *Psychotherapy and Psychosomatics*, *66*, 179–184.

Pope, H. G., Jr., & Yurgelun-Todd, D. (1996). The residual cognitive effects of heavy marijuana use in college students. *Journal of the American Medical Association*, *275*, 521–527.

Quinn, H. R., Matsumoto, I., Callaghan, P. D., Long, L. E., Arnold, J. C., Gunasekaran, N., . . . McGregor, I. S. (2008). Adolescent rats find repeated delta(9)-THC less aversive than adult rats but display greater residual cognitive deficits and changes in hippocampal protein expression following exposure. *Neuropsychopharmacology*, *33*, 1113–1126. http://dx.doi.org/10.1038/sj.npp.1301475

Rigucci, S., Marques, T. R., Di Forti, M., Taylor, H., Dell'Acqua, F., Mondelli, V., . . . Dazzan, P. (2016). Effect of high-potency cannabis on corpus callosum microstructure. *Psychological Medicine*, *46*, 841–854. http://dx.doi.org/10.1017/S0033291715002342

Rodriguez de Fonseca, F., Ramos, J. A., Bonnin, A., & Fernandez-Ruiz, J. J. (1993). Presence of cannabinoid binding sites in the brain from early postnatal ages. *Neuroreport*, *4*, 135–138.

Rogers, R. D., Wakeley, J., Robson, P. J., Bhagwagar, Z., & Makela, P. (2007). The effects of low doses of delta-9 tetrahydrocannabinol on reinforcement processing in the risky decision-making of young healthy adults. *Neuropsychopharmacology*, *32*, 417–428. http://dx.doi.org/10.1038/sj.npp.1301175

Roser, P., Gallinat, J., Weinberg, G., Juckel, G., Gorynia, I., & Stadelmann, A. M. (2009). Psychomotor performance in relation to acute oral administration of Delta9-tetrahydrocannabinol and standardized cannabis extract in healthy human subjects. *European Archives of Psychiatry and Clinical Neuroscience*, *259*, 284–292. http://dx.doi.org/10.1007/s00406-009-0868-5

Rubino, T., Realini, N., Braida, D., Guidi, S., Capurro, V., Vigano, D., . . . Parolaro, D. (2009). Changes in hippocampal morphology and neuroplasticity induced by adolescent THC treatment are associated with cognitive impairment in adulthood. *Hippocampus*, *19*, 763–772. http://dx.doi.org/10.1002/hipo.20554

Rubino, T., Vigano, D., Realini, N., Guidali, C., Braida, D., Capurro, V., . . . Parolaro, D. (2008). Chronic delta 9-tetrahydrocannabinol during adolescence provokes sex-dependent changes in the emotional profile in adult rats: Behavioral and biochemical correlates. *Neuropsychopharmacology*, *33*, 2760–2771. http://dx.doi.org/10.1038/sj.npp.1301664

Schneider, M., & Koch, M. (2003). Chronic pubertal, but not adult chronic cannabinoid treatment impairs sensorimotor gating, recognition memory, and the performance in a progressive ratio task in adult rats. *Neuropsychopharmacology*, *28*, 1760–1769. http://dx.doi.org/10.1038/sj.npp.1300225

Schneider, M., & Koch, M. (2007). The effect of chronic peripubertal cannabinoid treatment on deficient object recognition memory in rats after neonatal mPFC lesion. *European Neuropsychopharmacology*, *17*, 180–186. http://dx.doi.org/10.1016/j.euroneuro.2006.03.009

Schuster, R. M., Crane, N. A., Mermelstein, R., & Gonzalez, R. (2012). The influence of inhibitory control and episodic memory on the risky sexual behavior of young adult cannabis users. *Journal of the International Neuropsychological Society*, 18, 827–833. http://dx.doi.org/10.1017/S1355617712000586

Schuster, R. M., Crane, N. A., Mermelstein, R., & Gonzalez, R. (2015). Tobacco May Mask Poorer Episodic Memory Among Young Adult Cannabis Users. *Neuropsychology*, 29, 759–766. http://dx.doi.org/10.1037/neu0000173

Schwartz, R. H., Gruenewald, P. J., Klitzner, M., & Fedio, P. (1989). Short-term memory impairment in cannabis-dependent adolescents. *American Journal of Diseases of Children*, 143, 1214–1219.

Schweinsburg, A. D., Brown, S. A., & Tapert, S. F. (2008). The influence of marijuana use on neurocognitive functioning in adolescents. *Current Drug Abuse Reviews*, 1, 99–111.

Schweinsburg, A. D., Schweinsburg, B. C., Cheung, E. H., Brown, G. G., Brown, S. A., & Tapert, S. F. (2005). fMRI response to spatial working memory in adolescents with comorbid marijuana and alcohol use disorders. *Drug and Alcohol Dependence*, 79, 201–210. http://dx.doi.org/10.1016/j.drugalcdep.2005.01.009

Schweinsburg, A. D., Schweinsburg, B. C., Medina, K. L., McQueeny, T., Brown, S. A., & Tapert, S. F. (2010). The influence of recency of use on fMRI response during spatial working memory in adolescent marijuana users. *Journal of Psychoactive Drugs*, 42, 401–412. http://dx.doi.org/10.1080/02791072.2010.10400703

Silveri, M. M., Jensen, J. E., Rosso, I. M., Sneider, J. T., & Yurgelun-Todd, D. A. (2011). Preliminary evidence for white matter metabolite differences in marijuana-dependent young men using 2D J-resolved magnetic resonance spectroscopic imaging at 4 Tesla. *Psychiatry Research*, 191, 201–211. http://dx.doi.org/10.1016/j.pscychresns.2010.10.005

Solowij, N., Jones, K. A., Rozman, M. E., Davis, S. M., Ciarrochi, J., Heaven, P. C., . . . Yucel, M. (2011). Verbal learning and memory in adolescent cannabis users, alcohol users and nonusers. *Psychopharmacology*, 216, 131–144. http://dx.doi.org/10.1007/s00213-011-2203-x

Solowij, N., Jones, K. A., Rozman, M. E., Davis, S. M., Ciarrochi, J., Heaven, P. C., . . . Yucel, M. (2012). Reflection impulsivity in adolescent cannabis users: a comparison with alcohol-using and non-substance-using adolescents. *Psychopharmacology*, 219, 575–586. http://dx.doi.org/10.1007/s00213-011-2486-y

Sowell, E. R., Thompson, P. M., Holmes, C. J., Batth, R., Jernigan, T. L., & Toga, A. W. (1999). Localizing age-related changes in brain structure between childhood and adolescence using statistical parametric mapping. *Neuroimage*, 9, 587–597. http://dx.doi.org/10.1006/nimg.1999.0436

Spear, L. P. (2000). The adolescent brain and age-related behavioral manifestations. *Neuroscience and Biobehavioral Reviews*, 24, 417–463.

Stevens, B., Allen, N. J., Vazquez, L. E., Howell, G. R., Christopherson, K. S., Nouri, N., . . . Barres, B. A. (2007). The classical complement cascade mediates CNS synapse elimination. *Cell*, 131, 1164–1178. http://dx.doi.org/10.1016/j.cell.2007.10.036

Substance Abuse and Mental Health Services Administration. (2014). *Results from the 2013 National Survey on Drug Use and Health: Summary of national findings*. NSDUH Series H-48, HHS Publication No. (SMA) 14-4863. Rockville, MD: Author.

Sung, Y. H., Carey, P. D., Stein, D. J., Ferrett, H. L., Spottiswoode, B. S., Renshaw, P. F., & Yurgelun-Todd, D. A. (2013). Decreased frontal N-acetylaspartate levels in adolescents concurrently using both methamphetamine and marijuana. *Behavioural Brain Research*, *246*, 154–161. http://dx.doi.org/10.1016/j.bbr.2013.02.028

Tait, R. J., Mackinnon, A., & Christensen, H. (2011). Cannabis use and cognitive function: 8-year trajectory in a young adult cohort. *Addiction*, *106*, 2195–2203. http://dx.doi.org/10.1111/j.1360-0443.2011.03574.x

Tamm, L., Epstein, J. N., Lisdahl, K. M., Molina, B., Tapert, S., Hinshaw, S. P., . . . Group, M. T. A. N. (2013). Impact of ADHD and cannabis use on executive functioning in young adults. *Drug and Alcohol Dependence*, *133*, 607–614. http://dx.doi.org/10.1016/j.drugalcdep.2013.08.001

Tamnes, C. K., Ostby, Y., Fjell, A. M., Westlye, L. T., Due-Tonnessen, P., & Walhovd, K. B. (2010). Brain maturation in adolescence and young adulthood: regional age-related changes in cortical thickness and white matter volume and microstructure. *Cerebral Cortex*, *20*, 534–548. http://dx.doi.org/10.1093/cercor/bhp118

Tapert, S. F., Granholm, E., Leedy, N. G., & Brown, S. A. (2002). Substance use and withdrawal: neuropsychological functioning over 8 years in youth. *Journal of the International Neuropsychological Society*, *8*, 873–883.

Tapert, S. F., Schweinsburg, A. D., Drummond, S. P., Paulus, M. P., Brown, S. A., Yang, T. T., & Frank, L. R. (2007). Functional MRI of inhibitory processing in abstinent adolescent marijuana users. *Psychopharmacology*, *194*, 173–183. http://dx.doi.org/10.1007/s00213-007-0823-y

Teicher, M. H., Barber, N. I., Gelbard, H. A., Gallitano, A. L., Campbell, A., Marsh, E., & Baldessarini, R. J. (1993). Developmental differences in acute nigrostriatal and mesocorticolimbic system response to haloperidol. *Neuropsychopharmacology*, *9*, 147–156. http://dx.doi.org/10.1038/npp.1993.53

Tunbridge, E. M., Weickert, C. S., Kleinman, J. E., Herman, M. M., Chen, J., Kolachana, B. S., . . . Weinberger, D. R. (2007). Catechol-o-methyltransferase enzyme activity and protein expression in human prefrontal cortex across the postnatal lifespan. *Cerebral Cortex*, *17*, 1206–1212. http://dx.doi.org/10.1093/cercor/bhl032

Viveros, M. P., Llorente, R., Moreno, E., & Marco, E. M. (2005). Behavioural and neuroendocrine effects of cannabinoids in critical developmental periods. *Behavioural Pharmacology*, *16*, 353–362.

Viveros, M. P., Llorente, R., Suarez, J., Llorente-Berzal, A., Lopez-Gallardo, M., & de Fonseca, F. R. (2012). The endocannabinoid system in critical neurodevelopmental periods: sex differences and neuropsychiatric implications. *Journal of Psychopharmacology*, *26*, 164–176. http://dx.doi.org/10.1177/0269881111408956

Wager, T. D., & Smith, E. E. (2003). Neuroimaging studies of working memory: A meta-analysis. *Cognitive, Affective, and Behavioral Neuroscience*, *3*, 255–274.

Wilson, W., Mathew, R., Turkington, T., Hawk, T., Coleman, R. E., & Provenzale, J. (2000). Brain morphological changes and early marijuana use: a magnetic resonance and positron emission tomography study. *Journal of Addictive Diseases*, *19*, 1–22. http://dx.doi.org/10.1300/J069v19n01_01

Zalesky, A., Solowij, N., Yucel, M., Lubman, D. I., Takagi, M., Harding, I. H., . . . Seal, M. (2012). Effect of long-term cannabis use on axonal fibre connectivity. *Brain*, *135*, 2245–2255. http://dx.doi.org/10.1093/brain/aws136

5

The Impact of Marijuana on Mental Health

CHRISTINE L. MILLER

INTRODUCTION

There is an intriguing paradox in the public's perception of many drugs in that negative physical impacts are more easily understood and accepted than negative mental impacts. Marijuana provides a perfect case study of this phenomenon, accentuated all the more because there is often a time lag between its use and the negative mental health impacts when they occur and a stark contrast between acute and more lasting effects. The general public is quite familiar with the caricature of the mellow pot smoker; thus, there is a perception that only the weak of mind and spirit can develop long-term psychiatric problems from this drug or that if such symptoms do occur, the marijuana was likely spiked with other drugs. Through a rigorous review of the literature, this chapter will seek to address this common bias.

The primary topic covered will be the most well studied of its mental health effects, the risk for developing long-term psychosis, primarily schizophrenia spectrum disorders but also bipolar disorder with psychosis. Each section will highlight the challenges and limitations of studying the link between marijuana use and mental health. The chapter closes with a review of research concerning the impact of marijuana use on mood disorders and suicidal ideation. For the two most serious outcomes, chronic psychosis and suicidal ideation, the impact of marijuana will be compared to that of other recreational drugs, illustrating both common and unique effects.

PSYCHOTIC OUTCOMES FROM MARIJUANA USE

Reports of this serious side effect are nothing new, as made all too clear by accessing much older literature from different cultures. Dhunjibhoy et al. (1930) describe concerns about marijuana's mental effects dating to 14th-century Egypt, and the authors outline in detail their experience treating what they call "Indian

Hemp Insanity" or chronic manic-depressive psychosis thought to be caused by various forms of marijuana used in their region. But many decades would have to pass before rigorous epidemiology began to be applied in lieu of sporadic, anecdotal reports. It was in this realm that several European countries along with collaborators from the southern hemisphere surged to the forefront in the late 20th century. The United States was somewhat behind the curve in addressing the question, perhaps in part because we have lacked a centralized healthcare system to facilitate data collection, but perhaps also because epidemiology and public health received comparatively less attention and less funding during the molecular biology revolution that captivated American bioscience during that time. Another factor may have been the funneling of research funds toward blockbuster drugs to cure psychiatric disorders, rather than focusing attention on recreational drugs that might be causing them. For these and other reasons, psychiatrists in the United States have been very slow to catch on to emerging themes of marijuana's impact psychotic disorders more thoroughly explored by scientists in other countries.

At the cutting edge of the epidemiology on marijuana's impact has been Robin Murray of Great Britain and his protégé and collaborator, Jim van Os of the Netherlands. What began for Murray as a fielding of questions from parents about whether their children might have developed a psychotic disorder from their marijuana habit (no, unlikely, he would say at the time; Mohun, Ridout, & Suzuki, 2010) evolved into a full-fledged effort to explore the question of whether these parents could be right. A large Swedish study gave strength to the notion that the effort was worthwhile when the proportion of schizophrenia cases in military recruits was discovered to be much higher in marijuana users than in nonusers (Andréasson, Engström, Allebeck, & Rydberg, 1987). Murray's group and colleagues in other countries then began their own research in earnest, amassing a large collection of association studies that in bulk pointed to a strong correlation between marijuana use and the development of schizophrenia and other psychotic disorders, yet none definitively stating that marijuana had a casual role in these outcomes. Even as the number of large association studies grew around the world, including reports from New Zealand (Fergusson, Horwood, & Swain-Campbell, 2003), eventually the United States (Davis, Compton, Wang, Levin, & Blanco, 2013), and many others (meta-analysis by Moore et al., 2007), showing, on average, a doubling in risk associated with the lower strength marijuana prevalent in the 20th century, the lingering specter of reverse causation remained (i.e., perhaps those who were in the incipient stages of psychosis were more likely to use marijuana).

Yet it appears as though the critical mass of key reports has finally been reached, where it can be said that although no one type of research has definitively proven causation, collectively there can no longer be much doubt that marijuana is a causal factor. What follows will be an enumeration of the criteria for causation of chronic psychosis that have been tested in numerous epidemiologic and some case-control clinical studies. By way of acknowledging the magnitude of the prior controversy concerning this particular aspect of the question, the population sizes of each relevant study are specified in the following subsections.

A Dose–Response Effect in Risk for Schizophrenia

Barring unusual threshold-type effects, and U-shaped dose–response curves such as those that can be seen with radiation exposure and mutagenesis (Vilenchik & Knudson, 2000), the general rule of thumb is that a statistically significant dose response curve should be seen in the exposure of a subject to a drug if the drug is causing the outcome (Steenland & Deddens, 2004), and that is indeed what is seen with marijuana and psychotic disorders. If no dose–response is seen, the agent is much less likely to be causal. Several studies have shown such a dose–response, both in the frequency of use and the strength of the product (a) from a longitudinal study of 50,000 Swedish transcripts (Zammit, Allebeck, Andreasson, Lundberg, & Lewis, 2002); (b) in a longitudinal study of over 4,000 Dutch citizens, aged 18 to 84 (van Os et al., 2002); and (c) in a case-control study of 514 subjects conducted in Great Britain by Di Forti et al. (2009). In general, the risk rises to 2.1-fold with weekly use (meta-analysis by Moore et al., 2007) and is more pronounced with a high-strength product. The most recent estimate for use of high-strength skunk in a case control study of 780 subjects in Great Britain is a 2.7-fold increase in risk for psychosis with weekly use, whereas daily use conferred a 5.4-fold increase in risk (Di Forti et al., 2015).

Ruling Out Self-Medication or Reverse Causation

The evidence for the emergence of psychotic symptoms leading to the initiation of a marijuana habit is far outweighed by prospective studies showing marijuana use triggers psychosis. Prospective studies are regarded as the best way to address the issue of which comes first, because the investigators are not relying on retrospective self-report of the timing of psychotic symptoms relative to the subject's marijuana use. In a prospective study of more than 1,000 subjects reported by Arseneault et al. (2002), marijuana use was found to precede the psychosis, and not vice versa. Another prospective study of over 2,400 teens conducted by members of Jim van Os's team in the Netherlands, which involved clinical interviews, demonstrated that the most significant outcome was that those who were not exhibiting a liability for psychosis (including symptoms that might be deemed subclinical) at study onset were significantly more likely to experience psychotic symptoms if they began marijuana use, and whereas a liability for psychosis was associated with a trend toward initiating marijuana use, this trend did not reach significance (Henquet et al., 2005). Kuepper et al. (2011) then extended that work to more than 1,900 teens and young adults and found no evidence for self-medication in a prospective study. Subjects were first assessed for psychotic symptoms at the second time point of the study, and no association with marijuana initiation was seen at the subsequent (third) time point. Once again, those who had no pre-existing psychotic symptoms were more likely to develop them if they commenced marijuana use.

One prospective study of 2,120 adolescents did find a relatively equal bidirectional effect between psychosis and marijuana use; that is, those without psychotic symptoms at study onset were more likely to become psychotic if they started marijuana use, and those with psychotic symptoms at study onset were also more likely to start using marijuana (Griffith-Lendering et al., 2013). Lewis, Heron, and Zammit (2013) offered a critique of the Griffith-Lendering study, pointing out that the assessment of psychosis liability was made by self-reported questionnaires, where self-report of psychotic-like experiences can be high, and not clinical interviews, which tend to provide more conservative assessments of psychotic symptoms based on the experience the clinicians have in treating actual psychosis. Another report also indicated the psychotic symptoms generally preceded the marijuana use (Schiffman, Nakamura, Earleywine, & LaBrie, 2005), but that study was not prospective and was relatively small (189 subjects) as compared to the prospective investigations previously detailed.

Looking at the question from another angle, if psychotic symptoms were to lead to marijuana use, you would expect those with a family history of schizophrenia to be more likely to begin marijuana use than control subjects, but they are not, as demonstrated in a case-control study of 263 subjects in the Netherlands (Veling, Mackenbach, Os, & Hoek, 2008). Similarly, in a study of 282 subjects versus control subjects, Proal, Fleming, Galvez-Buccollini, and Delisi (2014) found that marijuana users were no more likely than nonusers to have a family history of schizophrenia. Finally, Fergusson Horwood, and Ridder (2005) have shown in a longitudinal of 1,265 youth in New Zealand, the development of psychotic symptoms while using marijuana often results in marijuana cessation. But this trend may be dependent on the severity of the psychosis, because obviously a point is reached in full psychosis where self-insight into the disorder is often lost. Indeed, Foti, Kotov, Guey, and Bromet (2010) found that in 229 subjects tracked for 10 years, those with milder symptoms (perhaps earlier in the course of their illness) were likely to quit their habit, while the more severe the symptoms were, the more likely an individual was to commence marijuana use.

Delta-9-Tetrahydrocannabinol and Psychotic Symptoms in Clinical Subjects

Purified delta-9-tetrahydrocannabinol (Δ^9-THC) has been administered intravenously in small clinical investigations. In such studies, significant psychotic symptoms could be measured by changes in the Positive and Negative Syndrome Scale (PANSS) or paranoia scores: (a) 5 mg administered to 22 subjects (screened to exclude those with a family history of psychosis) resulted in a 43% increase in positive PANSS scores and a 50% increase in PANSS negative scores (D'Souza et al., 2004); (b) 1.25 mg administered to 16 subjects (screened to exclude those with a family history of major mental illness) resulted in approximately a 64% increase in PANSS positive scores and a 43% increase in PANSS negative scores (Morrison et al., 2011); (c) 1.5 mg administered to 122 individuals with a personal history of psychotic symptoms randomized to either case or control status showed that most paranoia scores approximately doubled with administration of Δ^9-THC (Freeman et al., 2015). Another clinical investigation of PANSS scores (in 15 subjects apparently not screened for family history) utilized oral administration of 10 mg Δ^9-THC and observed a 36% average increase in positive scores and a 33% average increase in negative scores (Bhattacharyya et al., 2012). Only one of the resulting publications reported the data as the percentage of individual subjects who demonstrated positive psychotic symptoms (Morrison et al., 2011), and one other presented the individual data in figure form from which the percentage could be inferred (Bhattacharyya et al., 2012); for both studies the results were that approximately 40% of the subjects showed increases in PANSS positive scores. Note that none of the subjects in the studies as described were marijuana-naïve.

Other clinical studies have shown full-fledged psychotic breaks in subjects with a prior history of marijuana use (smokers) when oral formulations of Δ^9-THC were administered in those who had no personal history of a psychiatric diagnosis but were not screened for family history: in 1 out of 16 female subjects dosed with 20 mg (Kaufmann et al., 2010), in 2 out of 8 male subjects dosed with 16 to 20 mg (Favrat et al., 2005), and in 1 out of 17 male subjects dosed with ≤15 mg (Leweke, Schneider, Thies, Münte, & Emrich, 1999). Combining these studies of oral administration, nearly 10% of the treated subjects experienced a transient but nevertheless full marijuana-induced psychosis after a single dose. Favrat et al. (2005) measured the blood levels of both Δ9-THC and 11-hydroxy-THC and found that for the more severe of the two marijuana-induced psychosis cases in their investigation, the THC breakdown product, 11-hydroxy-THC level exceeded even that of Δ^9-THC (~6 ng/ml and ~5 ng/ml, respectively). Of note, 11-hydroxy-THC has been reported to be as psychoactive as Δ^9-THC in a clinical study involving intravenous administration of the at a rate of 0.02 mg/kg over 7 min (Perez-Reyes et al., 1972), while another study reported 11-hydroxy-THC to be 20% more potent when administered as 0.05 mg/kg in a 3-min intravenous bolus (Hollister & Gillespie, 1975), consistent with significantly more potent physiologic effects seen in an animal model (Karler & Turkanis, 1987).

The basis for blood levels of 11-hydroxy-THC being higher after oral administration of Δ^9-THC than after smoking or even intravenous administration is that oral administration involves a high degree of first pass metabolism through the liver (Ohlsson et al., 1980). Furthermore, the persistence of 11-hydroxy-THC in the blood can be of greater duration than Δ^9-THC itself, depending on the individual (see Schwilke et al., 2009, Fig. 5.1). Clearly, genetic variability in production of 11-hydroxy-THC by first pass metabolism in the liver (thought to be controlled in part by CYP2C9; Sachse-Seeboth et al., 2009) could contribute to the high variability in psychotomimetic response seen with recreational ingestion of Δ^9-THC. It has long been noted by psychiatrists in Asia that psychotic episodes from marijuana occur more frequently in that region of the world, and one reason thought to underlie this phenomenon is marijuana is often ingested rather than smoked there. Bhang, a beverage made from marijuana leaves and flowers, combined with fruit and nuts is quite popular in that culture and can be associated with psychotic breaks following ingestion (Chaudry, Moss, Bashir, & Suliman, 1991).

Age of Onset for Schizophrenia Spectrum Disorders in Marijuana Users

Similar to the connection between other etiologies causal for disease, such as suspected carcinogens and cancer, marijuana has been shown to generally decrease the age of onset of schizophrenia by 2.7 years (meta-analysis by Large. Sharma, Compton, Slade, & Nielssen, 2011). In contrast, although tobacco use rates are very high in schizophrenia, smoking tobacco does not lower the age of onset of schizophrenia (Myles et al., 2012) nor does alcohol use (Galvez-Buccollini et al., 2012). Similarly, other recreational drugs of abuse have been found to have no significant effect on the age of onset (Barnes, Mutsatsa, Hutton, Watt, & Joyce, 2006).

The caveat to this area of research is that the peak age of onset of schizophrenia varies quite a bit from study to study and that to have an impact on reducing the age of onset, marijuana use must obviously begin before the peak onset age for schizophrenia (age 21–24 years reported for men; age 22–28 years reported for women; Beratis, Gabriel, & Hoidas, 1994; Faraone, Chen, Goldstein, & Tsuang, 1994; Ganguli & Brar, 1992; Hafner et al., 1998; Kessler et al., 2007; Meltzer et al., 1997). If late onset psychosis is seen, say greater than age 25 or so for men and age 29 or so for women, then late onset marijuana use (or other drugs of abuse) might be suspected, thus confounding the possible role of marijuana in interpreting some temporal onset studies.

Risk for Chronic Psychosis Compared to Other Drugs

A very large landmark study in 2013 of 18,478 Finnish patients whose first inpatient hospital admission was based on a diagnosis of a substance-induced psychosis (Niemi-Pynttari et al., 2013) has cast significant doubt on the notion that marijuana has less impact on chronic psychosis than other drugs or that marijuana must be laced with common hallucinogens to cause schizophrenia. Patient discharge records were accrued for a period of 16 years, and the patients were followed for an additional 8 to 10 years to determine the prevalence of conversions of discharge diagnoses into schizophrenia spectrum disorders. The results revealed that of all the causes of substance-induced psychosis, marijuana cases most consistently converted from the initial diagnosis (which is potentially reversible) to a diagnosis of chronic psychosis (a schizophrenia spectrum disorder). For marijuana cases, the conversion occurred 46%of the time; for amphetamine and methamphetamine cases, 30% of the time; and for hallucinogens (e.g., LSD, PCP), 24%of the time. Similarly, in a large study of tens of thousands of drug users in a population-based cohort in California, Callaghan et al. (2012) found that a cocaine use disorder was not as great a risk factor for schizophrenia as was a marijuana or methamphetamine use disorder. A more recent study by a Danish team has confirmed that marijuana use carries the greatest risk for schizophrenia as compared to alcohol, hallucinogens, sedatives, opioids, cocaine, and amphetamines (Nielsen, Toftdahl, Nordentoft, & Hjorthøj, 2017).

This work followed on the heels of a smaller study (476 drug using subjects in St. Louis, Missouri) of the prevalence of psychotic symptoms (not full psychosis nor chronic psychosis) as a function of drug of abuse (Smith, Thirthalli, Abdallah, Murray, & Cottler, 2009). The results showed that among drug-dependent users, 80% of those dependent on cocaine, 63.5% dependent on marijuana, 56.1% dependent on amphetamines, and 53.1% dependent on opiates reported psychotic symptoms. But among users who were not diagnosed as dependent on their drug of choice, marijuana users had the highest prevalence of psychotic symptoms (12.4%). Compton, Chien, and Bollini (2009) conducted a small-scale investigation (60 subjects) into the impact of alcohol, marijuana, and cocaine use on symptoms of schizotypy in first-degree relatives patients with schizophrenia as compared to controls and found that marijuana use in those relatives had the strongest impact on the expression of symptoms.

Finally, Giordano et al. (2015) found that controlling for genetic background in a study of 5,456 Swedish patients meant that the increased risk for schizophrenia posed by the use of opiates, sedatives, and hallucinogens disappeared, whereas only that of marijuana use and cocaine/stimulants remained. Yet as compared to cocaine and other stimulants, marijuana use conveyed the highest risk in the co-relative comparisons.

Recovery Time Following a Psychotic Break

For the nearly 50% who recover from full-fledged marijuana-induced psychosis, the recovery is not immediate and can take months to years. González-Pinto et al. (2011) followed 52 patients who experienced a psychotic break following marijuana use and compared those who quit their habit after their first break to those who did not. The former group (n = 27) fared much better at the eight-year point (within about 30% of the optimal global functioning score), but those who did not quit (n = 25) fared significantly worse than first break psychosis cases who had never used at all. The recovery of those who quit was gradual, and it is clear from the error bars that much of the variation was between individuals. Restoring full function requires neurophysiological recovery, another indication that the impact of THC on these individuals is quite a bit more than an ephemeral change.

In a meta-analysis of publications looking at the question of marijuana cessation versus continuation after a psychosis diagnosis, those who continued to use were found to have higher relapse rates, longer hospital stays, and more severe positive symptoms than those who quit or those whose psychosis did not evolve in the context of marijuana use (Schoeler et al., 2016). Those who continued to use exhibited higher levels of positive psychotic symptoms than nonmarijuana using individuals admitted for psychosis. Although continuing users did not differ from nonusers with psychosis in terms of negative symptoms, they exhibited a trend for higher levels of negative symptoms than those who discontinued their marijuana use, illustrating a possible role for a perceived need for self-medication in the former group. The issue of potential confounding by initial severity of illness was partially addressed by the finding that those who ceased using marijuana experienced significantly higher levels of functioning on follow-up than those who had never used at all, illustrating that as a group the users at the time of admission were not likely to have had a more serious, unremitting form of the disease. More recently, Patel et al. (2016) found in a study of 2,026 first episode psychosis patients that those admitted to hospitals for marijuana-induced psychosis were more likely to be prescribed more than one antipsychotic over time, possibly attributable to poor efficacy of antipsychotic drugs in the more severe course of illness experienced by the users. However, marijuana-induced psychosis may contribute to neurophysiologic deficits not present among those whose schizophrenia is primarily derived from genetic risk, a factor that cannot be ruled out as a reason for the antipsychotic failure.

COUNTERARGUMENTS

Many important points about the likelihood for no causal role of marijuana in the onset of schizophrenia are raised during informal communications rather than scientific reports, yet conveying these arguments can be influential if it occurs at scientific conferences, in legislative hearings, in drug policy forums, or in interviews with the media. The following is a list of the most commonly held counterarguments to marijuana being causative for schizophrenia, followed by a presentation of the available data relevant to each.

Counterargument: Use Rates Differ Between Countries but Psychosis Rates the Same

Marijuana use has been historically more prevalent in the United States than in Europe. Is there any evidence that US schizophrenia prevalence rates are higher? The short answer is yes, based on prevalence studies conducted in the 1980s and 1990s. However, the question points to the problematic nature of population studies, either comparing different time points in the same population or, as is the issue here, making comparisons between populations. So many confounding variables cannot be controlled for, including but not limited to the different genetic make-up between groups of people separated by the Atlantic Ocean. Also, the generally very low prevalence rate of schizophrenia makes it problematic to determine whether there are significantly statistical differences when comparisons are made because large populations must be studied (though the advantage of low prevalence diseases is that large effect sizes can be measured). But in as much as the issue is raised by others considering whether this drug has impacts that are significant at the population level, what evidence there is should be presented. In the only comprehensive psychiatric epidemiology study of its kind to date in the United States, the one-month point prevalence rate for schizophrenia was found to be 0.7% from five U.S. epidemiologic catchment areas (Keith, Regier, & Rae, 1991). Keith et al. noted this was higher than the 0.25% to 0.53% point prevalence rates reported for Europe (Jablensky, 1986), where the use of marijuana has been, on average, less than in the United States (e.g., 1995 ESPAD report; European Monitoring Centre for Drugs and Drug Addiction, 1997).

Counterargument: With Increased Marijuana Popularity, No Change in Psychosis Rates

The rate of schizophrenia did not increase when the rate of marijuana use skyrocketed in the 1960s. At issue is the question of who was conducting longitudinal psychiatric epidemiology on populations during the 1960s, and if it wasn't being done for the population of interest, would the change have been great enough for the average practitioner to notice? A common misconception involves the assumption that because the risk for schizophrenia doubles with marijuana use, the incidence of schizophrenia itself would double (Degenhardt, Hall, & Lynskey, 2003), which would be true only if everyone in the country took up the habit. Whenever you are quantifying the impact of an environmental factor on disease prevalence, the evaluation should be limited to those who are likely to have been exposed to that factor. At its peak, the 1960s revolution resulted by 1976 to 1978 (Johnston, O'Malley, Bachman, & Schulenberg, 2012a, 2012b) in somewhat more than 11% of 12th graders and young adults using daily but less than 38% using monthly. Weekly use is the rate that appears to correspond to a doubling of the risk for schizophrenia (Moore et al., 2007). Therefore, roughly extrapolating for weekly use by splitting the difference in rates between daily and monthly use, the weekly use rate would have been in the vicinity of 24.5% (Johnston et al., 2012a, 2012b). To err on the side of maximizing the change in use, the trough in marijuana use rates preceding the 1960s impact could be assumed to be 0% (the data are unavailable for that time period, and, of course, it was unlikely to have been so low); thus, the difference would be predicted to have resulted in at most an 24.5% increase in the rate of schizophrenia, (24.5% − 0%) × twofold risk) + (75.5% × onefold risk) − 100% = 24.5%). To expect the average psychiatric practice to notice such a change over the period of time from the 1960s to the 1970s is clearly unrealistic. Only well-conducted epidemiology can be expected to discern such a difference. Most such studies began well after this time of rapid change in marijuana use (one exception in Britain reported by Der, Gupta, and Murray in 1990, is described in the following discussion), and even then, very few were longitudinal population studies, where the incidence in defined geographical areas was followed over time. In general, population epidemiology is considered to be of the weakest type because it is much more difficult to control for confounders that change over time, including (but certainly not limited to) the movement of different groups of people in and out of the area of interest. Much better are case control studies, which look at groups in one defined point in time and which can ascertain both marijuana use and psychiatric health, as well as attempt to exhaustively catalogue the factors that can potentially confound the outcome of interest. Moreover, many population studies of schizophrenia incidence over time did not have data on marijuana use over time, and others had data on marijuana use over time but not schizophrenia incidence.

Yet, a few sporadic, longitudinal comparisons of small populations were published in the 1970s and 1980s, which together are suggestive of interesting trends. For most, but not all, it is possible to relate the incidence data for schizophrenia to relevant marijuana use data. One such report utilized the catchment area for New York mental health hospitals and reported a roughly threefold decline in schizophrenia admissions from a 1976 peak to a trough by 1988 (Stoll et al., 1993). This time period corresponded to a sharp decline (by approximately 50%) in marijuana use by teens and young adults in the United States (Johnston et al., 2012a, 2012b, 2014), but the other major change reported by Stoll et al. was the switch from second edition of the DSM to the third edition in 1978, which made the criteria for schizophrenia diagnoses more strict and more in line with European standards. However, Loranger (1990) pointed out that for the same New York catchment study, adding back in the diagnoses lost with the stricter criteria cut the decline in schizophrenia cases by no more than half, leaving open the likelihood that a portion of the decline was a real change in disease incidence. Another other relevant study is one out of Denmark (Munk-Jorgensen, 1986), where detailed health data collection has a well-established history, showing a 10% decline in the incidence of schizophrenia in males aged 15 to 24 years at a time (1972–1974) when marijuana use in that age group had declined 20% (Retterstol, 1975). Indeed, it was reported that in most Western countries, the increase in drug use in the 1960s and early 1970s was followed by a decrease in the late 1970s and throughout the 1980s (van Solinge, 1998), perhaps attributable in part to increased interdictions, crop eradication efforts, and the resulting sharp decline in the supply in that time period (Chawla & Pichon, 2006). Thus, in Finland, which had experienced a rapid increase in marijuana use by youth in 1968–1970 to 85.5% "ever use" in the cities (Moser, 1974), by 1990s "ever use" was reported to be down to 21% (Poikolainen et al., 2000). During the same time period, schizophrenia incidence in Finland was reported to be in decline for birth cohorts born between 1954 and 1965 (Suvisaari, Haukka, Tanskanen, & Lönnqvist, 1999), such that the incidence was 33% lower in those born in 1965 than in those born in 1954. In Britain, Der et al. (1990), reported a sharp

33% rise in schizophrenia incidence in the late 1960s, followed by a remarkable decline in schizophrenia incidence in the 1970s into the 1980s (the title of the article was "Is Schizophrenia Disappearing?"). But, unfortunately, contemporaneous marijuana use numbers were not available for Britain at that time. The 33% rise in schizophrenia incidence over an eight-year period in the late 1960s was attributed by the authors to the possible incorporation of readmissions into the first admissions data, though a role for a spike in marijuana use driven by the 1960s revolution cannot be ruled out.

Because these studies from the United States and Europe are sparse and rudimentary, the relevance of these reports to the question at hand remains unclear. The situation is emblematic of the nature of the data available during that time period and reinforces the point that psychiatric epidemiology was not yet prepared to discern the role that marijuana may have played in changes in incidence of this major mental disease.

Counterargument: Studies Showing No Association between Use and Psychotic Disorders

Some studies show no association between marijuana use and the development of a psychotic disorder. Bechtold, Simpson, White, and Pardini (2015) recently reported on a longitudinal study from a cohort followed in Pittsburgh where the probability of a psychotic disorder was found to be equal between the marijuana users and the nonusers after the data were corrected for several co-variates. In a reanalysis submitted by the authors by way of a clarification to the journal (Clarification to Bechtold et al., 2015), the data actually showed a 2.5-fold higher risk for a psychotic disorder in the marijuana users, which reached significance in a one-tailed t-test, both with and without adjusting for race as a covariate. At issue is whether the study was adequately powered to detect the effect size seen historically in prior association studies (2 to 2.5-fold for the marijuana strength prevalent in the 20th century), and it was not. In addition, the original analysis applied corrections for covariates that had no valid theoretical basis: the presence or absence of health insurance and the current socioeconomic status of the subject at age 36. The flaw in this approach was twofold. One is that overadjustment bias is a problem in small studies (Arbogast & Ray, 2011), particularly if the adjustment has no theoretical basis (Schisterman, Cole, & Platt, 2009). Second, the covariates the authors employed are known as *collider variables* (Madigan et al., 2014); that is, marijuana use may be inextricably associated with lack of health insurance and low current socioeconomic status. Both a lack of health insurance and a low current socioeconomic status co-segregate with groups of individuals who are diagnosed with psychotic disorders because psychotic individuals have an extremely difficult time staying employed and, therefore, in keeping health insurance. In addition, low current socioeconomic status and a lack of health insurance also align with heavy marijuana use. Marijuana users are less likely to achieve educational and career goals (Arria, Caldeira, Bugbee, Vincent, & O'Grady, 2015; Cerdá et al., 2016) and thus more likely to be employed in jobs that did not provide health insurance during the pre-Obamacare time period encompassed by the study. Correcting for those covariates will not only obscure the marijuana effect, but there is also no theoretical basis to apply these correction factors as they have shown no independent association with psychotic disorders.

Another important report of a negative association between marijuana and psychosis demonstrated that for a small group (100 subjects) at very high risk of psychosis (positive family history, presence of one psychotic symptom of duration less than one week, etc.), the 22% who used marijuana at least once a month prior to assessment were not at greater risk for the development of full psychosis and/or schizophrenia (Phillips et al., 2002). Of the 100 total subjects, 32% received a diagnosis of full psychosis during the course of the study, and that rate was not significantly affected by cannabis use status. The authors themselves point to relatively small size as the main limitation of the study, but there are also other ways to understand the outcome. The primary issues of concern are that the length of follow-up was only 12 months, and the study was not designed to examine the difference in impact of marijuana on those with a family history of psychosis versus those without (in contrast, see Arendt, Mortensen, Rosenberg, Pedersen, & Waltoft, 2008; Shakoor et al., 2015) or whether marijuana use may have placed 22% of the group in the high risk category to begin with, a question best answered by prospective studies similar to Arseneault et al. (2002), Henquet et al., (2005), and Kuepper et al. (2011). Their results run contrary to the conclusions of a large meta-analysis (discussed in a preceding subsection) showing that once the first psychotic symptoms appear, there is no question that marijuana cessation improves the outcome (Schoeler et al., 2016).

Given the overwhelming number of studies showing a positive association between marijuana use and the development of schizophrenia, studies reporting negative results deserve special scrutiny to ensure they are adequately powered to detect effect sizes of interest, whether appropriate statistics are applied, if the research design permits a fair test of study hypotheses, and to determine whether the assumptions about possible confounding variables are based on sound logic and appropriate covariates.

Counterargument: Family History of Psychosis Is the Main Determinant

Some researchers are inclined to believe that if marijuana causes psychosis, it may only be in those with a family history. The first point to be made here is that surprisingly few individuals with schizophrenia have a first-degree family history for psychosis; for example, the proportion was determined to be 5.5% in Denmark (Mortensen et al., 1999). But, despite this relatively small proportion with family history, it is clear that the risk for developing a marijuana-induced psychosis is higher in those who do have a family history versus those who do not (Arendt et al., 2008), undoubtedly because of their vulnerability for psychosis no matter what the environmental trigger.

Yet, is a positive family history required to be susceptible to marijuana-induced psychosis? Actually, the degree of family history has been found to be lower in those who are diagnosed with schizophrenia following marijuana-induced psychosis than nonmarijuana users diagnosed with schizophrenia, and estimating that factor from the large Arendt et al. study (2008) combined with data from Pedersen and Mortensen (2001) on the proportion with a positive father, mother, and sibling family history yields a figure of about 0.7-fold. Similarly, a more recent study by Proal et al. (2014) reported a 0.7-fold degree of family history in schizophrenia patients who are marijuana users versus those who are not, although the study was underpowered to determine if the effect size seen was significant (Miller, 2014). The similarity of the two results (0.7-fold for both) gives strength to the concept that having a family history may not be a necessary component of risk for marijuana-induced psychosis.

Here, it must be made clear that the small proportion of probands with a family history of schizophrenia does not necessarily diminish the genetic contribution (roughly 50% concordance rate for schizophrenia between monozygotic twins; Gottesman & Shields, 1967) but rather points to the fact that schizophrenia is both a polygenic and heterogeneous genetic disorder, meaning more than one gene is required (Gottesman & Shields, 1967) and that the set of genes responsible for the disease can differ from population to population and from individual to individual (also in an environmentally specific manner due to gene–environment interplay). The bottom line is that family history can be negative, but the disease expression in an individual may still have a strong genetic component due to a unique combination of genes (Agerbo et al., 2015) coming in from different branches of the family tree interacting in a negative way (and with environmental factors like marijuana) to result in psychosis.

Controlling for the risk based on genetic background is partially accomplished by comparing siblings who use marijuana as compared to their paired siblings who do not; McGrath et al. (2010) have shown that doing so does not substantially diminish the marijuana effect (twofold increase in risk for those who started using before age 15 as compared to their nonusing sibling). A more recent study by Giordano et al. (2015) in a large Swedish cohort found that co-relative comparisons of risk conferred by marijuana use could be extrapolated to control for genetic background, and the elevation of risk attributable solely to marijuana for a schizophrenia diagnosis was 3.3-fold at the three-year point after a diagnosis of marijuana abuse, dropping to 1.67-fold for a diagnosis of schizophrenia at the seven-year point after a diagnosis of marijuana abuse.

In a study of monozygotic and dizygotic twins, Shakoor et al. (2015) reported that controlling for family history of psychosis did not significantly diminish the relationship between marijuana use and the development of psychosis. To further address the issue of family history of risk for psychosis being required for mediating the marijuana effect, a recent genetic association study has shown the gene AKT1 contributes to vulnerability to marijuana-induced psychosis even in those without a family history (Morgan, Freeman, Powell, & Curran, 2016). Because the effect size is relatively small, the results point toward AKT1 as being only one factor mediating the marijuana effect, in keeping with a heterogeneous, polygenic mediation of both schizophrenia and the marijuana effect.

The final point of importance in this subsection is that even in those with a heavy family history of schizophrenia for example, those with an identical twin who is diagnosed with schizophrenia—only about half the time will the other twin develop schizophrenia as well (reviewed by Gottesman & Shields, 1967; also see Shakoor et al., 2015). The genetic penetrance of this disease is far from complete. Thus, the impact of marijuana in an individual with high genetic risk for schizophrenia has both consequence and meaning because no one is destined to develop schizophrenia as a result of their genetic make-up alone. Even should the majority of those at risk prove to be those with a positive family history of psychosis in either first- or second-degree relatives, at least 10% of the population falls into that category. Given the lifetime prevalence of schizophrenia is on average 0.72% (Saha, Chant, Welham, & Mcgrath, 2005), though with considerable variation through space and time (Saha et al., 2006), when added to the 1% prevalence of psychotic bipolar disorder (Merikangas et al., 2011), the number of first- or second-degree relatives at risk can be calculated from data on the average family size (https://www.cia.gov/library/publications/the-world-factbook/fields/2127.html), while taking into account lowered fertility of the proband (Haukka, Suvisaari, & Lönnqvist, 2003). Some overlap in family member risk might occur between schizophrenia and bipolar 1 pedigrees but surely not enough to lower the total prevalence of those with a positive family history of psychosis to below 10%. This number represents a lot of individuals to put at risk.

Counterargument: Psychotic Symptoms Rare among Average Users

Actually, the prevalence of isolated psychotic symptoms at some point in time is about 12% to 15% in the average recreational user of the low-strength marijuana more common in the last century (Barkus, Stirling, Hopkins, & Lewis, 2006; Smith et al., 2009; Thomas, 1996). Not only was the marijuana lower in THC (<3% on average) during that time, hashish commonly used in that era was higher in cannabidiol (CBD; Mehmedic et al., 2010), a cannabinoid that may mitigate the risk of psychosis somewhat (Leweke et al., 2012). To compute the final expected percentage of schizophrenia cases in users starting with the average frequency who experience a psychotic symptom from typical use (selecting the average; i.e., 13.5%), on average, about 35% (Cannon et al., 2008) of those who experience such prodromal symptoms (i.e., 35% of the 13.5% in this case) can be expected to convert to full psychosis (a combination of psychotic symptoms at once). Of those who develop full marijuana-induced psychosis, about half (46%) will convert to a schizophrenia spectrum disorder over time (Arendt et al., 2008; Niemi-Pynttari et al., 2013), such that the final risk for schizophrenia is therefore 13.5% × 35% × 46% (i.e. on the order of 2.17%). Remarkably, this result is not far afield from the figure expected from the large-scale studies directly looking at the final association between marijuana use and schizophrenia spectrum disorders, where the lifetime morbid risk of the disorder is on the order of 0.72% (Saha et al., 2005) and weekly marijuana use increases that risk about 2.1-fold (Moore et al., 2007).

More recent studies of high-strength marijuana have found a 5.4-fold increase in risk for psychosis (Di Forti et al., 2015), such that marijuana users now constitute nearly 25% of all new cases of psychosis in one area of London, attributed to high-strength marijuana use being so prevalent in that district. Despite the common portrayal by the media of psychotic outcomes from marijuana use being rare, no one would consider a fivefold increase in risk, which results in this agent being associated with one fourth of new psychosis cases in a heavy use area, a rare event.

Counterargument: Restricting Marijuana Use in Many, Spares Few from Chronic Psychosis

That thousands of individuals would need to be kept from using marijuana to prevent one case of schizophrenia is a widely reported misinterpretation of a study by Hickman et al. (2009). The study authors had calculated, for example, that 2,800 young men aged 20 to 24 years would need to be kept from marijuana to spare one person from schizophrenia (or, because women are at lower risk, 5,282 if both genders are pooled, estimated from Hickman et al., 2009, Figure 3). The data were reported as "number needed to prevent" (NNP), analyzed in a similar manner to the "number needed to treat" factor used in studies of therapeutic drugs (e.g., Tripepi, Jager, Dekker, Wanner, & Zoccali, 2007). Unknown to many psychiatrists (Woolston, 2014), scientists publishing on the subject (Hall & Degenhardt, 2010; Hill, 2014; McGrath, 2012) and other readers of the paper, the figures the authors reported were misleading because they were based on yearly disease incidence rates (McCabe et al., 2010; Room & Rehm, 2009) relevant to the following scenario: Thousands must be prevented from using in just one year to spare one person from schizophrenia in that same year, meaning if you prevented that same group from using as they aged over the 24 years (the time represented by the age ranges covered in the study), you would have saved roughly one person per year or roughly 24 individuals from schizophrenia. But if the prevention only lasted one year, then indeed thousands would be required to spare just one. Imagine the hue and cry if such a strategy were applied to prevention of smoking cigarettes to spare one person from lung cancer. Prevention goals are always multiyear, if not a lifetime. Because the risk for schizophrenia changes with age, to more accurately calculate how many would need to be prevented from a few decades of use, the numbers Hickman et al. provided for each age group can be divided by the number of years of risk spanned by each age group (ages 16–19, 20–24, 25–19, 30–34, and 35–39; see Figure 5.1). Factoring in the greater risk for today's high strength marijuana as compared to the lower strength product Hickman et al. based their estimates on, the number of individuals (men and women) needed to prevent from use of high potency marijuana from age 16 to age 39, for example, is likely no more than 50 (Figure 5.1). Three other types of publications (see Figure 5.1) were utilized to generate NNP-24 years, and the resulting range in estimated values (19–50) is presented to illustrate the general framework in which to think about each analysis. Of course, the range in NNP-24 year values is fairly consistent with the risk of schizophrenia being increased 5.4-fold (Di Forti et al., 2015) from a lifetime morbid risk of 0.72% on average (Saha et al., 2005) to ~4% by daily high potency skunk use in London; that is, a 3.3% excess of users (about 1 out of 30) would be expected to develop schizophrenia in their lifetime from their high-strength marijuana habit.

Hickman et al. (2009) have since issued a clarification of the meaning of their NNP values, buried within the discussion section of another published paper (Gage et al., 2016): "These figures will be lower if calculating risk of schizophrenia over the entire lifespan" (p. 554). Unfortunately, they did not recalculate NNP based on a multiyear prevention strategy, leaving readers to formulate their own estimates. The widespread misunderstanding engendered by their original report illustrates the importance of thinking about numbers from a few different angles. Thousands never made sense, simply based on the lifetime morbid risk of schizophrenia being pegged at nearly 1 out of a 100 and knowing the factor by which marijuana increases the risk (Figure 5.1).

Further explanation of Figure 5.1 is necessary for the reader to understand the derivation of the calculations and the assumptions upon which they are based. These details are as follows: The calculated values will obviously change as risk estimates for h.s product are modified in the future. The NNP analyses for h.s. commencing from the Hickman et al. (2009) and Moore et al. (2007) results (upper and right panels) assume the percent conversion from a full psychotic break to schizophrenia does not differ according to the original cause of the psychosis. Should future studies make clear that conversion from a full psychotic break to schizophrenia differs for non-marijuana-induced psychosis (i.e. is not on the order of 46%), the final NNP-24yr estimate in the upper and right panels for high strength product would need to be adjusted accordingly (up if greater than 46% conversion, down if less). Four different starting points for the analyses of published data were utilized, commencing with the original NNP publication by Hickman et al. (2009) as the frame of reference for key criteria (i.e. definition of use rate; strength of cannabis used based on time period of the study; approx. age range of population for incidence; baseline incidence of schizophrenia over a 24-yr period). Note that the Hickman et al. publication (upper center box) utilized the average increase in risk for psychosis calculated for weekly use of cannabis (2.09-fold) reported by Moore et al. (2007), right box. Unless otherwise noted (see Arendt et al. data (2008) for Denmark), the mean 24-yr incidence of schizophrenia for ages 16-39 (0.0048) was derived from Figure 2 of Hickman et al. (2009). To calculate the NNP-24 yr for low-moderate strength marijuana from the Hickman et al. (2009) data (top box), for a population of men and women

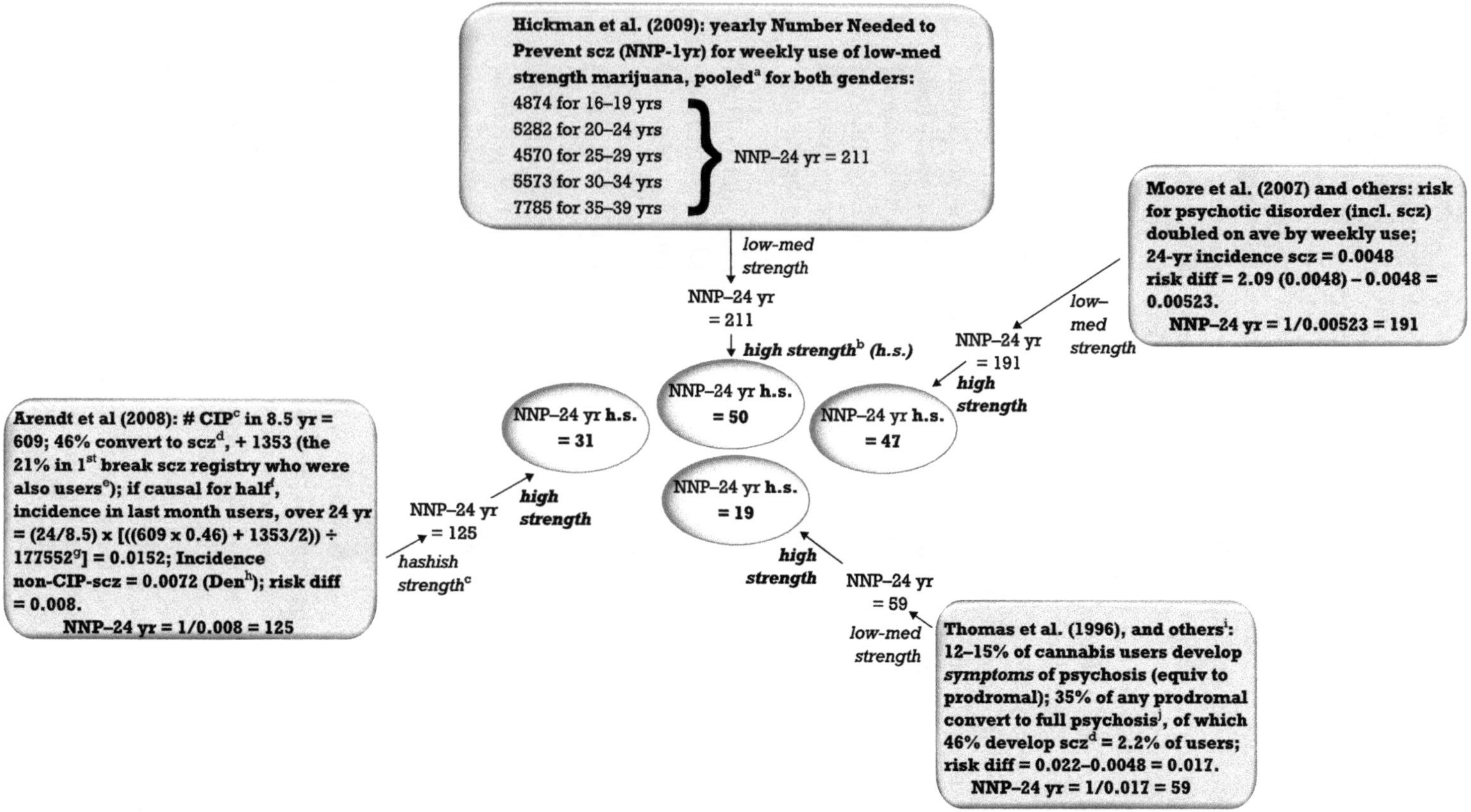
Hickman et al. (2009): yearly Number Needed to Prevent scz (NNP-1yr) for weekly use of low-med strength marijuana, pooled[a] for both genders:
4874 for 16–19 yrs
5282 for 20–24 yrs
4570 for 25–29 yrs
5573 for 30–34 yrs
7785 for 35–39 yrs
NNP–24 yr = 211
low-med strength
NNP–24 yr = 211
high strength[b] (h.s.)
NNP–24 yr h.s. = 50
Moore et al. (2007) and others: risk for psychotic disorder (incl. scz) doubled on ave by weekly use;
24-yr incidence scz = 0.0048
risk diff = 2.09 (0.0048) – 0.0048 = 0.00523.
NNP–24 yr = 1/0.00523 = 191
low–med strength
NNP–24 yr = 191
high strength
NNP–24 yr h.s. = 47
Arendt et al (2008): # CIP[c] in 8.5 yr = 609; 46% convert to scz[d], + 1353 (the 21% in 1st break scz registry who were also users[e]); if causal for half[f], incidence in last month users, over 24 yr = (24/8.5) x [((609 x 0.46) + 1353/2)) ÷ 177552[g]] = 0.0152; Incidence non-CIP-scz = 0.0072 (Den[h]); risk diff = 0.008.
NNP–24 yr = 1/0.008 = 125
hashish strength[c]
NNP–24 yr = 125
high strength
NNP–24 yr h.s. = 31
NNP–24 yr h.s. = 19
high strength
NNP–24 yr = 59
low-med strength
Thomas et al. (1996), and others[i]: 12–15% of cannabis users develop symptoms of psychosis (equiv to prodromal); 35% of any prodromal convert to full psychosis[j], of which 46% develop scz[d] = 2.2% of users;
risk diff = 0.022–0.0048 = 0.017.
NNP–24 yr = 1/0.017 = 59

Figure 5.1 Framework to estimate "number needed to prevent" from marijuana use over 24 years (NNP-24yr) to save one person from a schizophrenia spectrum disorder (scz), derived both for weekly use of low-medium strength cannabis and for daily use of high strength (h.s.) cannabis.[1]

[a]Averages estimated from Figure 3 of Hickman et al. (2009) as described in figure legend.

[b]High strength as defined by daily use of high strength "skunk" (Di Forti et al., 2015).

[c]CIP corresponds to cases of cannabis-induced psychosis, most of whom were hashish users (Arendt et al., 2008).

dApproximately 46% of cases of cannabis-induced psychosis convert to schizophrenia spectrum disorders (Arendt et al., 2008; Niemi-Pynttari et al., 2013).

eThe % underdiagnosed in schizophrenia registry with illegal drug use was assumed to be 37.3 (Hansen et al., 2000), and of those about 56% were likely cannabis users (Larsen et al., 2006); thus 0.56 × .373 = 21%.

fPsychosis liability and marijuana use have a roughly equivalent bi-directional interaction in some studies Griffith-Lendering et al. (2013).

gTo calculate incidence, the number of Danish residents who used cannabis in the last month was identified for the at risk population of young adults from an EMCDDA mongraph (7.8% of the Arendt et al. study population of 2,276,309; i.e., 177,552).

hThe incidence in non-CIP schizophrenia was available from Arendt et al. (2008): number of first break schizophrenia cases = 6476, the % underdiagnosed in scz registry with illegal drug use was assumed to be 37.3% (Hansen et al., 2000), and of those about 56% were likely cannabis users (Larsen et al., 2006); thus 0.56 × 37.3 = 21%; assuming that marijuana was causal for a maximum of half of those individuals, = 1,353/2, then 6476 − (1,353/2)= 5,800 were the likely maximum number of cases in which marijuana played no role. The population in the study of Arendt et al. was 2,276,309. Incidence of first break schizophrenia in which marijuana played no role was then = 5,800/2,276,309 for the 8.5 years of the study. For a 24-yr period, the incidence could be estimated to be (24/8.5)(5,800/2,276,309)= 0.0072.

iAlso Barkus et al. (2006) and Smith et al. (2009).

jCannon et al. (2008).

moving through the ages 16 through 39 years, the same age range covered by the Hickman et al. study (2009), the NNP-1yr for each age group was either specified in the text for the age groups or could be estimated from Figure 3 of their study (top panels of their Figure 3) for men and women. The NNP-1yr for each age group was then averaged for the genders so there would be an equal probability of yielding a male or female individual with schizophrenia (had they all been using marijuana). Based on the gender proportions presented by Hickman et al. (2009), the proportion of women to men NNP yearly values were on average 2:1 (i.e. you would need to prevent twice as many women as men in order to achieve an equal probability of sparing a female and a male from schizophrenia), a ratio that would therefore be represented in the gender compositions of the NNP-24yr values calculated from the Hickman et al. data (but not in the three other paths to NNP-24yr shown in Figure 5.1). Using the age range of 25–29 years as an example, the average NNP-1yr across males and females was 4570; that figure was then divided by the number of years in that age group (five) to yield NNP-5yr; the equivalent calculation was carried out for the other age groups; the average NNP-5yr for all age groups (or, in the case for those 16-19, NNP-4yr) was determined; and then that figure was divided by the number of age groups (five) to yield the final NNP-24yr (211 persons). Because by definition, NNP = 1/risk difference (where risk difference equals the incidence of the disease in the marijuana-using population minus the incidence of the disease in non-users), or alternatively, 1/NNP = risk difference, and the background incidence was determined to be 0.0048 as an average of the rate for each gender (Figure 2 of Hickman et al., 2009), 1/211 = incidence of the disease in the marijuana using population minus 0.0048. This then enables the calculation of the incidence of the disease in daily users of high strength marijuana which is 5.4-fold the risk as compared to non-users (Di Forti et al., 2015), or 5.4 ÷ 2.09 times the risk (Moore et al., 2007) posed to weekly users of low-moderate strength marijuana, i.e. 2.584-fold the value used by Hickman et al. (2009) in their analysis. Thus, 1/211 = z – 0.0048; where z = incidence of the disease in weekly users of low-mod strength marijuana = 0.00954. 1/NNP-24yr h.s. = 2.584 (0.00954)-0.0048; thus NNP-24-yr h.s. = 50. The calculations derived from the data of Arendt et al. (2008) in the lower left box of Figure 5.1, also require additional explanation: 1) The subjects are reported to have predominantly used hashish, a form relatively rich in cannabidiol but approximately the same THC content (Licata et al., 2005); and 2) It is the only publication presented which incorporates data on incident cannabis use and incident psychotic disorders (including cannabis-induced psychosis, CIP, for which full causality is assumed because of some remission seen when drug-free). As specified in Figure 5.1, approximately 46% who experience CIP will convert to a schizophrenia spectrum disorder (Arendt et al., 2008; Niemi-Pynttari et al., 2013).

MARIJUANA USE AND BIPOLAR DISORDER

As compared to the association with schizophrenia, the study of the relationship between marijuana use and bipolar disorder is in its infancy. Patients with bipolar disorder are generally able to function at a higher level than schizophrenia patients, and thus the potential seriousness of the impact on schizophrenia rates naturally focused the research attention in that direction. But the emerging literature does point toward a roughly equivalent impact of marijuana on bipolar disorder as on schizophrenia. For example, Agrawal, Nurnberger, and Lynskey (2012) found a 6.8-fold higher marijuana use rate in bipolar patients versus control subjects. The majority of the subjects 89.9%) were of the bipolar 1 (with psychotic features) diagnosis, and although there was no difference between the subtypes of patients (bipolar 1 vs. 2) in terms of their relative use rates, the marijuana-using patients were experiencing a greater level of disability in terms of life functioning. Henquet, Krabbendam, Graaf, Have, and Os (2006) found a 2.7-fold increased risk for mania at follow-up in a prospective study of marijuana users versus nonusers, independent of the development of psychosis. Similar to the finding of a reduction in age of onset of schizophrenia in marijuana users, there is a reduction in age of onset of bipolar disorder in the users. Research has shown a range of figures: 7.5 years earlier onset in excessive marijuana users as compared to excessive alcohol users (reviewed by Lagerberg et al., 2011), 5.1 years earlier onset for first depressive episode in marijuana users as compared to nonusers (Kvitland et al., 2016), and 2.6 years earlier as compared to those who reported no substance use (Agrawal et al., 2012). Similar to the age of onset in schizophrenia, the timing of the drug use under investigation should precede the peak age of onset of the disease. Yet, as compared to schizophrenia, the peak age of onset of bipolar disorder is more broad and includes more childhood onset cases and a significant proportion of adults over the age of 40 yrs (Baldessarini et al., 2012), which is not generally seen for schizophrenia, at least in males (reviewed by Hafner et al., 1998, Figure 2). Perhaps in keeping with the importance of the use occurring before the peak age of onset of the disease seen in the absence of drug use, Strakowski et al. (2007) did not find a reduction in age of onset of bipolar illness as a function of marijuana use but did find a greater association of marijuana use with psychotic symptoms, as well as a similar disease trajectory pattern seen by González-Pinto et al. (2011) for schizophrenia. Those whose bipolar disorder appeared to be triggered by marijuana use fared better after quitting their habit relatively soon after the first break than those whose onset of bipolar disorder followed marijuana abuse. As one might expect, Weiss et al. (2005) found that, in general, substance use continuation was associated with a worse outcome and those who eventually quit their habit (but not necessarily after the first break) fared worse than those who never used at all.

Finally, a very large study published more recently by Blanco et al. (2016) found no significant effect of past-year adult marijuana use on the development of bipolar disorder, but a closer inspection of the study's data makes clear that roughly 18% of control subjects (who had not used in the past year) had used at some point in the past; otherwise the total number of controls described in the study exceeded by several thousand a prior description of the study population (Blanco et al., 2014). Other explanations of this discrepancy are clearly possible but not obvious to the reader of either paper. Because the trajectory of marijuana's impact on bipolar disorder could theoretically outlast its time frame of use, particularly in those who did not quit marijuana use immediately after their first symptom of the disease (Strakowski et al., 2007), including in the control subjects, those exposed to marijuana in prior time periods potentially confounded their conclusion. Furthermore, because the unadjusted finding for marijuana's association with bipolar disorder demonstrated a large effect size (3.7-fold for bipolar 1 disorder) and was close to significance after adjustment for covariates in logistic regression analysis by Blanco et al. (2016), the association could well have been skewed away from significance by the authors' decision regarding the control subjects. Indeed, a prior analysis of the same study population found that regular marijuana use (not just past-year use limited to adulthood) uniquely predicted the development of bipolar disorder (Cougle, Hakes, Macatee, Chavarria, & Zvolensky, 2015).

MARIJUANA AND ANXIETY, PANIC ATTACKS, AND DEPRESSION

Anxiety and Panic

Anxiety as an acute outcome from marijuana use was recognized long before marijuana's association with psychosis became well accepted, and the type of anxiety it triggered was reported to be similar to the panic reactions seen in users of hallucinogens (reviewed by Hollister, 1986). In clinical administration of oral Δ^9-THC, Zuardi, Shirakawa, Finkelfarb, and Karniol (1982) reported a large increase in anxiety experienced by the subjects. Thomas (1996) reported that the most common physical or mental health symptoms experienced by regular users were anxiety and panic attacks. In population studies where covariates were controlled for, other authors (Hayatbakhsh et al., 2007; Medina & Shear, 2007) found a strong association between marijuana use and anxiety scores, independent of the use of other drugs. Another prospective study of over 7,000 subjects found a 1.6-fold increase in risk posed by marijuana use and the development of anxiety disorders after adjusting for sociodemographic variables but not after adjusting for additional confounding variables, specifically parental psychiatric history, traumatic childhood events, and symptoms of neuroticism in the subject (van Laar, Dorsselaer, Monshouwer, & Graaf, 2007). Whether marijuana has an anxiety-provoking effect in vulnerable subjects due to the presence of one or more of such background characteristics would nevertheless be of interest for further research.

The co-morbidity between experiences of panic episodes and marijuana use was investigated by Dannon, Lowengrub, Amiaz, Grunhaus, and Kotler (2004), and the outcome was that many who experienced isolated episodes of panic soon after their first use of the drug went on to develop full-fledged panic disorders. A prospective study of over 1,700 adolescents found that panic disorder was 4.9-fold more likely in those who developed cannabis dependence than in nonusers, whereas dependence on other drugs of abuse did not increase risk (Zvolensky et al., 2008) except for nicotine, the impact of which could not be disentangled from marijuana because of the strong co-variation between the two drugs.

Subsequent work in a much larger number of subjects (over 34,000; Cougle et al., 2015) revealed that among the substance use categories examined (alcohol, nicotine, and marijuana), regular marijuana use uniquely predicted the development of panic disorder with agoraphobia even after adjusting for potentially confounding covariates.

These studies raise particular concerns for the use of medical marijuana to treat victims of posttraumatic stress disorder (PTSD), who are already at greater risk for not only psychosis (Pepper & Agius, 2009; Pierre, 2010) but also severe anxiety and panic. In this regard, a recent study of a few thousand veterans with PTSD (Wilkinson, Stefanovics, & Rosenheck, 2015) found that marijuana users were less likely to make progress in overcoming their condition and were more likely to be violent.

Although Δ^9-THC may aid in the extinction of fearful memories in PTSD patients via modulation of the endocannabinoid system (Neumeister, 2013; Rabinak et al., 2013), it may also make positive emotional memory less well consolidated (Ballard, Gallo, & Wit, 2013) and is not good for memory in general (Solowij & Battisti, 2008; Wise, Thorpe, & Lichtman, 2009). CBD, the nonpsychoactive component of marijuana, holds equal promise for fearful memory extinction without many of the psychiatric risks (Das et al., 2013; Stern, Gazarini, Takahashi, Guimarães, & Bertoglio, 2012). In point of fact, CBD holds promise as a medication to reduce anxiety in humans (Blessing, Steenkamp, Manzanares, & Marmar, 2015; Schier et al., 2012), and, as discussed in Chapter 10, CBD may also have other medicinal value.

Depression

The data concerning the impact of this drug on depression include one prospective study of over 7,000 subjects of a wide age range showing an increase in covariate-adjusted risk (1.6-fold) for a first incidence of major depression (van Laar et al., 2007), less strong a risk than the 5.6-fold increase in risk for depression if used weekly in the past year by young adult women (Patton et al., 2002). One study showed no significant increase in risk (Harder et al., 2006), but these investigators considered only past-year marijuana use in adults as it relates to past seven-day depression (rather than past-year depression) and also relied solely on propensity score matching to adjust for covariates, either of which could underlie the difference in outcome as compared to the regression analysis of the other studies. Alternatively, the different outcome could possibly lie in the age of onset of the marijuana use, as past-year use by adults was also investigated by Blanco et al. (2016) and was not associated with depression after adjusting for covariates (with caveats noted previously for the Blanco et al. study), while early use was found to have more impact from an unadjusted analysis of a World Health Organization study (de Graaf et al., 2010). But further investigation of that question has revealed no impact of age of use onset on depression, finding, on average, a nearly 1.8-fold increase in covariate-adjusted risk independent of that factor (Fairman & Anthony,

2012). As one would expect, the effect size has been found to be sensitive to the degree of use, the lowest risk being associated with less than monthly and the highest with daily use, 1.2 versus 1.6-fold, respectively (Silins et al., 2014). A fairly recent meta-analysis concluded that an approximately 1.6-fold increase in risk in depression occurred with at least weekly cannabis use (Lev-Ran et al., 2013), and in a longitudinal study published in 2017, Feingold, Rehm, and Lev-Ran (2017) reported that more frequent marijuana use was significantly associated with having developed more depressive symptoms at follow-up,—for example, anhedonia, insomnia, or hypersomnia and psychomotor problems.

The possibility of self-medication was addressed in a small study of 119 marijuana-dependent subjects by Arendt et al. (2007), who found that dependent subjects who were depressed were no more likely to report they were using marijuana to relieve depression than were nondepressed subjects. Furthermore, subjects who experienced prior depressive episodes were less likely to report feelings of happiness and more likely to experience depressed symptoms while under the influence of marijuana.

To examine the influence of genetic risk for depression in mediating the potential effect of marijuana on depression, Agrawal, Nelson et al. (2017) studied a cohort of Australian twins. They found that even in monozygotic (identical) twins, the twin who used marijuana frequently or initiated use early was up to 1.5-fold more likely to meet the criteria for major depressive disorder than the twin who never used or used very little, and the difference between the impact seen in the identical twin group and the nonidentical twin group was not great. Thus, genetic differences between individuals could not explain the outcome of major depression in the marijuana users.

Marijuana, Anxiety and Depression, and Withdrawal

Unlike psychosis, there is strong evidence that marijuana withdrawal exacerbates underlying anxiety and depression, independent of any role in triggering these traits in the first place. Hasin et al. (2008) found depressed mood and anxiety to be an important part of the suite of the psychological withdrawal symptoms seen, coming in second and third relative to the number of subjects reporting hypersomnia. Cornelius, Chung, Martin, Wood, and Clark (2008) reported that increased anxiety and depression occurred in 55% and 52% of patients undergoing withdrawal, respectively. It should be noted that all of the subjects were diagnosed with major depressive disorder and cannabis dependence prior to their abstinence from cannabis. Levin et al. (2010) reported that 50% reported increased anxiety, and 45% reported increased depression during withdrawal with an average onset after quitting of 2.9 days and 4.2 days and an average duration of 95 days and 122 days, respectively. In contrast, Budney, Moore, Vandrey, and Hughes (2003) reported a faster onset of increased anxiety and depression during withdrawal, within 1.3 days on average for both.

The relatively short onset of the withdrawal symptoms in a matter of slightly more than a day or so raises the distinct possibility that the fluctuations seen in blood Δ^9-THC levels and the high degree of interindividual variability (Battistella et al., 2013) could easily lead to anxiety and depression during variations in weekly patterns of regular use. However, the long average duration of the symptoms during abstinence raise the possibility of a more enduring impact that could be considered less a part of withdrawal and more reflective of an enduring behavioral change. More longitudinal research on the order of the 7 to 10 years covered by the research on psychosis triggered by marijuana (Arendt et al., 2008; Gonzalez-Pinto et al., 2011; Niemi-Pynttari et al., 2013) will be required to separate out acute effects from withdrawal effects and any permanent impact of marijuana use on anxiety and depression syndromes.

MARIJUANA AND RISK FOR SUICIDE

The suspected link between marijuana use and suicide is not unexpected given the preponderance of its other mental health effects, all of which are associated with increased risk for suicide. The possible role for marijuana in triggering suicidal ideation and suicidal attempts was noted several decades ago by Andréasson and Allebeck (1990) in a large study of mortality in Swedish transcripts assessed at follow-up in 1983, but the association was not significant after potentially confounding variables were corrected for. Other reports pointed to a connection between suicidality and marijuana use, but the studies were often small and either observational only (increasingly marijuana use preceded the suicides in the Micronesian Island of Truk; Hezel, 1984), unadjusted for covariates (Garnefski & de Wilde, 1998), or the association diminished to a nonsignificant trend after adjustment for covariates (Beautrais, Joyce, & Mulder, 1999). In contrast, using case-control data from the US National Mortality Followback Survey in 1993, Kung, Pearson, and Liu (2003) found an increased risk of suicide in marijuana users, 2.3-fold for males and 4.8 fold for females. Yet, in a study of Swiss adolescents, reported to have one of the highest rates of suicide in Europe, Gex, Narring, Ferron, and Michaud (1998) found that, in contrast to other drugs, cannabis use was unrelated to suicide attempts after adjusting for covariates. Pedersen (2008) reported that subjects who had used cannabis 11 or more times in the past year were 2.9-fold more likely to attempt suicide after adjusting for confounding covariates. In Nova Scotia, Rasic, Weerasinghe, Asbridge, and Langille (2013) found that polydrug abuse was significantly associated with suicide attempts in a group of high school students, but cannabis use alone was only predictive of depression without suicidal features, possibly because the marijuana-only users were found to use it infrequently.

One of the most effective means to adjust a priori for genetic background and confounding environmental effects is to study the differential impact of marijuana in twins. Thus, Lynskey et al. (2004) investigated suicide risk in an Australian twin cohort (interviewed in the years 1996–2000) and found that adjusted risk for suicidal ideation and attempts were significantly elevated in the marijuana-using twin of the pair. For attempted suicide, marijuana increased the risk 3.4-fold and 2.5-fold for onset of use before or after turning 17 years of age, respectively. Of the covariates adjusted for (conduct disorder, childhood sex abuse, alcohol use, tobacco use, major depression), the co-predictive variables were alcohol use and conduct disorder. However, the study appears to have been underpowered to address the risk for monozygotic twins and dizygotic twins as separate categories. Delforterie et al. (2015) later investigated an expanded version of the same twin cohort, finding a doubling in suicide ideation only in those with a high degree of cannabis use disorder. The risk was slightly higher for marijuana than for other recreational drug use, but nicotine was protective and, unlike other studies (Arrias et al., 2016; reviewed by Norström & Rossow, 2016), alcohol was found to have no effect. In an even more recent follow-up study, Agrawal, Nelson et al. (2017) analyzed the updated Australian registry. They found that members of identical and nonidentical twin pairs who frequently used marijuana (defined as more than 100 times of use) were at a more than 3.6-fold increased odds of reporting suicidal ideation lasting more than one day and a more than sixfold odds of engaging in a suicide attempt (here, the nonidentical twin comparison only) than their nonusing twin. Because the impacts were generally similar in the nonidentical and identical twin pairs (with an exception being a difference in attempts), they concluded that genetic factors played a relatively small role in mediating the effects seen.

A meta-analysis of the association between marijuana use and suicide (Borges, Bagge, & Orozco, 2016) placed the odds ratio at 2.56-fold for death by suicide in marijuana users as compared to nonusers. Included were studies published in the 1990s through 2014, but it seems likely the risk reported for suicide may have increased as the potency for typical marijuana has increased in recent years. One of the recent covariate-adjusted studies reported the risk of completed suicide to be fivefold for marijuana users as compared to nonusers (Arendt, Munk-Jørgensen, Sher, & Jensen, 2013), and in two others, the risk of suicide attempts to be sevenfold (Clarke et al., 2014; Silins et al., 2014), even when a history of mood disorder was controlled for (Clarke et al., 2014).

The risk may be different or perhaps even more variable in populations already at high risk of suicidal behaviors. Kvitland et al. (2016) found a nearly 10-fold increase in recent onset bipolar 1 patients who used marijuana in the past six months versus bipolar 1 patients who had not done so. More recent research revealed no increase in suicide attempts in bipolar patients who used marijuana, but a 1.9-fold increase in completed suicides (Østergaard, Nordentoft, & Hjorthøj, 2017). Yet, for individuals affected with major depressive disorder, Feingold et al. (2017) reported no impact of cannabis use on suicidal ideation or attempts.

In a prospective study of unrelated individuals, Agrawal, Tillman et al. (2017) investigated the timing issue, comparing the role of marijuana in initiating suicidal behaviors versus suicidal behaviors initiating marijuana use. Their findings showed a significantly reduced likelihood of initiating marijuana use following a bout of suicidal ideation, but no significant difference in risk of suicidal ideation or attempt following the initiation of marijuana use. For the latter result, the sample size may have been underpowered for all the covariate adjustments made, given the effect size that appeared to have been present in the unadjusted values.

The increased risk of suicidal behaviors from marijuana is generally found in association with chronic use. Yet, acute, sudden onset suicidal ideation has also been known to occur following oral ingestion of more than one 10 mg dose of Δ^9-THC, as seen in three medical examiners' reports of three cases of psychosis with suicidal ideation, extensively covered by media outlets in a state where marijuana is legal (Nicholson, 2014; Reuter, 2015; Steffen, 2014). The descriptions make it clear that an impending sense of doom was dominating the thoughts of the unfortunate consumers. Another tragic case from Boulder, Colorado, was outlined in a 2015 documentary covering the mental health impacts of this drug, predominantly focusing on youth (Belsher, 2015).

Confirming these nonacademic reports, suicidal ideation following oral ingestion of Δ^9-THC in the clinic can also be found in the scientific literature (Russo et al., 2015; reviewed by Koppel et al., 2014). One academic paper reported suicidal ideation in 1 out of 14 subjects administered a liquid form of pure Δ^9-THC (20 mg doses) over a period of three days in a clinical setting, an outcome that preceded the administration of the marijuana "inverse agonist" subsequently tested (Gorelick et al., 2011). The particular cannabinoid "inverse agonist" (Rimonabant) was itself withdrawn from the market before the study was completed because of its link to increased risk for suicidal ideation (Robertson & Allison, 2009), which should not be interpreted to mean that direct (not "inverse") agonists are without those effects. As a partial agonist, Δ^9-THC (Mackie, 2008) could theoretically interfere with the full agonist action of endogenous cannabinoids, potentially leading to a neurophysiologic end result similar to Rimonobant's.

Marijuana is not unique among recreational drugs in terms of its impact on suicidal tendencies, as recreational drug use in general was found to substantially increase risk of suicide attempts in European youth (Kokkevi, Rotsika, Arapaki, & Richardson, 2012), with the risk of self-reported suicide attempts doubling for each additional drug used. Wong, Zhou, Goebert, and Hishinuma (2013) reported a significant association with suicidality in US youth for each of 10 substances used (heroin, methamphetamine, steroids, cocaine, ecstasy, hallucinogens, inhalants, marijuana, alcohol, and tobacco). Fowler, Rich, and Young (1986) found that fully 53% of suicide cases in the San Diego Suicide Study had received a substance abuse diagnosis of one type of another. O'Boyle and Brandon (1998) reported that suicide attempters were significantly more likely to abuse multiple drugs, including alcohol, than nonattempters. In Britain, polydrug use was shown to be significantly associated with lifetime suicide attempts, but the particular drugs of greatest risk were not identified (Smith, Farrell, Bunting, Houston, J. E., & Shevlin, 2011). A study of suicide in Benin (Randall, Doku, Wilson, & Peltzer, 2014) reported that after adjusting for confounding variables, illicit drug use of all kinds conferred a threefold elevation in risk. A postmortem survey of deaths by suicide in western Australia found alcohol to be the most prevalent drug in postmortem samples, followed by marijuana (Hillman, 2000).

Of the studies focused on specific types of other recreational drugs, cocaine abuse has unequivocally been associated with suicide over the years (Arias et al., 2016; Burge, Felts, Chenier, & Parrillo, 1995; Darke & Kaye, 2004; Kandel, Raveis, & Davies, 1991; Tondo et al., 1999), as high as ninefold in an unadjusted study (Marzuk et al., 1992). Heroin users were reported to be 14 times more likely than their nonusing peers to die from suicide (Darke & Ross, 2002), though separating out intentional from unintentional overdose can clearly be problematic. A long-term follow-up study demonstrated that suicide attempts are reported by 42% of a very large cohort of heroin users (Darke et al., 2015), a nearly 10-fold higher rate than the 4.6% reported to have attempted suicide in the general population (Kessler, Borges, & Walters, 1999). Abstinence from heroin in former addicts has been shown to be protective but polydrug use enhanced the suicide risk (Darke et al., 2015).

Thus, in contrast to marijuana increasing risk for chronic psychosis, the increased risk it conveys for suicide is not greater than for other recreational drugs of abuse, particularly as compared to cocaine and heroin. Potential confounders of apparent suicides from those other drugs are unintentional deaths from overdoses, which is not a factor with marijuana, although, in common with LSD and other hallucinogens, it may be difficult to separate out intentional suicide from unintended deaths due to physical behaviors induced by the drug. Furthermore, much more research must be conducted to determine whether the increased risk for suicide in marijuana users is merely the culmination of its effect to increase conditions of psychosis, anxiety, panic, and depression or whether it represents a risk factor for suicidal thoughts and actions in addition to the suicide risk intrinsically posed by those conditions. The acute onset of suicidal ideation with oral ingestion and the study by Clarke et al. (2014), where the investigators controlled for a history of mood disorders, suggests the latter scenario remains a possibility.

SUMMARY

The challenges facing epidemiological research on factors that influence mental health are enormous, in part because the brain is our most complex and finely tuned organ. From genetic factors to obstetrical complications, nutrition, infections, radiation exposure, chronic stress, and toxic insults, the plethora of variables that must be addressed can be daunting. These factors are not constant through time and space, and detrimental changes in one may be complemented by mitigating improvements in another. But within epidemiological studies lie clues to potentially solving some of our most crippling diseases, and the rewards of delving into the complexity are enormous. Such is the case with marijuana and mental disorders, and if policies derived from such explorations are to err, they should err on the side of public health rather than public opinion.

Much has been written about the need to place marijuana's health effects in the context of legal recreational drugs commonly used in our society today. Thus, for a drug like alcohol, there is no question that drinking too much can lead to fatal overdoses, whereas acute fatalities from marijuana are rare events, usually occurring as cardiotoxicities, not CNS toxicities (Dines et al., 2015; Hartung, Kauferstein, Ritz-Timme, & Daldrup, 2014). For cigarettes, there is also no question that long-term use is associated with a substantial risk of early death from lung cancer, and although marijuana-induced schizophrenia can result in early mortality (Olfson, Gerhard, Huang, Crystal, & Stroup, 2015), it is not necessarily an irrevocable sentence for early death.

Indeed, with both alcohol and cigarettes, there are important ways in which their harms to human health are more manageable than those caused by marijuana. Alcohol can be used responsibly with no lasting negative impact, for example, by drinking a single glass of wine or a beer a couple of times per week. Marijuana at that rate of use poses more than a doubling in risk for being diagnosed with a schizophrenia spectrum disorder. Apart from the human tragedy, the economic toll marijuana can cause through increasing risk for schizophrenia certainly represents no minor impact, as enumerated by Wu et al. (2005) who reported the annual cost of schizophrenia to the United States was $63 billion (2002 dollars). Moreover, determining precisely who is immune to this outcome, what rate of use is safe, and how protective marijuana cessation will be for an individual user is not possible at this point in time. Smoking cigarettes damages the respiratory system extensively, but if users quit before age 40, they can largely erase their increased risk for cancer (Thun et al., 2013). For marijuana, there is usually not such a long such grace period during which the user has a chance to learn from their mistakes. Full psychotic breaks and suicidal ideation can happen very early on, even in those with no family history, and full recovery is not guaranteed for those who quit.

The preponderance of evidence reviewed in this chapter substantiates not only a significant, causal role for marijuana in chronic psychotic syndromes but also a strong association with mood disorders and suicidal ideation. Thus, there can no longer be any doubt that the range of negative mental health impacts of this drug, too frequently dismissed as fear-mongering rhetoric, must be positioned at the front and center of international drug policy dialogue.

REFERENCES

Agerbo, E., Sullivan, P. F., Vilhjálmsson, B. J., Pedersen, C. B., Mors, O., Børglum, A. D., . . . Mortensen, P. B. (2015). Polygenic risk score, parental socioeconomic status, family history of psychiatric disorders, and the risk for schizophrenia. *JAMA Psychiatry*, *72*, 635–641. http://dx.doi.org/10.1001/jamapsychiatry.2015.0346

Agrawal, A., Nelson, E. C., Bucholz, K. K., Tillman, R., Grucza, R. A., Statham, D. J., . . . Lynskey, M. T. (2017). Major depressive disorder, suicidal thoughts and behaviours, and cannabis involvement in discordant twins: A retrospective cohort study. *The Lancet Psychiatry*, 4, 706–714. http://dx.doi.org/10.1016/S2215-0366(17)30280-8

Agrawal, A., Nurnberger, J. I., & Lynskey, M. T. (2012). Cannabis involvement in individuals with bipolar disorder. *Psychiatry Research*, 185, 459–461. http://dx.doi.org/10.1016/j.psychres.2010.07.007

Agrawal, A., Tillman, R., Grucza, R. A., Nelson, E. C., McCutcheon, V. V., Few, L., . . . & Hesselbrock, V. M. (2017). Reciprocal relationships between substance use and disorders and suicidal ideation and suicide attempts in the Collaborative Study of the Genetics of Alcoholism. *Journal of Affective Disorders*, 213, 96–104. http://dx.doi.org/10.1016/j.jad.2016.12.060

Andréasson, S., & Allebeck, P. (1990). Cannabis and mortality among young men: A longitudinal study of Swedish conscripts. *Scandinavian Journal of Social Medicine*, 18, 9–15.

Andréasson, S., Engström, A., Allebeck, P., & Rydberg, U. (1987). Cannabis and schizophrenia: A longitudinal study of Swedish conscripts. *The Lancet*, 330, 1483–1486. http://dx.doi.org/10.1016/s0140-6736(87)92620-1

Arbogast, P. G., & Ray, W. A. (2011). Performance of disease risk scores, propensity scores, and traditional multivariable outcome regression in the presence of multiple confounders. *American Journal of Epidemiology*, 174, 613–620. http://dx.doi.org/10.1093/aje/kwr143

Arendt, M., Mortensen, P. B., Rosenberg, R., Pedersen, C. B., & Waltoft, B. L. (2008). Familial predisposition for psychiatric disorder. *Archives of General Psychiatry*, 65, 1269–1274. http://dx.doi.org/10.1001/archpsyc.65.11.1269

Arendt, M., Munk-Jørgensen, P., Sher, L., & Jensen, S. O. (2013). Mortality following treatment for cannabis use disorders: Predictors and causes. *Journal of Substance Abuse Treatment*, 44, 400–406. http://dx.doi.org/10.1016/j.jsat.2012.09.007

Arendt, M., Rosenberg, R., Fjordback, L., Brandholdt, J., Foldager, L., Sher, L., & Munk-Jørgensen, P. (2007). Testing the self-medication hypothesis of depression and aggression in cannabis-dependent subjects. *Psychological Medicine*, 37, 935–945. http://dx.doi.org/10.1017/s0033291706009688

Arias, S. A., Orianne, D., Sullivan, A. F., Boudreaux, E. D., Miller, I., & Camargo, J. C. (2016). Substance use as a mediator of the association between demographics, suicide attempt history, and future suicide attempts in emergency department patients. *Crisis*, 37, 385–391. http://dx.doi.org/10.1027/0227-5910/a000380

Arria, A. M., Caldeira, K. M., Bugbee, B. A., Vincent, K. B., & O'Grady, K. E. (2015). The academic consequences of marijuana use during college. *Psychology of Addictive Behaviors*, 29, 564–575. http://dx.doi.org/10.1037/adb0000108

Arseneault, L., Cannon, M., Poulton, R., Murray, R., Caspi, A., & Moffitt, T. E. (2002). Cannabis use in adolescence and risk for adult psychosis: Longitudinal prospective study. *British Medical Journal*, 325, 1212–1213. http://dx.doi.org/10.1136/bmj.325.7374.1212

Baldessarini, R. J., Tondo, L., Vazquez, G. H., Undurraga, J., Bolzani, L., Yildiz, A., . . . Tohen M. (2012). Age at onset versus family history and clinical outcomes in 1,665 international bipolar-I disorder patients. *World Psychiatry*, 11, 40–46.Ballard, M. E., Gallo, D. A., & Wit, H. D. (2013). Pre-encoding administration of amphetamine or THC preferentially modulates emotional memory in humans. *Psychopharmacology, 226,* 515–529. http://dx.doi.org/10.1007/s00213-012-2924-5

Barkus, E., Stirling, J., Hopkins, R., & Lewis, S. (2006). Cannabis-induced psychosis-like experiences are associated with high schizotypy. *Psychopathology, 39,* 175–178. http://dx.doi.org/10.1159/000092678

Barnes, T. R., Mutsatsa, S., Hutton, S., Watt, H., & Joyce, E. (2006). Comorbid substance use and age at onset of schizophrenia. *British Journal of Psychiatry, 188,* 237–242. http://dx.doi.org/10.1192/bjp.bp.104.007237

Battistella, G., Fornari, E., Thomas, A., Mall, J., Chtioui, H., Appenzeller, M., . . . Giroud, C. (2013). Weed or wheel! fMRI, behavioural, and toxicological investigations of how cannabis smoking affects skills necessary for driving. *PLoS ONE, 8,* e52545. http://dx.doi.org/10.1371/journal.pone.0052545

Beautrais, A. L., Joyce, P. R., & Mulder, R. T. (1999). Cannabis abuse and serious suicide attempts. *Addiction, 94,* 1155–1164. http://dx.doi.org/10.1046/j.1360-0443.1999.94811555.x

Bechtold, J., Simpson, T., White, H. R., & Pardini, D. (2015). Chronic adolescent marijuana use as a risk factor for physical and mental health problems in young adult men. *Psychology of Addictive Behaviors, 29,* 552–563. http://dx.doi.org/10.1037/adb0000103

Belsher, J. (dir.). (2015). *The other side of cannabis.* San Luis Obispo, CA: J. Belsher Creative.

Beratis, S., Gabriel, J., & Hoidas, S. (1994). Age at onset in subtypes of schizophrenic disorders. *Schizophrenia Bulletin, 20,* 287–296. http://dx.doi.org/10.1093/schbul/20.2.287

Bhattacharyya, S., Crippa, J., Allen, P., Martin-Santos, R., Borgwardt, S., Fusar-Poli, P., . . . McGuire, P. (2012). Induction of psychosis by Δ9-Tetrahydrocannabinol reflects modulation of prefrontal and striatal function during attentional salience processing. *Archives of General Psychiatry, 69,* 27–36. http://dx.doi.org/10.1001/archgenpsychiatry.2011.161

Blanco, C., Hasin, D. S., Wall, M. M., Flórez-Salamanca, L., Hoertel, N., Wang, S., . . . Olfson, M. (2016). Cannabis use and risk of psychiatric disorders: Prospective evidence from a US national longitudinal study. *JAMA Psychiatry, 73,* 388–395. http://dx.doi.org/10.1001/jamapsychiatry.2015.3229

Blanco, C., Rafful, C., Wall, M. M., Ridenour, T. A., Wang, S., & Kendler, K. S. (2014). Towards a comprehensive developmental model of cannabis use disorders. *Addiction, 109,* 284–294. http://dx.doi.org/10.1111/add.12382

Blessing, E. M., Steenkamp, M. M., Manzanares, J., & Marmar, C. R. (2015). Cannabidiol as a potential treatment for anxiety disorders. *Neurotherapeutics, 12,* 825–836. http://dx.doi.org/10.1007/s13311-015-0387-1

Borges, G., Bagge, C. L., & Orozco, R. (2016). A literature review and meta-analyses of cannabis use and suicidality. *Journal of Affective Disorders, 195,* 63–74. http://dx.doi.org/10.1016/j.jad.2016.02.007

Budney, A. J., Moore, B. A., Vandrey, R. G., & Hughes, J. R. (2003). The time course and significance of cannabis withdrawal. *Journal of Abnormal Psychology, 112,* 393–402. http://dx.doi.org/10.1037/0021-843x.112.3.393

Burge, V., Felts, M., Chenier, T., & Parrillo, A. V. (1995). Drug use, sexual activity, and suicidal behavior in U.S. high school students. *Journal of School Health, 65,* 222–227. http://dx.doi.org/10.1111/j.1746-1561.1995.tb03366.x

0

Callaghan, R. C., Cunningham, J. K., Allebeck, P., Arenovich, T., Sajeev, G., Remington, G., . . . Kish, S. J. (2012). Methamphetamine use and schizophrenia: A population-based cohort study in California. *American Journal of Psychiatry, 169,* 389–396. http://dx.doi.org/10.1176/appi.ajp.2011.10070937

Cannon, T. D., Cadenhead, K., Cornblatt, B., Woods, S. W., Addington, J., Walker, E., . . . Heinssen, R. (2008). Prediction of psychosis in youth at high clinical risk. *Archives of General Psychiatry, 65,* 28–37. http://dx.doi.org/10.1001/archgenpsychiatry.2007.3

Cerda, M., Moffitt, T. E., Meier, M. H., Harrington, H., Houts, R., Ramrakha, S., . . . Caspi, A. (2016). Persistent cannabis dependence and alcohol dependence represent risks for midlife economic and social problems: A longitudinal cohort study. *Clinical Psychological Science, 4,* 1028–1046. http://dx.doi.org/10.1177/2167702616630958

Chaudry, H. R., Moss, H. B., Bashir, A., & Suliman, T. (1991). Cannabis psychosis following bhang ingestion. *Addiction, 86,* 1075–1081. http://dx.doi.org/10.1111/j.1360-0443.1991.tb01874.x

Chawla, S., & Pichon, T. L. (2006). *2006 world drug report.* Vienna, Austria: United Nations Office on Drugs and Crime.

Clarification to Bechtold et al. (2015). *Psychology of Addictive Behaviors, 29,* lx–x. http://dx.doi.org/10.1037/adb0000153

Clarke, M. C., Coughlan, H., Harley, M., Connor, D., Power, E., Lynch, F., . . . Cannon, M. (2014). The impact of adolescent cannabis use, mood disorder and lack of education on attempted suicide in young adulthood. *World Psychiatry, 13,* 322–323. http://dx.doi.org/10.1002/wps.20170

Compton, M. T., Chien, V. H., & Bollini, A. M. (2009). Associations between past alcohol, cannabis, and cocaine use and current schizotypy among first-degree relatives of patients with schizophrenia and non-psychiatric controls. *Psychiatric Quarterly, 80,* 143–154. http://dx.doi.org/10.1007/s11126-009-9102-x

Cornelius, J. R., Chung, T., Martin, C., Wood, D. S., & Clark, D. B. (2008). Cannabis withdrawal is common among treatment-seeking adolescents with cannabis dependence and major depression, and is associated with rapid relapse to dependence. *Addictive Behaviors, 33,* 1500–1505. http://dx.doi.org/10.1016/j.addbeh.2008.02.001

Cougle, J. R., Hakes, J. K., Macatee, R. J., Chavarria, J., & Zvolensky, M. J. (2015). Quality of life and risk of psychiatric disorders among regular users of alcohol, nicotine, and cannabis: An analysis of the National Epidemiological Survey on Alcohol and Related Conditions (NESARC). *Journal of Psychiatric Research, 66-67,* 135–141. http://dx.doi.org/10.1016/j.jpsychires.2015.05.004

Dannon, P. N., Lowengrub, K., Amiaz, R., Grunhaus, L., & Kotler, M. (2004). Comorbid cannabis use and panic disorder: Short term and long term follow-up study. *Human Psychopharmacology: Clinical and Experimental, 19,* 97–101. http://dx.doi.org/10.1002/hup.560

Darke, S., & Kaye, S. (2004). Attempted suicide among Injecting and noninjecting cocaine users in Sydney, Australia. *Journal of Urban Health: Bulletin of the New York Academy of Medicine, 81,* 505–515. http://dx.doi.org/10.1093/jurban/jth134

Darke, S., & Ross, J. (2002). Suicide among heroin users: Rates, risk factors and methods. *Addiction, 97,* 1383–1394. http://dx.doi.org/10.1046/j.1360-0443.2002.00214.x

Darke, S., Ross, J., Marel, C., Mills, K. L., Slade, T., Burns, L., & Teesson, M. (2015). Patterns and correlates of attempted suicide amongst heroin users: 11-year follow-up of the Australian treatment outcome study cohort. *Psychiatry Research, 227,* 166–170. http://dx.doi.org/10.1016/j.psychres.2015.04.010

Das, R. K., Kamboj, S. K., Ramadas, M., Yogan, K., Gupta, V., Redman, E., . . . Morgan, C. J. (2013). Cannabidiol enhances consolidation of explicit fear extinction in humans. *Psychopharmacology, 226,* 781–792. http://dx.doi.org/10.1007/s00213-012-2955-y

Davis, G. P., Compton, M. T., Wang, S., Levin, F. R., & Blanco, C. (2013). Association between cannabis use, psychosis, and schizotypal personality disorder: Findings from the National Epidemiologic Survey on Alcohol and Related Conditions. *Schizophrenia Research, 151,* 197–202. http://dx.doi.org/10.1016/j.schres.2013.10.018

Degenhardt, L., Hall, W., & Lynskey, M. (2003). Testing hypotheses about the relationship between cannabis use and psychosis. *Drug and Alcohol Dependence, 71,* 37–48. http://dx.doi.org/10.1016/s0376-8716(03)00064-4

de Graaf, R., Radovanovic, M., van Laar, M., Fairman, B., Degenhardt, L., Aguilar-Gaxiola, S., . . . Anthony, J. C. (2010). Early cannabis use and estimated risk of later onset of depression spells: Epidemiologic evidence from the population-based World Health Organization World Mental Health Survey Initiative. *American Journal Epidemiology, 172,* 149–159. http://dx.doi.org/10.1093/aje/kwq096

Delforterie, M., Lynskey, M., Huizink, A., Creemers, H., Grant, J., Few, L., . . . Agrawal, A. (2015). The relationship between cannabis involvement and suicidal thoughts and behaviors. *Drug and Alcohol Dependence, 150,* 98–104. http://dx.doi.org/10.1016/j.drugalcdep.2015.02.019

Der, G., Gupta, S., & Murray, R. (1990). Is schizophrenia disappearing? *The Lancet, 335,* 513–516. http://dx.doi.org/10.1016/0140-6736(90)90745-q

Dhunjibhoy, J. E. (1930). A brief resume of the types of insanity commonly met with in India, with a fully description of "Indian hemp insanity" peculiar to the country. *Journal of Mental Science, 76,* 254–264. http://dx.doi.org/10.1192/bjp.76.313.254

Di Forti, M. D., Marconi, A., Carra, E., Fraietta, S., Trotta, A., Bonomo, M., . . . Murray, R. M. (2015). Proportion of patients in south London with first-episode psychosis attributable to use of high potency cannabis: A case-control study. *The Lancet Psychiatry, 2,* 233–238. http://dx.doi.org/10.1016/s2215-0366(14)00117-5

Di Forti, M. D., Morgan, C., Dazzan, P., Pariante, C., Mondelli, V., Marques, T. R., . . . Murray, R. M. (2009). High-potency cannabis and the risk of psychosis. *British Journal of Psychiatry, 195,* 488–491. http://dx.doi.org/10.1192/bjp.bp.109.064220

Dines, A. M., Wood, D. M., Galicia, M., Yates, C. M., Heyerdahl, F., Hovda, K. E., . . . Dargan, P. I. (2015). Presentations to the emergency department following cannabis use—a multi-centre case series from ten European countries. *Journal of Medical Toxicology, 11,* 415–421. http://dx.doi.org/10.1007/s13181-014-0460-x

D'Souza, D. C., Perry, E., Macdougall, L., Ammerman, Y., Cooper, T., Wu, Y., . . . Krystal, J. H. (2004). The psychotomimetic effects of intravenous delta-9-Tetrahydrocannabinol in healthy individuals: implications for psychosis. *Neuropsychopharmacology, 29,* 1558–1572. http://dx.doi.org/10.1038/sj.npp.1300496

European Monitoring Centre for Drugs and Drug Addiction. (1997). *The 1995 ESPAD report.* Retrieved from http://www.espad.org/sites/espad.org/files/ESPAD_report_2015.pdf

Fairman, B. J., & Anthony, J. C. (2012). Are early-onset cannabis smokers at an increased risk of depression spells? *Journal of Affective Disorders, 138,* 54–62. http://dx.doi.org/10.1016/j.jad.2011.12.031

Faraone, S. V., Chen, W. J., Goldstein, J. M., & Tsuang, M. T. (1994). Gender differences in age at onset of schizophrenia. *British Journal of Psychiatry*, 164, 625–629. http://dx.doi.org/10.1192/bjp.164.5.625

Favrat, B., Ménétrey, A., Augsburger, M., Rothruizen, L., Appenzeller, M., Bouclin, T., . . . Giroud, C. (2005). Two cases of "cannabis acute psychosis" following the administration of oral cannabis. *BMC Psychiatry*, 5, 17. http://dx.doi.org/10.1186/1471-244X-5-17

Feingold, D., Rehm, J., & Lev-Ran, S. (2017). Cannabis use and the course and outcome of major depressive disorder: A population based longitudinal study. *Psychiatry Research*, 251, 225–234. http://dx.doi.org/ 10.1016/j.psychres.2017.02.027

Fergusson, D. M., Horwood, L. J., & Ridder, E. M. (2005). Tests of causal linkages between cannabis use and psychotic symptoms. *Addiction*, 100, 354–366. http://dx.doi.org/10.1111/j.1360-0443.2005.01001.x

Fergusson, D., Horwood, L., & Swain-Campbell, N. (2003). Cannabis dependence and psychotic symptoms in young people. *Psychological Medicine*, 33, 15–21. http://dx.doi.org/10.1017/s0033291702006402

Foti, D. J., Kotov, R., Guey, L. T., & Bromet, E. J. (2010). Cannabis use and the course of schizophrenia: 10-Year follow-up after first hospitalization. *American Journal of Psychiatry*, 167, 987–993. http://dx.doi.org/10.1176/appi.ajp.2010.09020189

Fowler, R. C., Rich, C. L., & Young, D. (1986). San Diego Suicide Study. Substance abuse in young cases *Archives of General Psychiatry*, 43, 962–965. http://dx.doi.org/10.1001/archpsyc.1986.01800100056008

Freeman, D., Dunn, G., Murray, R. M., Evans, N., Lister, R., Antley, A., . . . Morrison, P. D. (2015). How cannabis causes paranoia: using the intravenous administration of 9-Tetrahydrocannabinol (THC) to identify key cognitive mechanisms leading to paranoia. *Schizophrenia Bulletin*, 41, 391–399. http://dx.doi.org/10.1093/schbul/sbu098

Gage, S. H., Hickman, M., & Zammit, S. (2016). Association between cannabis and psychosis: epidemiologic evidence. *Biological Psychiatry*, 79, 549–556. http://dx.doi.org/10.1016/j.biopsych.2015.08.001

Galvez-Buccollini, J. A., Proal, A. C., Tomaselli, V., Trachtenberg, M., Coconcea, C., Chun, J., . . . Delisi, L. E. (2012). Association between age at onset of psychosis and age at onset of cannabis use in non-affective psychosis. *Schizophrenia Research*, 139, 157–160. http://dx.doi.org/10.1016/j.schres.2012.06.007

Ganguli, R., & Brar, J. S. (1992). Generalizability of first-episode studies in schizophrenia. *Schizophrenia Bulletin*, 18, 463–469. http://dx.doi.org/10.1093/schbul/18.3.463

Garnefski, N., & Wilde, E. J. (1998). Addiction-risk behaviours and suicide attempts in adolescents. *Journal of Adolescence*, 21, 135–142. http://dx.doi.org/10.1006/jado.1997.0137

Gex, C. R., Narring, F., Ferron, C., & Michaud, P. (1998). Suicide attempts among adolescents in Switzerland: Prevalence, associated factors and comorbidity. *Acta Psychiatrica Scandinavica*, 98, 28–33. http://dx.doi.org/10.1111/j.1600-0447.1998.tb10038.x

Giordano, G. N., Ohlsson, H., Sundquist, K., Sundquist, J., & Kendler, K. S. (2015). The association between cannabis abuse and subsequent schizophrenia: A Swedish national co-relative control study. *Psychological Medicine*, 45, 407–414. http://dx.doi.org/10.1017/s0033291714001524

Gonzalez-Pinto, A., Alberich, S., Barbeito, S., Gutierrez, M., Vega, P., Ibanez, B., . . . Arango, C. (2011). Cannabis and first-episode psychosis: different long-term outcomes depending on continued or discontinued use. *Schizophrenia Bulletin, 37,* 631–639. http://dx.doi.org/10.1093/schbul/sbp126

Gorelick, D. A., Goodwin, R. S., Schwilke, E., Schwope, D. M., Darwin, W. D., Kelly, D. L., . . . Huestis, M. A. (2011). Antagonist-elicited cannabis withdrawal in humans. *Journal of Clinical Psychopharmacology, 31,* 603–612. http://dx.doi.org/10.1097/jcp.0b013e31822befc1

Gottesman, I. I., & Shields, J. (1967). A polygenic theory of schizophrenia. *Proceedings of the National Academy of Sciences, 58,* 199–205. http://dx.doi.org/10.1073/pnas.58.1.199

Griffith-Lendering, M. F., Wigman, J. T., Leeuwen, A. P., Huijbregts, S. C., Huizink, A. C., Ormel, J., . . . Vollebergh, W. A. (2013). Cannabis use and vulnerability for psychosis in early adolescence-a TRAILS study. *Addiction, 108,* 733–740. http://dx.doi.org/10.1111/add.12050

Hafner, H., Heiden, W. A., Behrens, S., Gattaz, W. F., Hambrecht, M., Loffler, W., . . . Stein, A. (1998). Causes and consequences of the gender difference in age at onset of schizophrenia. *Schizophrenia Bulletin, 24,* 99–113. http://dx.doi.org/10.1093/oxfordjournals.schbul.a033317

Hall, W., & Degenhardt, L. (2010). What are the policy implications of the evidence on cannabis use and psychosis? *Addiction, 105,* 1332–1333. http://dx.doi.org/10.1111/j.1360-0443.2010.02919.x

Hansen, S., Munk-Jorgensen, P., Guldbaek, B., Solgard, T., Lauszus, K., Albrechtsen, N., . . . Bertelsen, A. (2000). Psychoactive substance use diagnoses among psychiatric in-patients. *Acta Psychiatrica Scandinavica, 102,* 432–438. http://dx.doi.org/10.1034/j.1600-0447.2000.102006432.x

Harder, V. S., Morral, A. R., & Arkes, J. (2006). Marijuana use and depression among adults: Testing for causal associations. *Addiction, 101,* 1463–1472. http://dx.doi.org/10.1111/j.1360-0443.2006.01545.x

Hartung, B., Kauferstein, S., Ritz-Timme, S., & Daldrup, T. (2014). Sudden unexpected death under acute influence of cannabis. *Forensic Science International, 237,* e11–e13. http://dx.doi.org/10.1016/j.forsciint.2014.02.001

Hasin, D. S., Keyes, K. M., Alderson, D., Wang, S., Aharonovich, E., & Grant, B. F. (2008). Cannabis withdrawal in the United States. *Journal of Clinical Psychiatry, 69,* 1354–1363. http://dx.doi.org/10.4088/jcp.v69n0902

Haukka, J., Suvisaari, J., & Lönnqvist, J. (2003). Fertility of patients with schizophrenia, their siblings, and the general population: a cohort study from 1950 to 1959 in Finland. *American Journal of Psychiatry, 160,* 460–463. http://dx.doi.org/10.1176/appi.ajp.160.3.460

Hayatbakhsh, M. R., Najman, J. M., Jamrozik, K., Mamun, A. A., Alati, R., & Bor, W. (2007). Cannabis and anxiety and depression in young adults: a large prospective study. *Journal of the American Academy of Child & Adolescent Psychiatry, 46,* 408–417. http://dx.doi.org/10.1097/chi.0b013e31802dc54d

Henquet, C., Krabbendam, L., Graaf, R. D., Have, M. T., & Os, J. V. (2006). Cannabis use and expression of mania in the general population. *Journal of Affective Disorders, 95,* 103–110. http://dx.doi.org/10.1016/j.jad.2006.05.002

Henquet, C., Krabbendam, L., Spauwen, J., Kaplan, C., Lieb, R., Wittchen, H., & Van Os, J. (2005). Prospective cohort study of cannabis use, predisposition for psychosis, and psychotic symptoms in young people. *British Medical Journal, 330*, 11–15. http://dx.doi.org/10.1136/bmj.38267.664086

Hezel, F. X. (1984). Cultural patterns in Trukese suicide. *Ethnology, 23*, 193–206. http://dx.doi.org/10.2307/3773746

Hickman, M., Vickerman, P., Macleod, J., Lewis, G., Zammit, S., Kirkbride, J., & Jones, P. (2009). If cannabis caused schizophrenia-how many cannabis users may need to be prevented in order to prevent one case of schizophrenia? England and Wales calculations. *Addiction, 104*, 1856–1861. http://dx.doi.org/10.1111/j.1360-0443.2009.02736.x

Hill, M. N. (2014). Clearing the smoke: What do we know about adolescent cannabis use and schizophrenia? *Journal of Psychiatry & Neuroscience 39*, 75–77. http://dx.doi.org/10.1503/jpn.140028

Hillman, S. D. (2000). *Youth suicide in Western Australia involving cannabis and other drugs: A literature review and research report.* Perth: Western Australian Drug Abuse Strategy Office.

Hollister, L. E. (1986). Health aspects of cannabis. *Pharmacology Reviews, 38*, 1–20.

Hollister, L. E., & Gillespie, H. K. (1975). Action of delta-9-tetrahydrocannabinol. An approach to the active metabolite hypothesis. *Clinical Pharmacology & Therapeutics, 18*, 714–719.

Jablensky, A. (1986). Epidemiology of Schizophrenia: A European perspective. *Schizophrenia Bulletin, 12*, 52–73. http://dx.doi.org/10.1093/schbul/12.1.52-73

Johnston, L. D., O'Malley, P. M., Bachman, J. G., & Schulenberg, J. E. (2012a). *Monitoring the Future national survey results on drug use, 1975–2011. Vol. 1: Secondary school students.* Ann Arbor: Institute for Social Research, University of Michigan.

Johnston, L. D., O'Malley, P. M., Bachman, J. G., & Schulenberg, J. E. (2012b). *Monitoring the Future national survey results on drug use, 1975–2011. Vol. 2: College students and adults ages 19–50.* Ann Arbor: Institute for Social Research, University of Michigan.

Johnston, L. D., O'Malley, P. M., Bachman, J. G., Schulenberg, J. E., & Miech, R. A. (2014). *Monitoring the Future national survey results on drug use, 1975–2013: Vol. 2. College students and adults ages 19–55.* Ann Arbor: Institute for Social Research, University of Michigan.

Kandel, D. B., Raveis, V. H., & Davies, M. (1991). Suicidal ideation in adolescence: Depression, substance use, and other risk factors. *Journal of Youth and Adolescence, 20*, 289–309. http://dx.doi.org/10.1007/bf01537613

Karler, R., & Turkanis, S. A. (1987). Different cannabinoids exhibit different pharmacological and toxicological properties. *NIDA Research Monograph, 79*, 96–107. http://dx.doi.org/10.1037/e496672006-009

Kaufmann, R. M., Kraft, B., Frey, R., Winkler, D., Weiszenbichler, S., Bäcker, C., . . . Kress, H. G. (2010). Acute psychotropic effects of oral cannabis extract with a defined content of Δ 9-tetrahydrocannabinol (THC) in healthy volunteers. *Pharmacopsychiatry, 43*, 24–32. http://dx.doi.org/10.1055/s-0029-1237397

Keith, S. J., Regier, D. A., & Rae, D. S. (1991). Schizophrenic disorders. In L. N. Robins & D. A. Regier (Eds.), *Psychiatric disorders in America: The epidemiologic catchment area study* (pp. 33–52). New York: Free Press.

Kessler, R. C., Amminger, G. P., Aguilar-Gaxiola, S., Alonso, J., Lee, S., & Üstün, T. B. (2007). Age of onset of mental disorders: A review of recent literature. *Current Opinion in Psychiatry, 20*, 359–364. http://dx.doi.org/10.1097/yco.0b013e32816ebc8c

Kessler, R. C., Borges, G., & Walters, E. E. (1999). Prevalence of and risk factors for lifetime suicide attempts in the National Comorbidity Survey. *Archives of General Psychiatry, 56*, 617–626. http://dx.doi.org/10.1001/archpsyc.56.7.617

Kokkevi, A., Rotsika, V., Arapaki, A., & Richardson, C. (2012). Adolescents' self-reported suicide attempts, self-harm thoughts and their correlates across 17 European countries. *Journal of Child Psychology and Psychiatry, 53*, 381–389. http://dx.doi.org/10.1111/j.1469-7610.2011.02457.x

Koppel, B. S., Brust, J. C., Fife, T., Bronstein, J., Youssof, S., Gronseth, G., & Gloss, D. (2014). Systematic review: Efficacy and safety of medical marijuana in selected neurologic disorders: Report of the Guideline Development Subcommittee of the American Academy of Neurology. *Neurology, 82*, 1556–1563. http://dx.doi.org/10.1212/wnl.0000000000000363

Kuepper, R., Os, J. V., Lieb, R., Wittchen, H., Hofler, M., & Henquet, C. (2011). Continued cannabis use and risk of incidence and persistence of psychotic symptoms: 10 year follow-up cohort study. *British Medical Journal, 342*, d738. http://dx.doi.org/10.1136/bmj.d738

Kung, H. C., Pearson, J. L., & Liu, X. (2003). Risk factors for male and female suicide decedents ages 15?64 in the United States. *Social Psychiatry and Psychiatric Epidemiology, 38*, 419–426. http://dx.doi.org/10.1007/s00127-003-0656-x

Kvitland, L. R., Melle, I., Aminoff, S. R., Lagerberg, T. V., Andreassen, O. A., & Ringen, P. A. (2016). Cannabis use in first-treatment bipolar I disorder: Relations to clinical characteristics. *Early Intervention in Psychiatry, 10*, 36–44. http://dx.doi.org/10.1111/eip.12138

Lagerberg, T. V., Sundet, K., Aminoff, S. R., Berg, A. O., Ringen, P. A., Andreassen, O. A., & Melle, I. (2011). Excessive cannabis use is associated with earlier age at onset in bipolar disorder. *European Archives of Psychiatry and Clinical Neuroscience, 261*, 397–405. http://dx.doi.org/10.1007/s00406-011-0188-4

Large, M., Sharma, S., Compton, M. T., Slade, T., & Nielssen, O. (2011). Cannabis use and earlier onset of psychosis: A systematic meta-analysis. *Archives of General Psychiatry, 68*, 555–561. http://dx.doi.org/10.1001/archgenpsychiatry.2011.5

Larsen, T. K., Melle, I., Auestad, B., Friis, S., Haahr, U., Johannessen, J. O., . . . Mcglashan, T. H. (2006). Substance abuse in first-episode non-affective psychosis. *Schizophrenia Research, 88*, 55–62. http://dx.doi.org/10.1016/j.schres.2006.07.018

Lev-Ran, S., Roerecke, M., Foll, B. L., George, T. P., Mckenzie, K., & Rehm, J. (2013). The association between cannabis use and depression: A systematic review and meta-analysis of longitudinal studies. *Psychological Medicine, 44*, 797–810. http://dx.doi.org/10.1017/s0033291713001438

Levin, K. H., Copersino, M. L., Heishman, S. J., Liu, F., Kelly, D. L., Boggs, D. L., & Gorelick, D. A. (2010). Cannabis withdrawal symptoms in non-treatment-seeking adult cannabis smokers. *Drug and Alcohol Dependence, 111*, 120–127. http://dx.doi.org/10.1016/j.drugalcdep.2010.04.010

Leweke, F. M., Piomelli, D., Pahlisch, F., Muhl, D., Gerth, C. W., Hoyer, C., . . . Koethe, D. (2012). Cannabidiol enhances anandamide signaling and alleviates psychotic symptoms of schizophrenia. *Translational Psychiatry, 2*, e94. http://dx.doi.org/10.1038/tp.2012.15

Leweke, F. M., Schneider, U., Thies, M., Münte, T. F., & Emrich, H. M. (1999). Effects of synthetic Δ9-tetrahydrocannabinol on binocular depth inversion of natural and artificial objects in man. *Psychopharmacology, 142,* 230–235. http://dx.doi.org/ 10.1007/s002130050884

Lewis, G., Heron, J., & Zammit, S. (2013). Commentary on Griffith-Lendering et al. (2013): Cross-lagging cannabis and psychosis vulnerability. *Addiction, 108,* 741–742. http://dx.doi.org/10.1111/add.12101

Licata, M., Veri, P., & Beduschi, G. (2005). Δ9-THC content in illicit cannabis products over the period 1997-2004 (first four months). *Annali Dell'Istituto Superiore Di Sanità, 41,* 483–485.

Loranger, A. W. (1990). The impact of DSM-III on diagnostic practice in a university hospital. *Archives of General Psychiatry, 47,* 672–675. http://dx.doi.org/10.1001/ archpsyc.1990.01810190072010

Lynskey, M. T., Glowinski, A. L., Todorov, A. A., Bucholz, K. K., Madden, P. A., Nelson, E. C., . . . Heath, A. C. (2004). Major depressive disorder, suicidal ideation, and suicide attempt in twins discordant for cannabis dependence and early-onset cannabis use. *Archives General Psychiatry, 61,* 1026–1032. http://dx.doi.org/ 10.1001/ archpsyc.61.10.1026

Maccabe, J. H. (2010). Estimates of how many cannabis users need to be prevented in order to prevent one case of schizophrenia. *Evidence-Based Mental Health, 13,* 57. http://dx.doi.org/10.1136/ebmh.13.2.57

Mackie, K. (2008). Cannabinoid Receptors: Where they are and what they do. *Journal of Neuroendocrinology, 20*(Suppl 1), 10–14. http://dx.doi.org/10.1111/ j.1365-2826.2008.01671.x

Madigan, D., Stang, P. E., Berlin, J. A., Schuemie, M., Overhage, J. M., Suchard, M. A., . . . Ryan, P. B. (2014). A systematic statistical approach to evaluating evidence from observational studies. *Annual Review of Statistics and Its Application, 1,* 11–39. http://dx.doi.org/10.1146/annurev-statistics-022513-115645

Marzuk, P. M., Tardiff, K., Lepn, A. C., Stajic, M., Morgan, E. B., & Mann, J. J. (1992). Prevalence of cocaine use among residents of New York City who committed suicide during a one-year period. *American Journal of Psychiatry, 149,* 371–375. http:// dx.doi.org/10.1176/ajp.149.3.371

Mcgrath, J., Welham, J., Scott, J., Varghese, D., Degenhardt, L., Hayatbakhsh, M. R., . . . Najman, J. M. (2010). Association between cannabis use and psychosis-related outcomes using sibling pair analysis in a cohort of young adults. *Archives of General Psychiatry, 67,* 440–447. http://dx.doi.org/10.1001/ archgenpsychiatry.2010.6

Mcgrath, J. (2012). [Review of the book *Marijuana and madness,* by R. M. Murray, D. C. D'Souza, & D. Castle]. *Psychological Medicine, 42,* 1785. http://dx.doi.org/10.1017/ S0033291712001237Medina, K. L., & Shear, P. K. (2007). Anxiety, depression, and behavioral symptoms of executive dysfunction in ecstasy users: Contributions of polydrug use. *Drug and Alcohol Dependence, 87,* 303–311. http://dx.doi.org/10.1016/ j.drugalcdep.2006.09.003

Mehmedic, Z., Chandra, S., Slade, D., Denham, H., Foster, S., Patel, A. S., . . . ElSohly, M. A. (2010). Potency trends of Δ9-THC and other cannabinoids in confiscated cannabis preparations from 1993 to 2008. *Journal Forensic Science, 55,* 1209–1217. http://dx.doi.org/10.1111/j.1556-4029.2010.01441.x

Melzer, H. Y., Rabinowitz, J., Lee, M. A., Cola, P. A., Ranjan, R., Findling, R. L., & Thompson, P. A. (1997). Age at onset and gender of schizophrenic patients in relation to neuroleptic resistance. *American Journal of Psychiatry, 154*, 475–482. http://dx.doi.org/10.1176/ajp.154.4.475

Merikangas, K. R., Jin, R., He, J., Kessler, R. C., Lee, S., Sampson, N. A., . . . Zarkov, Z. (2011). Prevalence and correlates of bipolar spectrum disorder in the World Mental Health Survey Initiative. *Archives of General Psychiatry, 68*, 241–251. http://dx.doi.org/10.1001/archgenpsychiatry.2011.12

Miller, C. L. (2014). Caution urged in interpreting a negative study of cannabis use and schizophrenia. *Schizophrenia Research, 154*, 119–120. http://dx.doi.org/10.1016/j.schres.2014.02.014

Mohun, B. (dir.), Ridout, S. (writer), & Suzuki, D. T. (prod.). (2010). *The downside of high* [film]. Toronto, ON: CBC Learning.

Moore, T. H., Zammit, S., Lingford-Hughes, A., Barnes, T. R., Jones, P. B., Burke, M., & Lewis, G. (2007). Cannabis use and risk of psychotic or affective mental health outcomes: A systematic review. *The Lancet, 370*, 319–328. http://dx.doi.org/10.1016/s0140-6736(07)61162-3

Morgan, C. J., Freeman, T. P., Powell, J., & Curran, H. V. (2016). AKT1 genotype moderates the acute psychotomimetic effects of naturalistically smoked cannabis in young cannabis smokers. *Translational Psychiatry, 6*, e738. http://dx.doi.org/10.1038/tp.2015.219

Morrison, P. D., Nottage, J., Stone, J. M., Bhattacharyya, S., Tunstall, N., Brenneisen, R., . . . Ffytche, D. H. (2011). Disruption of frontal theta coherence by Δ9-tetrahydrocannabinol is associated with positive psychotic symptoms. *Neuropsychopharmacology, 36*, 827–836. http://dx.doi.org/10.1038/npp.2010.222

Mortensen, P. B., Pedersen, C. B., Westergaard, T., Wohlfahrt, J., Ewald, H., Mors, O., . . . Melbye, M. (1999). Effects of family history and place and season of birth on the risk of schizophrenia. *New England Journal of Medicine, 340*, 603–608. http://dx.doi.org/10.1056/nejm199902253400803

Moser, J. (1974). *Problems and programmes related to alcohol and drug dependence in 33 countries.* Geneva: World Health Organization.

Munk-Jørgensen, P. (1986). Decreasing first-admission rates of schizophrenia among males in Denmark from 1970 to 1984. *Acta Psychiatrica Scandinavica, 73*, 645–650. http://dx.doi.org/10.1111/j.1600-0447.1986.tb02738.x

Myles, N., Newall, H., Compton, M. T., Curtis, J., Nielssen, O., & Large, M. (2012). The age at onset of psychosis and tobacco use: A systematic meta-analysis. *Social Psychiatry and Psychiatric Epidemiology, 47*, 1243–1250. http://dx.doi.org/10.1007/s00127-011-0431-3

Neumeister, A. (2013). The endocannabinoid system provides an avenue for evidence-based treatment development for PTSD. *Depression and Anxiety, 30*, 93–96. http://dx.doi.org/10.1002/da.22031

Nicholson, K. (2014, April 17). Man who plunged from Denver balcony ate 6× recommended amount of pot cookie. *Denver Post.*

Nielsen, S. M., Toftdahl, N. G., Nordentoft, M., & Hjorthøj, C. (2017). Association between alcohol, cannabis, and other illicit substance abuse and risk of developing schizophrenia: a nationwide population based register study. *Psychological Medicine, 47*, 1668–1677. http://dx.doi.org/10.1017/S0033291717000162

Niemi-Pynttäri, J. A., Sund, R., Putkonen, H., Vorma, H., Wahlbeck, K., & Pirkola, S. P. (2013). Substance-induced psychoses converting into schizophrenia. *Journal of Clinical Psychiatry, 74*, e94–e99. http://dx.doi.org/10.4088/jcp.12m07822

Norström, T., & Rossow, I. (2016). Alcohol consumption as a risk factor for suicidal behavior: A systematic review of associations at the individual and at the population level. *Archives of Suicide Research, 20,* 489–506. http://dx.doi.org/10.1080/13811118.2016.1158678

O'Boyle, M., & Brandon, E. A. (1998). Suicide attempts, substance abuse, and personality. *Journal of Substance Abuse Treatment, 15,* 353–356. http://dx.doi.org/10.1016/s0740-5472(97)00224-9

Ohlsson, A., Lindgren, J., Wahlen, A., Agurell, S., Hollister, L. E., & Gillespie, H. K. (1980). Plasma delta-9-tetrahydrocannabinol concentrations and clinical effects after oral and intravenous administration and smoking. *Clinical Pharmacology and Therapeutics, 28,* 409–416. http://dx.doi.org/10.1038/clpt.1980.181

Olfson, M., Gerhard, T., Huang, C., Crystal, S., & Stroup, T. S. (2015). Premature mortality among adults with schizophrenia in the United States. *JAMA Psychiatry, 72,* 1172–1181. http://dx.doi.org/10.1001/jamapsychiatry.2015.1737

Østergaard, M. L., Nordentoft, M., & Hjorthøj, C. (2017). Associations between substance use disorders and suicide or suicide attempts in people with mental illness: A Danish nation-wide, prospective, register-based study of patients diagnosed with schizophrenia, bipolar disorder, unipolar depression or personality disorder. *Addiction, 112,* 1250–1259. http://dx.doi.org/ 10.1111/add.13788

Patel, R., Wilson, R., Jackson, R., Ball, M., Shetty, H., Broadbent, M., . . . Bhattacharyya, S. (2016). Association of cannabis use with hospital admission and antipsychotic treatment failure in first episode psychosis: An observational study. *British Medical Journal Open, 6,* e009888. http://dx.doi.org/10.1136/bmjopen-2015-009888

Patton, G. C., Coffey, C., Carlin, J. B., Degenhardt, L., Lynskey, M., & Hall, W. (2002). Cannabis use and mental health in young people: cohort study. *British Medical Journal, 325,*1195–1198.

Pedersen, C. B., & Mortensen, P. B. (2001). Family history, place and season of birth as risk factors for schizophrenia in Denmark: A replication and reanalysis. *British Journal of Psychiatry, 179,* 46–52. http://dx.doi.org/10.1192/bjp.179.1.46

Pedersen, W. (2008). Does cannabis use lead to depression and suicidal behaviours? A population-based longitudinal study. *Acta Psychiatrica Scandinavica, 118,* 395–403. http://dx.doi.org/10.1111/j.1600-0447.2008.01259.x

Pepper, H., & Agius, M. (2009). Phenomenology of PTSD and psychotic symptoms. *Psychiatria Danubina, 21,* 82–84.

Perez-Reyes, M., Timmons, M. C., Lipton, M. A., Davis, K. H., & Wall, M. E. (1972). Intravenous injection in man of delta-9-Tetrahydrocannabinol and 11-OH-delta-9-Tetrahydrocannabinol. *Science, 177,* 633–635. http://dx.doi.org/10.1126/science.177.4049.633

Phillips, L. J., Curry, C., Yung, A. R., Yuen, H. P., Adlard, S., & Mcgorry, P. D. (2002). Cannabis use is not associated with the development of psychosis in an "ultra" high-risk group. *Australian and New Zealand Journal of Psychiatry, 36,* 800–806. http://dx.doi.org/10.1046/j.1440-1614.2002.01089.x

Pierre, J. M. (2010). Psychosis associated with medical marijuana: risk vs. benefits of medicinal cannabis Use. *American Journal of Psychiatry, 167,* 598–599. http://dx.doi.org/10.1176/appi.ajp.2010.09121762

Poikolainen, K., Tuulio-Henriksson, A., Aalto-Setälä, T., Marttunen, M., Anttila, T., & Lönnqvist, J. (2001). Correlates of initiation to cannabis use: A 5-year follow-up of 15–19-year-old adolescents. *Drug and Alcohol Dependence, 62,* 175–180. http://dx.doi.org/10.1016/s0376-8716(00)00176-9

Proal, A. C., Fleming, J., Galvez-Buccollini, J. A., & Delisi, L. E. (2014). A controlled family study of cannabis users with and without psychosis. *Schizophrenia Research, 152,* 283–288. http://dx.doi.org/10.1016/j.schres.2013.11.014

Rabinak, C. A., Angstadt, M., Sripada, C. S., Abelson, J. L., Liberzon, I., Milad, M. R., & Phan, K. L. (2013). Cannabinoid facilitation of fear extinction memory recall in humans. *Neuropharmacology, 64,* 396–402. http://dx.doi.org/10.1016/j.neuropharm.2012.06.063

Randall, J. R., Doku, D., Wilson, M. L., & Peltzer, K. (2014). Suicidal behaviour and related risk factors among school-aged youth in the Republic of Benin. *PLoS ONE, 9,* e88233. http://dx.doi.org/10.1371/journal.pone.0088233

Rasic, D., Weerasinghe, S., Asbridge, M., & Langille, D. B. (2013). Longitudinal associations of cannabis and illicit drug use with depression, suicidal ideation and suicidal attempts among Nova Scotia high school students. *Drug and Alcohol Dependence, 129,* 49–53. http://dx.doi.org/10.1016/j.drugalcdep.2012.09.009

Retterstol, N. (1975). Er marijuanastoffene pa retur i Danmark? *Bilag til Tidsskrift for Den norske loegeforening nr, 34–36,* 842.

Reuter, E. (2015, March 30). Keystone visitor commits suicide after eating marijuana candies. *Summit Daily.*

Robertson, H. T., & Allison, D. B. (2009). Drugs associated with more suicidal ideations are also associated with more suicide attempts. *PLoS ONE, 4,* e7312 http://dx.doi.org/10.1371/journal.pone.0007312

Room, R., & Rehm, J. (2009). Commentary on Hickman et al. (2009): The place of risk in drug policies. *Addiction, 104,* 1862–1863. http://dx.doi.org/10.1111/j.1360-0443.2009.02794.x

Russo, M., Rifici, C., Sessa, E., D'Aleo, G., Bramanti, P., & Calabrò, R. S. (2015). Sativex-induced neurobehavioral effects: Causal or concausal? A practical advice! *DARU Journal of Pharmaceutical Sciences, 23,* 25. http://dx.doi.org/10.1186/s40199-015-0109-6

Sachse-Seeboth, C., Pfeil, J., Sehrt, D., Meineke, I., Tzvetkov, M., Bruns, E., . . . Brockmöller, J. (2009). Interindividual variation in the pharmacokinetics of Δ9-tetrahydrocannabinol as related to genetic polymorphisms in CYP2C9. *Clinical Pharmacology & Therapeutics, 85,* 273–276. http://dx.doi.org/10.1038/clpt.2008.213

Saha, S., Chant, D., Welham, J., & Mcgrath, J. (2005). A systematic review of the prevalence of schizophrenia *PLoS Medicine, 2,* e141. http://dx.doi.org/10.1371/journal.pmed.0020141

Saha, S., Chant, D., Welham, J., & Mcgrath, J. (2006). The incidence and prevalence of schizophrenia varies with latitude. *Acta Psychiatrica Scandinavica, 114,* 36–39. http://dx.doi.org/10.1111/j.1600-0447.2005.00742.x

Schier, A. R., Ribeiro, N. P., De Oliveira E Silva, A. C. Hallak, J. E., Crippa, J. A., Nardi, A. E., & Zuardi, A. W. (2012). Cannabidiol, a cannabis sativa constituent, as an anxiolytic drug. *Revista Brasileira De Psiquiatria, 34* (Suppl 1), 104–110. http://dx.doi.org/10.1016/s1516-4446(12)70057-0

Schiffman, J., Nakamura, B., Earleywine, M., & LaBrie, J. (2005). Symptoms of schizotypy precede cannabis use. *Psychiatry Research, 134,* 37–42. http://dx.doi.org/10.1016/j.psychres.2005.01.004

Schisterman, E. F., Cole, S. R., & Platt, R. W. (2009). Overadjustment bias and unneces-sary adjustment in epidemiologic studies. *Epidemiology, 20,* 488–495. http://dx.doi.org/10.1097/ede.0b013e3181a819a1

Schoeler, T., Monk, A., Sami, M. B., Klamerus, E., Foglia, E., Brown, R., . . . Bhattacharyya, S. (2016). Continued versus discontinued cannabis use in patients with psychosis: A systematic review and meta-analysis. *The Lancet Psychiatry, 3,* 215–225. http://dx.doi.org/10.1016/s2215-0366(15)00363-6

Schwilke, E. W., Schwope, D. M., Karschner, E. L., Lowe, R. H., Darwin, W. D., Kelly, D. L., . . . Huestis, M. A. (2009). 9-tetrahydrocannabinol (THC), 11-hydroxy-THC, and 11-nor-9-carboxy-THC plasma pharmacokinetics during and after continuous high-dose oral THC. *Clinical Chemistry, 55,* 2180–2189. http://dx.doi.org/10.1373/clinchem.2008.122119 9

Shakoor, S., Zavos, H. M., Mcguire, P., Cardno, A. G., Freeman, D., & Ronald, A. (2015). Psychotic experiences are linked to cannabis use in adolescents in the community because of common underlying environmental risk factors. *Psychiatry Research, 227,* 144–151. http://dx.doi.org/10.1016/j.psychres.2015.03.041

Silins, E., Horwood, L. J., Patton, G. C., Fergusson, D. M., Olsson, C. A., Hutchinson, D. M., . . . Mattick, R. P. (2014). Young adult sequelae of adolescent cannabis use: An integrative analysis. *The Lancet Psychiatry, 1,* 286–293. http://dx.doi.org/10.1016/s2215-0366(14)70307-4

Smith, G. W., Farrell, M., Bunting, B. P., Houston, J. E., & Shevlin, M. (2011). Patterns of polydrug use in Great Britain: Findings from a national household population survey. *Drug and Alcohol Dependence, 113,* 222–228. http://dx.doi.org/10.1016/j.drugalcdep.2010.08.010

Smith, M. J., Thirthalli, J., Abdallah, A. B., Murray, R. M., & Cottler, L. B. (2009). Prevalence of psychotic symptoms in substance users: A comparison across substances. *Comprehensive Psychiatry, 50,* 245–250. http://dx.doi.org/10.1016/j.comppsych.2008.07.009

Solowij, N., & Battisti, R. (2008). The chronic effects of cannabis on memory in humans: A review. *Current Drug Abuse Reviews, 1,* 81–98. http://dx.doi.org/10.2174/1874473710801010081

Steenland, K., & Deddens, J. A. (2004). A practical guide to dose–response analyses and risk assessment in occupational epidemiology. *Epidemiology, 15,* 63–70. http://dx.doi.org/10.1097/01.ede.0000100287.45004.e7

Steffen, J. (2014, August 22). Richard Kirk hearing: Suspect asked boy, 7, to kill him. *Denver Post.*

Stern, C. A., Gazarini, L., Takahashi, R. N., Guimarães, F. S., & Bertoglio, L. J. (2012). On disruption of fear memory by reconsolidation blockade: Evidence from cannabidiol treatment. *Neuropsychopharmacology, 37,* 2132–2142. http://dx.doi.org/10.1038/npp.2012.63

Stoll, A. L., Tohen, M., Baldessarini, R. J., Goodwin, D. C., Stein, S., Katz, S., . . . McGlashan, T. (1993). Shifts in diagnostic frequencies of schizophrenia and major affective disorders at six North American psychiatric hospitals, 1972–1988. *American Journal of Psychiatry, 150,* 1668–1673. http://dx.doi.org/10.1176/ajp.150.11.1668

Strakowski, S. M., Delbello, M. P., Fleck, D. E., Adler, C. M., Anthenelli, R. M., Keck, P. E., . . . Amicone, J. (2007). Effects of co-occurring cannabis use disorders on the course of bipolar disorder after a first hospitalization for mania. *Archives of General Psychiatry, 64*, 57–64. http://dx.doi.org/10.1001/archpsyc.64.1.57

Suvisaari, J. M., Haukka, J. K., Tanskanen, A. J., & Lönnqvist, J. K. (1999). Decline in the incidence of schizophrenia in Finnish cohorts born from 1954 to 1965. *Archives of General Psychiatry, 56*, 733–740. http://dx.doi.org/10.1001/archpsyc.56.8.733

Thomas, H. (1996). A community survey of adverse effects of cannabis use. *Drug and Alcohol Dependence, 42*, 201–207. http://dx.doi.org/10.1016/s0376-8716(96)01277-x

Thun, M. J., Carter, B. D., Feskanich, D., Freedman, N. D., Prentice, R., Lopez, A. D., . . . Gapstur, S. M. (2013). 50-year trends in smoking-related mortality in the United States. *New England Journal of Medicine, 368*, 351–364. http://dx.doi.org/10.1056/nejmsa1211127

Tondo, L., Baldessarini, R. J., Hennen, J., Minnai, G. P., Salis, P., Scamonatti, L, . . . Mannu, P. (1999) Suicide attempts in major affective disorder patients with co-morbid substance use disorders. *Journal of Clinical Psychiatry, 60*(Suppl 2), 63–69.

Tripepi, G., Jager, K., Dekker, F., Wanner, C., & Zoccali, C. (2007). Measures of effect: Relative risks, odds ratios, risk difference, and "number needed to treat." *Kidney International, 72*, 789–791. http://dx.doi.org/10.1038/sj.ki.5002432

van Laar, M. V., Dorsselaer, S. V., Monshouwer, K., & Graaf, R. D. (2007). Does cannabis use predict the first incidence of mood and anxiety disorders in the adult population? *Addiction, 102*, 1251–1260. http://dx.doi.org/10.1111/j.1360-0443.2007.01875.x

van Os, J., Bak, M., Hanssen, M., Bijl, R. V., De Graf, R., & Verdoux, H. (2002). Cannabis use and psychosis: A longitudinal population-based study. *American Journal of Epidemiology, 156*, 319–327. http://dx.doi.org/10.1093/aje/kwf043

van Solinge, T. B. (1998). Drug Use and Drug Trafficking in Europe. *Tijdschrift Voor Economische En Sociale Geografie, 89*, 100–105. http://dx.doi.org/10.1111/1467-9663.00010

Veling, W., Mackenbach, J., Os, J. V., & Hoek, H. (2008). Cannabis use and genetic predisposition for schizophrenia: A case-control study. *Psychological Medicine, 38*, 1251–1256. http://dx.doi.org/10.1017/s0033291708003474

Vilenchik, M. M., & Knudson, A. G. (2000). Inverse radiation dose-rate effects on somatic and germ-line mutations and DNA damage rates. *Proceedings of the National Academy of Sciences, 97*, 5381–5386. http://dx.doi.org/10.1073/pnas.090099497

Weiss, R. D., Ostacher, M. J., Otto, M. W., Calabrese, J. R., Fossey, M., Wisniewski, S. R., . . . Sachs, G. S. (2005). Does recovery from substance use disorder matter in patients with bipolar disorder? *Journal of Clinical Psychiatry, 66*, 730–735. http://dx.doi.org/10.4088/jcp.v66n0609

Wilkinson, S. T., Stefanovics, E., & Rosenheck, R. A. (2015). Marijuana use is associated with worse outcomes in symptom severity and violent behavior in patients with posttraumatic stress disorder. *Journal of Clinical Psychiatry, 76*, 1174–1180. http://dx.doi.org/10.4088/jcp.14m09475

Wise, L. E., Thorpe, A. J., & Lichtman, A. H. (2009). Hippocampal CB1 receptors mediate the memory impairing effects of Δ9-Tetrahydrocannabinol. *Neuropsychopharmacology, 34*, 2072–2080. http://dx.doi.org/10.1038/npp.2009.31

Woolston, C. (2014, February 15). As marijuana laws change, health risks of pot use are weighed. *Los Angeles Times.*

Wong, S. S., Zhou, B., Goebert, D., & Hishinuma, E. S. (2013). The risk of adolescent suicide across patterns of drug use: a nationally representative study of high school students in the United States from 1999 to 2009. *Social Psychiatry and Psychiatric Epidemiology, 48*, 1611–1620. http://dx.doi.org/ 10.1007/s00127-013-0721-z

Wu, E. Q., Birnbaum, H. G., Shi, L., Ball, D. E., Kessler, R. C., Moulis, M., & Aggarwal, J. (2005). The economic burden of schizophrenia in the United States in 2002. *Journal of Clinical Psychiatry, 66*, 1122–1129. http://dx.doi.org/10.4088/jcp.v66n0906

Zammit, S., Allebeck, P., Andreasson, S., Lundberg, I., & Lewis, G. (2002). Self reported cannabis use as a risk factor for schizophrenia in Swedish conscripts of 1969: Historical cohort study. *British Medical Journal, 325*, 1195–1199. http://dx.doi.org/10.1136/bmj.325.7374.1199 1199

Zuardi, A. W., Shirakawa, I., Finkelfarb, E., & Karniol, I. G. (1982). Action of cannabidiol on the anxiety and other effects produced by 9-THC in normal subjects. *Psychopharmacology, 76*, 245–250. http://dx.doi.org/10.1007/bf00432554

Zvolensky, M. J., Lewinsohn, P., Bernstein, A., Schmidt, N. B., Buckner, J. D., Seeley, J., & Bonn-Miller, M. O. (2008). Prospective associations between cannabis use, abuse, and dependence and panic attacks and disorder. *Journal of Psychiatric Research, 42*, 1017–1023. http://dx.doi.org/10.1016/j.jpsychires.2007.10.012

6

Impact of Marijuana Smoking on Lung Health

DONALD P. TASHKIN

INTRODUCTION

Since both the gas and particulate phase components within the smoke of marijuana and tobacco have many similarities apart for the presence of delta-9 tetrahydrocannabinol (THC) and approximately 60 other cannabinoid compounds within the smoke of marijuana and the presence of nicotine in tobacco smoke (Hoffmann, Brunnemann, Gori, & Wynder, 1975; Moir et al., 2007; Novotný, Merli, Wiesler, Fencl, & Saeed, 1982), there is concern that regular smoking of marijuana could be a risk factor for the well-known respiratory consequences of regular tobacco smoking. The most serious of these include chronic obstructive pulmonary disease (COPD) and respiratory cancer. COPD is characterized by persistent abnormalities in lung function, specifically airflow obstruction that is not fully reversible in response to bronchodilator therapy and that usually becomes progressively more pronounced with age. This review will focus on (a) the acute and chronic effects of marijuana on lung function and/or chronic respiratory symptoms, as indicators of the possible risk of regular marijuana smoking for the development of COPD; (b) the association of marijuana smoking with respiratory (lung and upper airway) cancer; (c) marijuana as a risk factor for lower respiratory infection; and (d) marijuana smoking as a possible contributor to pneumothorax/pneumomediastinum and bullous lung disease.

ACUTE EFFECTS OF MARIJUANA ON LUNG FUNCTION

Smoking a single marijuana cigarette (~900 mg, 1% or 2% THC) by healthy habitual users of marijuana was followed by a significant reduction in airway resistance and increase in specific airway conductance (SGaw), indicating bronchodilation (Tashkin, Shapiro, & Frank, 1973). This finding is at variance with the acute bronchoconstrictor effect of tobacco smoking, as previously reported in the literature (Nadel & Comroe, 1961). The bronchodilator effect of smoked marijuana was rapid in onset, persisted for at least 1 hr and showed dose dependency. Moreover, the magnitude of the effect was greater than that of a commercially available inhaled bronchodilator agent. When THC was removed from the marijuana cigarette by elution with ethanol, the bronchodilator effect was no longer evident, indicating that this effect was specifically related to THC. In view of the fact that the marijuana that is smoked today generally has a much higher concentration than the 1% to 2% that was made available by the National Institute on Drug Abuse to conduct the latter studies, it is possible that a greater magnitude of acute bronchodilation could result from the more potent preparations that are currently available. But the issue is complicated by the fact some dose–response studies with conventional inhaled bronchodilators have shown diminishing effects at higher doses. Moreover, some current marijuana smokers may titrate their inhalation behavior to achieve a desired level of high, which would mitigate the effects of smoking more potent preparations. When THC was administered in oral form, dose-dependent bronchodilation was also observed (Tashkin et al., 1973), but the onset of action was delayed (due to the time required for absorption from the intestine into the systemic circulation) and more prolonged (as long as 6 hr with highest dose) due to the longer half-life of THC in the plasma when ingested than inhaled. Similar findings were noted in patients with mild asthma (Tashkin, Shapiro & Frank, 1974). In addition, smoked marijuana was effective in rapidly reversing experimentally induced bronchospasm in asthmatic subjects. (Tashkin et al., 1975). Other investigators have also observed a bronchodilator effect of THC administered in nebulized form (Williams, Hartley, & Graham, 1976). These findings may explain the use of marijuana as a treatment for bronchial asthma in the 19th century (Grinspoon, 1969). On the other hand, marijuana contains a number of substances that are injurious to respiratory tissue (Hoffmann et al., 1975; Moir et al., 2007; Novotný et al., 1982), rendering it an unsuitable product for treating asthma, despite its bronchodilator properties. However, because of the latter, it may be better tolerated than tobacco by asthmatic individuals, given the bronchoconstrictor effect of tobacco. Thus, asthmatics may be tempted to adopt the habit of smoking marijuana as an alternative to tobacco. The mechanism of THC-induced bronchodilation appears to be due to binding to cannabinoid type 1 (CB1) receptors on vagal efferent nerve endings in the airways that are juxtaposed to airway smooth muscle, resulting in inhibition of release of acetylcholine from the nerve endings thereby reducing bronchomotor tone (Calignano et al., 2000; Grassin-Delyle et al., 2014). A similar parasympatholytic effect probably explains the inhibitory effect of THC on intestinal smooth muscle contractile activity (Rosell & Agurell, 1975).

CHRONIC EFFECTS OF MARIJUANA ON LUNG FUNCTION

Effects on Respiratory Symptoms

COPD is an obstructive pulmonary disorder that is frequently associated with chronic respiratory symptoms, including chronic cough, phlegm production,

Table 6.1 ASSOCIATION BETWEEN REGULAR MARIJUANA USE WITHOUT TOBACCO
AND SYMPTOMS OF CHRONIC BRONCHITIS COMPARED WITH NONSMOKERS OF
ANY SUBSTANCE

Author	Cough	Sputum	Wheeze	Shortness of Breath
Bloom[13]	↑*	↑	↑	ns
Tashkin[14]	↑	↑	↑	ns
Taylor[15]	↑*	↑*	↑*	↑*
Moore[16]	↑	↑	↑	ns
Aldington[17]	↑	↑	↑	N.R.
Tan[18]	No significant ↑ in any symptoms consistent with COPD			

NOTES: ↑ = significant increase compared with nonsmokers of any substance.
↑* = numeric increase compared with nonsmokers. ns = not significant.
N.R. = not reported.

wheeze, and shortness of breath, although these symptoms may also be present in tobacco smokers who have not developed COPD. Six cross-sectional
studies conducted using smokers and nonsmokers of marijuana and/or tobacco
recruited from the general community have examined the association of marijuana with self-reported chronic respiratory symptoms in the absence of concomitant tobacco smoking (Table 6.1; Aldington et al., 2007; Bloom et al., 1987;
Moore, Augustson, Moser, & Budney, 2005; Tan et al., 2009; Tashkin et al., 1987;
Taylor, Poulton, Moffitt, Ramankutty, & Sears, 2000). All but one of these studies
(Tan et al., 2009) found a significant increase in the proportion of marijuana
smokers who reported symptoms of chronic cough and sputum production and
wheeze compared to nonsmokers ($p < 0.05$), while increased shortness of breath
was not found to be associated with regular marijuana smoking. Two studies
have shown that the symptoms of chronic bronchitis associated with marijuana
smoking tend to resolve upon cessation of marijuana use (Hancox, Shin, Gray,
Poulton, & Sears, 2015; Tashkin, Simmons, & Tseng, 2012), similar to the improvement in cough, sputum, and wheeze after quitting tobacco smoking.

Cross-Sectional and Longitudinal Studies of Lung Function in Relation to Marijuana Smoking

Studies by nearly a dozen groups of investigators have systematically evaluated
the association of regular marijuana use alone with lung function abnormality
in comparison with nonsmokers. Participants in these studies were recruited
from the general population either randomly and/or through advertisements
(Aldington et al., 2007; Bloom et al., 1987; Moore et al., 2005; Tan et al., 2009;
Tashkin, Calvarese, Simmons, & Shapiro, 1980; Tashkin et al., 1987) or were
participants in established cohort or survey studies (Table 6.2; Hancox et al.,

Table 6.2 ASSOCIATION OF REGULAR MARIJUANA USE WITHOUT TOBACCO AND LUNG FUNCTION ABNORMALITY COMPARED WITH NONSMOKERS OF ANY SUBSTANCE

Author	FEV_1	FVC	FEV_1/FVC	TLC	FRC	RV	SG_{aw}	D_LCO
Tashkin[21]	ns	ns	N.R.	ns	ns	N.R.	↓	ns
Bloom[13]	ns	N.R.	↓	N.R.	N.R.	N.R.	N.R.	N.R.
Tashkin[14]	ns	ns	ns	ns	ns	ns	↑	ns
Sherrill[25]	↓*	ns	↓*	N.R.	N.R.	N.R.	N.R.	N.R.
Taylor[15]	N.R.	N.R.	↓	N.R.	N.R.	N.R.	N.R.	N.R.
Moore[16]	N.R.	N.R.	ns	N.R.	N.R.	N.R.	N.R.	N.R.
Aldington[17]	ns	N.R.	ns	ns	ns	ns	↓	ns
Hancox[22]	ns	↑†	↑	↑	↑	↑	↓	ns
Tan[18]	N.R.	N.R.	ns	N.R.	N.R.	N.R.	N.R.	N.R.
Pletcher[23]	↑‡	‡	N.R.	N.R.	N.R.	N.R.	N.R.	N.R.
Kempker[24]	ns	↑	↓	N.R.	N.R.	N.R.	N.R.	N.R.

NOTES: FEV_1 = forced expired volume in 1 sec. FVC = forced vital capacity. FEV_1/FVC = ratio of FEV_1 to FVC. TLC = total lung capacity. FRC = functional residual capacity. RV = residual volume. SG_{aw} = specific airway conductance. D_LCO = single-breath diffusing capacity of the lung for carbon monoxide. ns = no significant difference from nonsmokers. N.R. = not reported. ↓ = significant decrease compared to nonsmokers ($p < 0.05$). ↓* = significant decrease over time among previous but not current marijuana smokers, adjusted for tobacco cigarette smoking. = significant increase compared to nonsmokers ($p < 0.05$). ↑† = nonsignificant compared to nonsmokers. ↑‡ = significant increase compared to nonsmokers based on assessments over 20 years of follow-up (model includes lifetime exposure in joint-years).

2010; Kempker, Honig, & Marlin, 2015; Pletcher et al., 2012). Notably, the forced expired volume in 1 sec (FEV1; a measure of airflow) was not significantly different in seven of the eight studies in which this spirometric measure was recorded, and in the one study in which it was reported as abnormal, it was significantly reduced in previous but not current marijuana smokers (Sherrill, Krzyzanowski, Bloom, & Lebowitz, 1991). Interestingly, the forced vital capacity (FVC) was found to be significantly elevated in three of the six studies in which it was reported (Hancox et al., 2010; Kempker et al., 2015; Pletcher et al., 2012). In one of these three studies, the increase in FVC was accompanied by increases in other subdivisions of lung volume, namely, total lung capacity, functional residual capacity, and residual volume (Hancox et al., 2010). The reason for these elevations in lung volume among marijuana smokers is unclear but could be due to stretching of the lung due to the stylized technique of smoking marijuana that involves taking a deeper inhalation of the smoke followed by holding one's breath about four times longer than is the usual practice when smoking a tobacco cigarette. This breathing regimen might be analogous to that of competitive swimmers, among whom elevated vital capacity measurements have also been reported (Sable, Vaidya, & Sable, 2012). The most specific and sensitive marker of airflow obstruction in COPD is the ratio of FEV1 to FVC. This ratio was reported to be significantly reduced in four of the nine studies in which it was reported (Bloom, Kaltenborn, Paoletti, Camilli, & Lebowitz, 1987; Kempker et al., 2015; Sherrill et al., 1991; Taylor et al., 2000). However, in one of these four studies, the decrease was found only in previous and not in current smokers (Sherrill et al., 1991), and in one other of the four studies, it was reduced only in the heaviest users (i.e., those who reported more than 20 joint-years of smoking, with a joint-year defined as the number of joints smoked per day times the number of years smoked; Pletcher et al., 2012). Moreover, it has been suggested that the decrease in FEV1/FVC ratio could be spurious due to the effect of the elevated FVC in reducing the ratio in the face of a normal FEV1 (Hancox et al., 2010). Of the five studies that did not find a significant decrease in FEV1/FVC ratio, this ratio was significantly increased in one (Hancox et al., 2010) and not significantly different from nonsmokers in the other four (Aldington et al., 2007; Moore et al., 2005; Tan et al., 2009; Tashkin et al., 1987). In four studies, SGaw, the inverse of airway resistance adjusted for the lung volume at which it was obtained, was measured by wholebody plethysmography and in all of these studies was found to be modestly but significantly reduced, indicating the presence of airway obstruction (Aldington et al., 2007; Hancox et al., 2015; Tashkin et al., 1980, 1987). However, the degree of reduction in SGaw was relatively small (~25%) and not likely to be of clinical significance or to be associated with breathlessness on exertion. Indeed, shortness of breath has not been consistently reported in surveys of smokers of marijuana, and it is not clear that even chronic marijuana smokers experience breathlessness (Pletcher et al., 2012). Moreover, a reduced SGaw reflects obstruction in the larger airways, whereas the major site of obstruction in COPD is the small airways, and sensitive indices of small airways function have been found to be normal in marijuana smokers (Tashkin et al., 1987). The reductions in SGaw noted in these studies most likely reflects the increased edema, vascular congestion, and increased secretions observed in the central airways during videobronchoscopy of smokers of marijuana either alone or with tobacco, as reported by Roth et al. (1998). One might expect that the latter changes would increase the resistance to flow in these larger airways.

The diffusing capacity of the lung for carbon monoxide (DLCO) is a measure of gas transfer in the lung across the alveolar capillary membrane and is reduced when the membrane is thickened (as in interstitial lung disease) or destroyed (as in emphysema). The DLCO is the most sensitive (albeit a nonspecific) indicator of emphysema. In the four studies in which the DLCO was measured in smokers of marijuana without tobacco, the DLCO was found to be wellpreserved, arguing against an association between marijuana smoking and emphysema (Aldington et al., 2007; Hancox et al., 2015; Tashkin et al., 1980, 1987).

COPD is a progressive disease characterized by an accelerated loss of lung function (FEV1) with age. Three studies have examined lung function change over time in smokers of marijuana adjusted for tobacco (Hancox et al., 2010; Sherrill et al., 1991; Tashkin et al., 1997). In one of these studies, FEV1 and FEV1/FVC ratio were found to be significantly reduced only in those who had smoked marijuana in the past but not in those who reported using marijuana currently (Sherrill et al., 1991), findings that are difficult to interpret given the possible variability in chronicity of use and marijuana potency. In a later study, lung function was measured serially over eight years in smokers of marijuana and/or tobacco and nonsmokers (Tashkin et al., 1997). In this study, the smokers of marijuana alone had age-related declines in FEV1 that were not significantly different from the nonsmokers, irrespective of the amount of marijuana smoked (range of 1–10 joints daily for ≥ 5 years), while the tobacco smokers showed a significantly accelerated rate of decline that was dose-dependent. In the third study, lung function was measured serially in a birth cohort between ages 15 and 32 with adjustments for gender, height at age 32 years, and changes in height between ages 15 and 32 (Hancox et al., 2010). Over time, marijuana use was associated with a nonsignificant increase in FEV1, a significant increase in FVC, and a nonsignificant decrease in FEV1/FVC ratio. In contrast, tobacco smoking was associated with a significant decrease in FEV1, no change in FVC, and a significant decrease in FEV1/FVC ratio (Hancox et al., 2010). Taken together, the findings from these longitudinal studies do not suggest that marijuana use, in the absence of tobacco, is associated with an accelerated age-related decline in lung function as is characteristic of individuals who develop COPD. However, only a limited number of studies have addressed the impact of regular marijuana smoking on lung function and lung function change over time and these have been carried out mainly in younger individuals, many of whom were comparatively light smokers. Consequently, additional research is warranted to more clearly define the impact of habitual smoking of marijuana, especially long-term heavy smoking in older individuals, to more clearly the potential risks to lung health.

Effects on High-Resolution Computed Tomograph

Radiographic lung imaging with thoracic high-resolution computed tomography (HRCT) has been systematically performed in marijuana smokers in only one study (Aldington et al., 2007). In that study, HRCT slices in the apical region of the lungs of marijuana-only smokers were found to have a reduced lung density in the emphysema range (Hounsfield units less than −950) compared to nonsmokers, but no evidence of macroscopic emphysema was apparent in the marijuana smokers (1.3% prevalence in the marijuana smokers compared to 18.5% prevalence in the smokers of tobacco and 0% in the nonsmokers).

EFFECTS ON AIRWAY PATHOLOGY

To assess the impact of regular marijuana smoking on airway pathology, fiberoptic bronchoscopy with bronchial biopsies was performed according to a standard protocol in 40 smokers of marijuana alone, 31 smokers of tobacco alone, 44 smokers of both substances, and 53 nonsmokers (Fligiel et al., 1997). Smokers of marijuana alone had widespread histopathological abnormalities in their bronchial mucosa compared to nonsmokers, including replacement of the normal ciliated epithelial cells with increased numbers of mucus-secreting surface epithelial (goblet) cells (68% vs. 29%, respectively), reserve, cells (73 vs. 12%, respectively), and metaplastic squamous cells (33% vs. 6%, respectively). The extent of these alterations was similar to that found in the tobacco smokers. The loss of ciliated epithelium and the propensity to secrete an excessive amount of mucus into the airway (due to the increased numbers of goblet cells) might explain the increased prevalence of symptoms of chronic bronchitis in habitual marijuana smokers since the loss of ciliated epithlium is likely to impair mucociliary clearance so that cough might be an alternative mechanism to clear the excess amount of mucus from the airways.

INFERENCES CONCERNING THE RELATION BETWEEN MARIJUANA AND COPD

Despite the visual and histologic evidence of injury and inflammation in the large central airways and the increased prevalence of symptoms of chronic bronchitis in regular smokers of marijuana, the absence of evidence of significant airflow obstruction in most studies in which lung function was systematically measured argues against a definitive connection between smoking of marijuana and the occurrence of COPD, the defining feature of which is persistent airflow obstruction. Possible reasons for the lack of evidence implicating marijuana use, in contrast to tobacco smoking, as a risk factor for COPD include the generally smaller quantity of marijuana smoked on a daily basis compared to tobacco and the well-described observations that THC has immunosuppressive/anti-inflammatory properties (Klein, Friedman, & Specter, 1998; Roth, Baldwin, & Tashkin, 2002; Roth et al., 2004), including inhibition of the production/release of pro-inflammatory mediators by alveolar macrophages (Baldwin et al., 1997; Shay et al., 2003), the primary immune effector cell that resides in lung. Since activation of alveolar macrophages by components within the smoke of tobacco is believed to be crucial to the pathogenesis of COPD (Barnes & Celli, 2009), the inhibitory effect of THC within marijuana on alveolar macrophage function might exert a protective effect.

In sum, most studies show an adverse effect of marijuana smoking on symptoms of chronic bronchitis, consistent with the endoscopic and histopathological findings of large airway inflammation and injury in the large airways, but fail to show a significant impact of marijuana smoking on airway dynamics in the absence of concomitant tobacco use. However, the effect of very heavy

marijuana smoking on lung function is unclear, as is the impact of the more potent preparations of marijuana that are now available.

ASSOCIATION OF REGULAR MARIJUANA USE WITH RESPIRATORY CANCER

Several lines of evidence suggest that habitual marijuana smokers might be at
increased risk for the development of respiratory cancer, including cancers of the
lung and upper aerodigestive tract (UAT; tongue, oral cavity, oropharynx, larynx,
proximal esophagus). First, known carcinogens are present within the smoke of
marijuana (including the polycyclic aromatic hydrocarbon benz(a)pyrene, one of
the most important human carcinogens) in concentrations comparable to those
in tobacco smoke (Hoffmann et al., 1975; Moir et al., 2007; Novotný et al., 1982).
Second, although fewer cigarettes (joints) of marijuana than tobacco cigarettes
are generally smoked, four times the quantity of insoluble particulates (tar) are
deposited in the lower respiratory tract from the smoke of marijuana compared
to that of the same quantity of tobacco, thereby amplifying the exposure of the
lungs to the carcinogens within the inhaled tar from marijuana (Wu, Tashkin,
Djahed, & Rose, 1988). Third, exposure of hamster lung explants to the smoke
from marijuana over a two-year period led to accelerated malignant transforma-
tion compared to sham exposure and to a degree at least comparable to that from
exposure to the same quantity of tobacco (Leuchtenberger & Leuchtenberger,
1976). Fourth, bronchial biopsies obtained from habitual smokers of marijuana without tobacco revealed histopathologic alterations in the bronchial epithelium (e.g., squamous metaplasia, cellular atypia, cellular disorganization,
increased nuclear/cytoplasmic ratio) that have been shown to be precursors
to the subsequent development of lung cancer in tobacco smokers (Auerbach,
Stout, Hammond, & Garfinkel, 1961). Fifth, immunohistochemical assays from
bronchial biopsies obtained from marijuana-only smokers revealed significant
overexpression of the protein products of two of the genes known to be involved
prelung tumor progression, namely, epidermal growth factor receptor and KI-
67, a nuclear proliferation antigen, and this overexpression was numerically even
greater than that observed in the tobacco-only smokers (Barsky, Roth, Kleerup,
Simmons, & Tashkin, 1998). More recently, epidermal growth factor receptor
and downstream onco-proteins (Akt, P50, COX-2) were found to be significantly
overexpressed ($p < 0.01$) in laryngeal cancer specimens from smokers of marijuana compared to nonsmokers (Bhattacharyya et al., 2015). Sixth, several small
case series have indicated an unusually high proportion of regular marijuana
smokers among young persons (<40–50 yrs. of age) with lung or upper airway
cancer (Donald, 1991; Endicott, Skipper, & Hernandez, 1993; Fung, Gallagher, &
Machtay, 1998; Sridhar et al., 1994; Taylor, 1988).

A few older case-control epidemiologic studies showed a positive association
between marijuana use and UAT and lung cancers (Berthiller et al., 2008; Hsairi
et al., 1993; Sasco et al., 2002; Zhang et al., 1999), but there are caveats. In the

study showing a positive association with UAT cancer, the controls were not properly matched to the cases (Zhang et al., 1999). Moreover, the two studies that demonstrated a positive association with lung cancer (Hsairi et al., 1993; Sasco et al., 2002), as subsequently reviewed by Berthiller et al., 2008, were conducted in North Africa, where marijuana is usually admixed with tobacco, and the mixture is smoked in the form of a kiff, thus rendering it impossible to disentangle the effect of tobacco from that of marijuana (Table 6.3).

In contrast, there are several lines of evidence that argue against a link between marijuana and tobacco-related cancers. First, several groups of investigators have demonstrated an antitumoral effect of THC and other cannabinoids on a variety of malignancies (lung, glioma, thyroid, lymphoma, skin, pancreas, uterus, breast, and prostate) in both cell culture systems and animal models, as

Table 6.3 ASSOCIATION OF MARIJUANA USE WITH LUNG CANCER COMPARED TO NEVER SMOKING: EPIDEMIOLOGIC STUDIES

Author	Study Type	N	Relative Risk (95% CI)
Sidney[50]	Cohort (up to 8 years follow-up)	64,855	0.8 (0.5–1.2)
Hsairi[46]	Case/Control	110/110	8.2 (1.3–15.5)
Sasco[47]	Case/Control	118/235	5.6 (1.6–20.5)
Hashibe[55]	Case/Control	610/1026	0.63 (0.29–1.4)[a] 0.56 (0.29–1.1)[b]
Aldington[56]	Case/Control	79/324	1.2 (0.5–2.6)[c] 5.7 (1.5–21.6)[d]
Zhang[54]	Pooled analysis of 6 case-control studies	2159/2985	0.95 (0.66–1.38)
Callaghan[57]	Cohort (up to 40 years follow-up)	49,321	1.25 (0.84–1.87)[e] 2.12 (1.08–4.14)[f]

[a]Model compares those reporting ≥1 joint-year of marijuana use with never smokers and adjusts for age, tobacco cigarette smoking, race/ethnicity, education level and alcohol consumption.

[b]Adjusted odds ratio for the subgroup with the heaviest history of marijuana smoking (≥ 60 joint-years).

[c]Relative risk for all marijuana smokers compared to nonsmokers.

[d]Relative risk for the tertile with the heaviest history of marijuana smokers (≥10.5 joint-years).

[e]Hazard ratio for all self-reported ever marijuana smokers and nonsmokers adjusted for frequency of marijuana use up to age 19–20 years.

[f]Hazard ratio for those with a cumulative frequency of marijuana use >50 times up to age 19–20 years.

reviewed by Bifulco, Laezza, Pisanti, and Gazzerro (2006). Second, most well-designed epidemiologic studies that adequately controlled for tobacco use have failed to find a significant association between marijuana use and respiratory cancer (Table 6.3). For, example, a large cohort study of nearly 65,000 health plan participants in California followed for eight years did not show any association between marijuana use and any tobacco-related cancer, OR 0.8, 95% CI [0.5–1.2] (Sidney, Quesenberry, Friedman, & Tekawa, 1997). However, it is important to keep in mind that this sample consisted of a very heterogeneous group of marijuana users, including infrequent smokers and ex-smokers (Sidney et al., 1997). Three case-control studies in which the controls were properly matched to the cases showed null relationships between marijuana and oral cancer, OR 0.3–1.0, 95% CIs spanned 1.0 (Llewellyn, Johnson, & Warnakulasuriya, 2004; Llewellyn, Linklater, Bell, Johnson, & Warnak, 2004; Rosenblatt, Daling, Chen, Sherman, & Schwartz, 2004). A pooled analysis of six case-control studies failed to show an association between marijuana smoking and lung cancer, pooled OR 0.95, 95% CI [0.66–1.38], $p = 0.807$ (Zhang et al., 2015). Five of these six studies, including the one with the largest numbers of cases and controls (Hashibe et al., 2006) showed null associations, ORs0.57–1.06, while one showed a significantly positive association, OR 2.17, 95% CI [1.04–4.52], $p = 0.039$ (Aldington et al., 2008). However, in the latter study, while a significant association was noted in the heaviest smokers, relative risk 5.7, 95% CI [1.5–21.6], this subgroup contained only four controls, suggesting that the risk estimates were imprecise and probably inflated. A recently published cohort study of nearly 50,000 men aged 18 to 20 years conscripted into the Swedish military in 1969–1970 reported a significant relationship between self-reported cumulative use of marijuana on >50 occasions (designated as heavy use) up to the time of conscription (i.e., by age 19–20 years) and the occurrence of lung cancer over a subsequent 40-year follow-up period adjusted for cumulative lifetime tobacco use only up to age 19–20, hazard ratio 2.12, 95% CI [1.08–4.14] (Callaghan, Allebeck, & Sidorchuk, 2013). However, this study is flawed since 91% of the heavy marijuana users also smoked tobacco, and the authors were unable to neither determine true lifetime use of marijuana nor to adjust for true lifetime use of tobacco. While the evidence concerning possible associations of marijuana use with respiratory cancer is somewhat mixed, the weight of evidence tends to argue against the concept that habitual marijuana smoking in the absence of concomitant tobacco use is a significant risk factor for the development of respiratory cancer.

DOES REGULAR MARIJUANA SMOKING PREDISPOSE TO LOWER RESPIRATORY TRACT INFECTION?

The regular marijuana smoker's host defenses against lower respiratory tract infection are compromised by two factors. One of these is an increase of mucous secretions in the airway that are less likely to be adequately cleared from the lung due to the replacement of ciliated bronchial epithelium by hyperplastic goblet and basal cells or disordered squamous-like cells (Fligiel et al., 1997; Roth et al., 1998), consistent with an accumulation of mucus that could serve as a substrate for microbial pathogens. The other factor is the THC-related impairment in the phagocytic and microbicidal activity of alveolar macrophages, the principal immune-effector cell in the lung that protects the lung against infection (Baldwin et al., 1997; Roth, Whittaker, Salehi, Tashkin, & Baldwin, 2004; Shay et al., 2003). Some clinical evidence does implicate marijuana use as a possible risk factor for lower respiratory tract infection. For example, a large cohort study demonstrated an increased frequency of outpatient visits for respiratory illnesses in relation to self-reported marijuana use (Polen, Sidney, Tekawa, Sadler, & Friedman, 1993). Moreover, marijuana may be contaminated with Aspergillus fumigatus (Kurup, Resnick, Kagen, Cohen, & Fink, 1983), as well as potentially pathogenic gram-negative bacteria (Ungerleider, Andrysiak, Tashkin, & Gale, 1982), and isolated cases of Aspergillus pneumonia have been reported in marijuana smokers immunocompromised by AIDS (Denning et al., 1991), chronic granulomatous disease (Chusid, Gelfand, Nutter, & Fauci, 1975), bone marrow or renal transplantation (Hamadeh, Ardehali, Locksley, & York, 1988; Marks et al., 1996), or chemotherapy for lung cancer (Sutton, Lum, & Torti, 1986). More recently, clusters of tuberculosis have been reported in individuals who smoked marijuana using a shared water pipe with unsuspected cases of active cavitary tuberculosis (Munckhof, Konstantinos, Wamsley, Mortlock, & Gilpin, 2003; Thu, Hayes, Miles, Tierney, & Foy, 2013). In addition, older observational studies suggest a possible association between marijuana use and pneumonia (Caiaffa et al., 1994; Newell et al., 1985; Tindall et al., 1988). However, analysis of data in the late 1980s from the longitudinal Multicenter AIDS Cohort Study of gay men failed to demonstrate a significant association between self-reported marijuana use and either HIV seroconversion, the development of opportunistic pneumonia, or progression to full-blown AIDS (Kaslow et al., 1989). A further analysis of updated data from the Multicenter AIDS Cohort Study is underway to reevaluate the possible relationship between marijuana smoking and pneumonia risk.

ASSOCIATION OF MARIJUANA USE WITH OTHER RESPIRATORY DISORDERS

Several isolated cases of pneumothorax and pneumomediastinum have been reported in marijuana smokers (Beshay, Kaiser, Niedhart, Reymond, & Schmid, 2007; Birrer & Calderon, 1984; Feldman, Sullivan, Passero, & Lewis, 1993; Goodyear, Laws, & Turner, 2004; Hazouard et al., 2001; Herrejón et al., 1992; Luque, Cavallaro, Torres, Emmanual, & Hillman, 1987; Mattox, 1976; Miller, Spiekerman, & Hepper, 1972). It is possible that the special smoking technique employed by marijuana users—namely, a deep inhalation followed by a prolonged breathhold at high lung volumes—might predispose the marijuana users to leakage of air into the pleural space due to rupture of subpleural air spaces or blebs, especially if a Valsalva or Mueller maneuver is performed near total lung capacity against a closed glottis. Marijuana-related increases in lung volume, as previously noted (Hancox et al., 2010), could also be a predisposing factor. Several cases of bullous lung disease have also been reported in smokers of varying amounts of marijuana, usually along with tobacco (Hii, Tam, Thompson, & Naughton, 2008; Johnson, Smith, Morrison, Laszlo, & White, 2000; Phan, Lau, & Li, 2005). However, in the absence of studies that control for tobacco use, causality due to marijuana use cannot be inferred from these isolated observations (Tan, Hatam, & Treasure, 2006).

SUMMARY

Regular marijuana smoking is associated with symptoms of acute and chronic bronchitis and evidence of microscopic injury to the cells lining the central airways. However, the cross-sectional and longitudinal literature is relatively small, and some do not adequately control for tobacco use or are based on marijuana potencies that are not commonly available to current smokers. Thus, we cannot definitively say at this point that smoking marijuana predisposes the user to clinically significant COPD. Similarly, despite the fact that marijuana smoke contains many of the same carcinogens that are found in tobacco smoke, most adequately controlled epidemiologic studies have failed to find a significant association with respiratory cancer. Yet these studies are limited in number, and some of the findings are conflicting, underscoring the need for additional research about the association between marijuana smoking and respiratory cancer. Evidence of large airway injury and inflammation in habitual marijuana smokers and the immunosuppressive properties of THC suggest a predisposition to respiratory tract infection. However, while case series and older observational studies suggest a possible association between marijuana and pneumonia, large-scale epidemiologic studies testing for a significant association are largely lacking. Several cases of pneumothorax, pneumomediastinum, and bullous lung disease have been reported in marijuana smokers (often with tobacco), but a causal relationship to marijuana has not been established.

Whether the higher potency of currently available marijuana adversely affects the lung, as a consequence of the toxic respiratory irritants in the particulate and gaseous phases of the smoke and the carcinogenic polycyclic aromatic hydrocarbons in the tar phase that have the potential to injure the lung and cause cancer, is an open research question. While the concentration of THC may not be directly related to lung health, it is still possible that greater THC levels may increase the addictive potential of marijuana and thus also increase the likelihood of continued use, the cumulative effect of which could have a negative effect on the lung. In this light, THC concentration may have an indirect effect on respiratory health, a possibility that warrants further study.

REFERENCES

Aldington, S., Harwood, M., Cox, B., Weatherall, M., Beckert, L., Hansell, A., . . . Beasley, R. (2008). Cannabis use and risk of lung cancer: A case–control study. *European Respiratory Journal, 31*, 280–286. http://dx.doi.org/10.1183/09031936.00065707

Aldington, S., Williams, M., Nowitz, M., Weatherall, M., Pritchard, A., McNaughton, A., . . . Beasley, R. (2007). Effects of cannabis on pulmonary structure, function and symptoms. *Thorax, 62*, 1058–1063. http://dx.doi.org/10.1136/thx.2006.077081

Auerbach, O., Stout, A. P., Hammond, E. C., & Garfinkel, L. (1961). Changes in bronchial epithelium in relation to cigarette smoking and in relation to lung cancer. *New England Journal of Medicine, 265*, 253–267. http://dx.doi.org/10.1056/NEJM196108102650601

Baldwin, G. C., Tashkin, D. P., Buckley, D. M., Park, A. N., Dubinett, S. M., & Roth, M. D. (1997). Marijuana and cocaine impair alveolar macrophage function and cytokine production. *American Journal of Respiratory and Critical Care Medicine, 156*, 1606–1613. http://dx.doi.org/10.1164/ajrccm.156.5.9704146

Barnes, P. J., & Celli, B. R. (2009). Systemic manifestations and comorbidities of COPD. *European Respiratory Journal, 33*, 1165–1185. http://dx.doi.org/10.1183/09031936.00128008

Barsky, S. H., Roth, M. D., Kleerup, E. C., Simmons, M., & Tashkin, D. P. (1998). Histopathologic and molecular alterations in bronchial epithelium in habitual smokers of marijuana, cocaine, and/or tobacco. *Journal of the National Cancer Institute, 90*, 1198–1205. http://dx.doi.org/10.1093/jnci/90.16.1198

Berthiller, J., Straif, K., Boniol, M., Voirin, N., Benhaïm-Luzon, V., Ayoub, W. B., . . . Ayed, F. B. (2008). Cannabis smoking and risk of lung cancer in men: a pooled analysis of three studies in Maghreb. *Journal of Thoracic Oncology, 3*, 1398–1403. http://dx.doi.org/10.1097/JTO.0b013e31818ddcde

Beshay, M., Kaiser, H., Niedhart, D., Reymond, M. A., & Schmid, R. A. (2007). Emphysema and secondary pneumothorax in young adults smoking cannabis. *European Journal of Cardio-Thoracic Surgery, 32*, 834–838. http://dx.doi.org/10.1016/j.ejcts.2007.07.039

Bhattacharyya, S., Mandal, S., Banerjee, S., Mandal, G. K., Bhowmick, A. K., & Murmu, N. (2015). Cannabis smoke can be a major risk factor for early-age laryngeal cancer: A molecular signaling-based approach. *Tumor Biology, 36*, 6029–6036. http://dx.doi.org/10.1007/s13277-015-3279-4

Bifulco, M., Laezza, C., Pisanti, S., & Gazzerro, P. (2006). Cannabinoids and cancer: pros and cons of an antitumour strategy. *British Journal of Pharmacology, 148*, 123–135. http://dx.doi.org/10.1038/sj.bjp.0706632

Birrer, R. B., & Calderon, J. (1984). Pneumothorax, pneumomediastinum, and pneumopericardium following Valsalva's maneuver during marijuana smoking. *New York State Journal of Medicine, 84*, 619–620. http://dx.doi.org/10.1513/AnnalsATS.201212-127FR

Bloom, J. W., Kaltenborn, W. T., Paoletti, P., Camilli, A., & Lebowitz, M. D. (1987). Respiratory effects of non-tobacco cigarettes. *British Medical Journal, 295*, 1516–1518.

Caiaffa, W. T., Vlahov, D., Graham, N. M., Astemborski, J., Solomon, L., Nelson, K. E., & Munoz, A. (1994). Drug smoking, pneumocystis carinii pneumonia, and immunosuppression increase risk of bacterial pneumonia in human immunodeficiency virus-seropositive injection drug users. *American Journal of Respiratory and Critical Care Medicine, 150*, 1493–1498. http://dx.doi.org/10.1164/ajrccm.150.6.7952605

Calignano, A., Katona, I., Desarnaud, F., Giuffrida, A., La Rana, G., Mackie, K., . . . Piomelli, D. (2000). Bidirectional control of airway responsiveness by endogenous cannabinoids. *Nature, 408*, 96–101. http://dx.doi.org/10.1038/35040576

Callaghan, R. C., Allebeck, P., & Sidorchuk, A. (2013). Marijuana use and risk of lung cancer: A 40-year cohort study. *Cancer Causes & Control, 24*, 1811–1820. http://dx.doi.org/10.1007/s10552-013-0259-0

Chusid, M. J., Gelfand, J. A., Nutter, & Fauci, A. S. (1975). Letter: Pulmonary aspergillosis, inhalation of contaminated marijuana smoke, chronic granulomatous disease. *Annals of Internal Medicine, 82*, 682–683.

Denning, D. W., Follansbee, S. E., Scolaro, M., Norris, S., Edelstein, H., & Stevens, D. A. (1991). Pulmonary aspergillosis in the acquired immunodeficiency syndrome. *New England Journal of Medicine, 324*, 654–662. http://dx.doi.org/10.1056/NEJM199103073241003

Donald, P. J. (1991). Advanced malignancy in the young marijuana smoker. In H. Friedman (Ed.), *Drugs of abuse, immunity, and immunodeficiency* (pp. 33–46). New York: Plenum.

Endicott, J. N., Skipper, P., & Hernandez, L. (1993). Marijuana and head and neck cancer. In H. Friedman (Ed.), *Drugs of abuse, immunity, and AIDS* (pp. 107–113). New York: Plenum.

Feldman, A. L., Sullivan, J. T., Passero, M. A., & Lewis, D. C. (1993). Pneumothorax in polysubstance-abusing marijuana and tobacco smokers: Three cases. *Journal of Substance Abuse, 5*, 183–186. http://dx.doi.org/10.1016/0899-3289(93)90061-F

Fligiel, S. E., Roth, M. D., Kleerup, E. C., Barsky, S. H., Simmons, M. S., & Tashkin, D. P. (1997). Tracheobronchial histopathology in habitual smokers of cocaine, marijuana, and/or tobacco. *Chest, 112*, 319–326. http://dx.doi.org/10.1378/chest.112.2.319

Fung, M., Gallagher, C., & Machtay, M. (1998). Lung and aero-digestive cancers in young marijuana smokers. *Tumori, 85*, 140–142.

Goodyear, K., Laws, D., & Turner, J. (2004). Bilateral spontaneous pneumothorax in a cannabis smoker. *Journal of the Royal Society of Medicine, 97*, 435–436. http://dx.doi.org/10.1258/jrsm.97.9.435

Grassin-Delyle, S., Naline, E., Buenestado, A., Faisy, C., Alvarez, J. C., Salvator, H., . . . Devillier, P. (2014). Cannabinoids inhibit cholinergic contraction in human airways through prejunctional CB1 receptors. *British Journal of Pharmacology, 171*, 2767–2777. http://dx.doi.org/10.1111/bph.12597

Grinspoon, L. (1969). Marijuana. *Scientific American, 221*, 17–25.

Hamadeh, R., Ardehali, A., Locksley, R. M., & York, M. K. (1988). Fatal aspergillosis associated with smoking contaminated marijuana, in a marrow transplant recipient. *Chest, 94*, 432–433.

Hancox, R. J., Poulton, R., Ely, M., Welch, D., Taylor, D. R., McLachlan, C. R., . . . Sears, M. R. (2010). Effects of cannabis on lung function: a population-based cohort study. *European Respiratory Journal, 35*, 42–47. http://dx.doi.org/10.1183/09031936.00065009

Hancox, R. J., Shin, H. H., Gray, A. R., Poulton, R., & Sears, M. R. (2015). Effects of quitting cannabis on respiratory symptoms. *European Respiratory Journal, 46*, 80–87. http://dx.doi.org/10.1183/09031936.00228914

Hashibe, M., Morgenstern, H., Cui, Y., Tashkin, D. P., Zhang, Z. F., Cozen, W., . . . Greenland, S. (2006). Marijuana use and the risk of lung and upper aerodigestive tract cancers: Results of a population-based case-control study. *Cancer Epidemiology Biomarkers & Prevention*, *15*, 1829–1834. http://dx.doi.org/10.1158/1055-9965. EPI-06-0330

Hazouard, E., Koninck, J. C., Attucci, S., Fauchier-Rolland, F., Brunereau, L., & Diot, P. (2001). Pneumorachis and pneumomediastinum caused by repeated Müller's maneuvers: Complications of marijuana smoking. *Annals of Emergency Medicine*, *38*, 694–697. http://dx.doi.org/10.1067/mem.2001.118016

Herrejón, S. A., Blanquer, O. J., Simo, M. M., Ruiz, M. F., Núñez, S. C., & Chiner, V. E. (1992). Neumotorax por inhalacion de drogas [Pneumothorax due to drug inhalation]. *Anales de Medicina Interna*, *9*, 137–139.

Hii, S. W., Tam, J. D., Thompson, B. R., & Naughton, M. T. (2008). Bullous lung disease due to marijuana. *Respirology*, *13*, 122–127. http://dx.doi.org/10.1111/j.1440-1843.2007.01186.x

Hoffmann, D., Brunnemann, K. D., Gori, G. B., & Wynder, E. L. (1975). On the carcinogenicity of marijuana smoke. In V. C. Runeckles (Ed.), *Recent Advances in Phytochemistry* (pp. 63–81). New York: Plenum.

Hsairi, M., Achour, N., Zouari, B., Ben, R. H., Achour, A., Maalej, M., & Nacef, T. (1993). Facteurs étiologiques du cancer bronchique primitif en Tunisie [Etiologic factors in primary bronchial carcinoma in Tunisia]. *La Tunisie Medicale*, *71*, 265–268.

Johnson, M. K., Smith, R. P., Morrison, D., Laszlo, G., & White, R. J. (2000). Large lung bullae in marijuana smokers. *Thorax*, *55*, 340–342. http://dx.doi.org/10.1136/thorax.55.4.340

Kaslow, R. A., Blackwelder, W. C., Ostrow, D. G., Yerg, D., Palenicek, J., Coulson, A. H., & Valdiserri, R. O. (1989). No evidence for a role of alcohol or other psychoactive drugs in accelerating immunodeficiency in HIV-1—positive individuals: A report from the Multicenter AIDS Cohort Study. *JAMA*, *261*, 3424–3429. http://dx.doi.org/10.1001/jama.1989.03420230078030

Kempker, J. A., Honig, E. G., & Martin, G. S. (2015). The effects of marijuana exposure on expiratory airflow: A study of adults who participated in the US National Health and Nutrition Examination Study. *Annals of the American Thoracic Society*, *12*, 135–141. http://dx.doi.org/10.1513/AnnalsATS.201407-333OC

Klein, T. W., Friedman, H., & Specter, S. (1998). Marijuana, immunity and infection. *Journal of Neuroimmunology*, *83*, 102–115. http://dx.doi.org/10.1016/S0165-5728(97)00226-9

Kurup, V. P., Resnick, A., Kagen, S. L., Cohen, S. H., & Fink, J. N. (1983). Allergenic fungi and actinomycetes in smoking materials and their health implications. *Mycopathologia*, *82*, 61–64.

Leuchtenberger, C., & Leuchtenberger, R. (1976). Cytological and cytochemical studies of the effects of fresh marihuana cigarette smoke on growth and DNA metabolism of animal and human lung cultures (pp. 595–612). In M. C. Braude & S. Szara (Eds.), *The Pharmacology of Marijuana*. New York: Raven.

Llewellyn, C. D., Johnson, N. W., & Warnakulasuriya, K. A. A. S. (2004). Risk factors for oral cancer in newly diagnosed patients aged 45 years and younger: A case-control study in Southern England. *Journal of Oral Pathology & Medicine*, *33*, 525–532. http://dx.doi.org/10.1111/j.1600-0714.2004.00222.x

Llewellyn, C. D., Linklater, K., Bell, J., Johnson, N. W., & Warnakulasuriya, S. (2004). An analysis of risk factors for oral cancer in young people: a case-control study. *Oral Oncology, 40*, 304–313. http://dx.doi.org/10.1016/j.oraloncology.2003.08.015

Luque, M. A., III, Cavallaro, D. L., Torres, M., Emmanual, P., & Hillman, J. V. (1987). Pneumomediastinum, pneumothorax, and subcutaneous emphysema after alternate cocaine inhalation and marijuana smoking. *Pediatric Emergency Care, 3*, 107–109.

Marks, W. H., Florence, L., Lieberman, J., Chapman, P., Howard, D., Roberts, P., & Perkinson, D. (1996). Successfully treated invasive pulmonary aspergillosis associated with smoking marijuana in a renal transplant recipient. *Transplantation, 61*, 1771–1774.

Mattox, K. L. (1976). Pneumomediastinum in heroin and marijuana users. *Journal of the American College of Emergency Physicians, 5*, 26–28.

Miller, W. E., Spiekerman, R. E., & Hepper, N. G. (1972). Pneumomediastinum resulting from performing Valsalva maneuvers during marihuana smoking. *Chest, 62*, 233–234.

Moir, D., Rickert, W. S., Levasseur, G., Larose, Y., Maertens, R., White, P., & Desjardins, S. (2007). A comparison of mainstream and sidestream marijuana and tobacco cigarette smoke produced under two machine smoking conditions. *Chemical Research in Toxicology, 21*, 494–502. http://dx.doi.org/10.1021/tx700275p

Moore, B. A., Augustson, E. M., Moser, R. P., & Budney, A. J. (2005). Respiratory effects of marijuana and tobacco use in a US sample. *Journal of General Internal Medicine, 20*, 33–37. http://dx.doi.org/10.1111/j.1525-1497.2004.40081.x

Munckhof, W. J., Konstantinos, A., Wamsley, M., Mortlock, M., & Gilpin, C. (2003). A cluster of tuberculosis associated with use of a marijuana water pipe. *International Journal of Tuberculosis and Lung Disease, 7*, 860–865.

Nadel, J. A., & Comroe, J. H. (1961). Acute effects of inhalation of cigarette smoke on airway conductance. *Journal of Applied Physiology, 16*, 713–716.

Newell, G. R., Mansell, P. W., Wilson, M. B., Lynch, H. K., Spitz, M. R., & Hersh, E. M. (1985). Risk factor analysis among men referred for possible acquired immune deficiency syndrome. *Preventive Medicine, 14*, 81–91.

Novotný, M., Merli, F., Wiesler, D., Fencl, M., & Saeed, T. (1982). Fractionation and capillary gas chromatographic: Mass spectrometric characterization of the neutral components in marijuana and tobacco smoke condensates. *Journal of Chromatography A, 238*, 141–150.

Phan, T. D., Lau, K. K. P., & Li, X. (2005). Lung bullae and pulmonary fibrosis associated with marijuana smoking. *Australasian Radiology, 49*, 411–414. http://dx.doi.org/10.1111/j.1440-1673.2005.01472.x

Pletcher, M. J., Vittinghoff, E., Kalhan, R., Richman, J., Safford, M., Sidney, S., . . . Kertesz, S. (2012). Association between marijuana exposure and pulmonary function over 20 years. *JAMA, 307*, 173–181. http://dx.doi.org/10.1001/jama.2011.1961

Polen, M. R., Sidney, S., Tekawa, I. S., Sadler, M., & Friedman, G. D. (1993). Health care use by frequent marijuana smokers who do not smoke tobacco. *Western Journal of Medicine, 158*, 596–601.

Rosell, S., & Agurell, S. (1975). Effects of 7-hydroxy-delta-6=tetrahydrocannabinol and some related cannabinoids on the guinea pig isolated ilieum. *Acta Physiologica Scandinavica, 94*, 142–144.

Rosenblatt, K. A., Daling, J. R., Chen, C., Sherman, K. J., & Schwartz, S. M. (2004). Marijuana use and risk of oral squamous cell carcinoma. *Cancer Research, 64*, 4049–4054. http://dx.doi.org/10.1158/0008-5472.CAN-03-3425

Roth, M. D., Arora, A., Barsky, S. H., Kleerup, E. C., Simmons, M., & Tashkin, D. P. (1998). Airway inflammation in young marijuana and tobacco smokers. *American Journal of Respiratory and Critical Care Medicine, 157*, 928–937. http://dx.doi.org/10.1164/ajrccm.157.3.9701026

Roth, M. D., Baldwin, G. C., & Tashkin, D. P. (2002). Effects of delta-9-tetrahydrocannabinol on human immune function and host defense. *Chemistry and Physics of Lipids, 121*, 229–239. http://dx.doi.org/10.1016/S0009-3084(02)00159-7

Roth, M. D., Whittaker, K., Salehi, K., Tashkin, D. P., & Baldwin, G. C. (2004). Mechanisms for impaired effector function in alveolar macrophages from marijuana and cocaine smokers. *Journal of Neuroimmunology, 147*, 82–86. http://dx.doi.org/10.1016/j.jneuroim.2003.10.017

Sable, M., Viadya, S. M., & Sable, S. S. (2012). Comparative study of lung functions in swimmers and runners. *Indian Journal of Physiology & Pharmacology, 56*, 100–104.

Sasco, A. J., Merrill, R. M., Dari, I., Benhaïm-Luzon, V., Carriot, F., Cann, C. I., & Bartal, M. (2002). A case–control study of lung cancer in Casablanca, Morocco. *Cancer Causes & Control, 13*, 609–616. http://dx.doi.org/10.1023/A:1019504210176

Shay, A. H., Choi, R., Whittaker, K., Salehi, K., Kitchen, C. M., Tashkin, D. P., . . . Baldwin, G. C. (2003). Impairment of antimicrobial activity and nitric oxide production in alveolar macrophages from smokers of marijuana and cocaine. *Journal of Infectious Diseases, 187*, 700–704. http://dx.doi.org/10.1086/368370

Sherrill, D. L., Krzyzanowski, M., Bloom, J. W., & Lebowitz, M. D. (1991). Respiratory effects of non-tobacco cigarettes: a longitudinal study in general population. *International Journal of Epidemiology, 20*, 132–137. http://dx.doi.org/10.1093/ije/20.1.132

Sidney, S., Quesenberry, C. P., Jr., Friedman, G. D., & Tekawa, I. S. (1997). Marijuana use and cancer incidence (California, United States). *Cancer Causes & Control, 8*, 722–728.

Sridhar, K. S., Raub, W. A., Weatherby, N. L., Metsch, L. R., Surratt, H. L., Inciardi, J. A., . . . McCoy, C. B. (1994). Possible role of marijuana smoking as a carcinogen in the development of lung cancer at a young age. *Journal of Psychoactive Drugs, 26*, 285–288.

Sutton, S., Lum, B. L., & Torti, F. M. (1986). Possible risk of invasive pulmonary aspergillosis with marijuana use during chemotherapy for small cell lung cancer. *Annals of Pharmacotherapy, 20*, 289–291.

Tan, C., Hatam, N., & Treasure, T. (2006). Bullous disease of the lung and cannabis smoking: insufficient evidence for a causative link. *Journal of the Royal Society of Medicine, 99*, 77–80. http://dx.doi.org/10.1177/014107680609900220

Tan, W. C., Lo, C., Jong, A., Xing, L., FitzGerald, M. J., Vollmer, W. M., . . . Vancouver Burden of Obstructive Lung Disease (BOLD) Research Group. (2009). Marijuana and chronic obstructive lung disease: a population-based study. *Canadian Medical Association Journal, 180*, 814–820. http://dx.doi.org/10.1503/cmaj.081040

Tashkin, D. P., Calvarese, B. M., Simmons, M. S., & Shapiro, B. J. (1980). Respiratory status of seventy-four habitual marijuana smokers. *Chest, 78*, 699–706.

Tashkin, D. P., Coulson, A. H., Clark, V. A., Simmons, M., Bourque, L. B., Duann, S., . . . Gong, H. (1987). Respiratory Symptoms and Lung Function in Habitual Heavy Smokers of Marijuana Alone, Smokers of Marijuana and Tobacco, Smokers of Tobacco Alone, and Nonsmokers 1–3. *American Review of Respiratory Disease, 135*, 209–216.

Tashkin, D. P., Shapiro, B. J., & Frank, I. M. (1973). Acute pulmonary physiologic effects of smoked marijuana and oral Δ9-tetrahydrocannabinol in healthy young men. *New England Journal of Medicine, 289*, 336–341.

Tashkin, D. P., Shapiro, B. J., & Frank, I. M. (1974). Acute Effects of Smoked Marijuana and Oral Δ9-Tetrahydrocannabinol on Specific Airway Conductance in Asthmatic Subjects 1–3. *American Review of Respiratory Disease, 109*, 420–428.

Tashkin, D. P., Shapiro, B. J., Lee, Y. E., & Harper, C. E. (1975). Effects of Smoked Marijuana in Experimentally Induced Asthma 1, 2. *American Review of Respiratory Disease, 112*, 377–386.

Tashkin, D. P., Simmons, M. S., Sherrill, D. L., & Coulson, A. H. (1997). Heavy habitual marijuana smoking does not cause an accelerated decline in FEV1 with age. *American Journal of Respiratory and Critical Care Medicine, 155*, 141–148.

Tashkin, D. P., Simmons, M. S., & Tseng, C. H. (2012). Impact of changes in regular use of marijuana and/or tobacco on chronic bronchitis. *COPD: Journal of Chronic Obstructive Pulmonary Disease, 9*, 367–374. http://dx.doi.org/10.3109/15412555.2012.671868

Taylor, F. M., III. (1988). Marijuana as a potential respiratory tract carcinogen: a retrospective analysis of a community hospital population. *Southern Medical Journal, 81*, 1213–1216.

Taylor, D. R., Poulton, R., Moffitt, T. E., Ramankutty, P., & Sears, M. R. (2000). The respiratory effects of cannabis dependence in young adults. *Addiction, 95*, 1669–1677. http://dx.doi.org/10.1046/j.1360-0443.2000.951116697.x

Thu, K., Hayes, M., Miles, S., Tierney, L., & Foy, A. (2013). Marijuana "bong" smoking and tuberculosis. *Internal Medicine Journal, 43*, 456–458.

Tindall, B., Cooper, D. A., Donovan, B., Barnes, T., Philpot, C. R., Gold, J., & Penny, R. (1988). The Sydney AIDS Project: development of acquired immunodeficiency syndrome in a group of HIV seropositive homosexual men. *Australian and New Zealand Journal of Medicine, 18*, 8–15. http://dx.doi.org/10.1111/imj.12089

Ungerleider, J. T., Andrysiak, T., Tashkin, D. P., & Gale, R. P. (1982). Contamination of marihuana cigarettes with pathogenic bacteria: Possible source of infection in cancer patients. *Cancer Treatment Reports, 66*, 589–591.

Williams, S. J., Hartley, J. P., & Graham, J. D. (1976). Bronchodilator effect of delta1-tetrahydrocannabinol administered by aerosol of asthmatic patients. *Thorax, 31*(6), 720–723.

Wu, T. C., Tashkin, D. P., Djahed, B., & Rose, J. E. (1988). Pulmonary hazards of smoking marijuana as compared with tobacco. *New England Journal of Medicine, 318*, 347–351.

Zhang, L. R., Morgenstern, H., Greenland, S., Chang, S. C., Lazarus, P., Teare, M. D., . . . Liu, G. (2015). Cannabis smoking and lung cancer risk: Pooled analysis in the International Lung Cancer Consortium. *International Journal of Cancer, 136*, 894–903. http://dx.doi.org/10.1002/ijc.29036

Zhang, Z. F., Morgenstern, H., Spitz, M. R., Tashkin, D. P., Yu, G. P., Marshall, J. R., . . . Schantz, S. P. (1999). Marijuana use and increased risk of squamous cell carcinoma of the head and neck. *Cancer Epidemiology Biomarkers & Prevention, 8*, 1071–1078.

7

Marijuana-Impaired Driving

A Path through the Controversies

ROBERT L. DUPONT, ERIN A. HOLMES,
STEPHEN K. TALPINS, AND J. MICHAEL WALSH

INTRODUCTION

The United States has long recognized that alcohol impairs driving performance (Gouvin, 1987; DuPont, 2000; Sewell, Poling, & Sofuoglu, 2009). Nonetheless, alcohol-related driving was not only tolerated but seen as a source of humor in earlier decades. In 1973, 35.9% of all weekend nighttime drivers tested positive for alcohol in the National Roadside Survey (NRS), and 7.5% had blood alcohol concentrations (BAC) of 0.08 g/dl or higher (Berning, Compton, & Wochinger, 2015).

In 1980, Candace Lightner brought national attention to the alcohol-impaired driving problem when she founded Mothers Against Drunk Driving (MADD). The public responded. Law enforcement agencies prioritized alcohol-impaired driving, state legislatures passed new laws, including raising the minimum legal drinking age to 21 and lowering the illegal per se limit to 0.08 g/dl, and agencies produced countless public service announcements. American culture and social norms subsequently changed. The simple standard "Don't drink and drive" became widely accepted and the incidence of alcohol-related and alcohol-impaired driving plummeted. In 2013–2014, 1.5% of weekend nighttime drivers had BACs of 0.08 g/dl or higher, an astounding 80% decline from 1973. The dramatic reduction in alcohol-impaired driving has saved tens of thousands of lives. In 1982, an estimated 21,113 people were killed in crashes where at least one driver had a BAC of 0.08 g/dl or higher; in 2014, less than half that number, 9,967 people, were killed in crashes where at least one driver had a BAC of 0.08 g/dl or higher (National Highway Traffic Safety Administration [NHTSA], 2015). While no one is ready to declare victory in combating alcohol-impaired driving, these results represent an impressive 53% reduction in fatalities since 1982.

Unfortunately, while society learned to appreciate the dangers of alcohol-impaired driving over recent decades, it has ignored the growing dangers of drug-impaired driving. The results were predictable. In 2007, the first year that the NRS surveyed drivers for illicit drugs and medications, 16.3% of weekend nighttime drivers tested positive, while in 2013–2014, 22.5% were positive for drugs (Berning et al., 2015). Like alcohol, illicit drugs or medications can impair a person's ability to drive safely. The number of people killed in drug-related crashes increases with the drug use prevalence rate. Many were surprised when the percentage of fatally injured drivers with known positive drug test results increased from 28% in 2005 to 33% in 2009 (NHTSA, 2010); however, since that time the percentage has continued to rise. In 2013, 40% of fatally injured drivers tested positive (Fatality Analysis Reporting System, 2015).

The reduction in alcohol-related crashes is a remarkable triumph for the fields of public health and traffic safety but this progress did not happen quickly and was fraught with intense controversy, including litigation. Today's success in reducing alcohol-impaired driving has been realized through a comprehensive approach including the passage of strong policy, sustained and high visibility of enforcement efforts, implementation of evidence-based programs, targeting high-risk offenders for interventions, and public education and awareness campaigns. The lessons learned from the fight to eliminate drunk driving can now be employed to address the burgeoning drugged driving problem.

While many people are just beginning to appreciate the dangers of drugged driving, efforts to identify and reduce the problem actually began more than four decades ago. Despite these efforts, policymakers, practitioners, and advocates continue to encounter challenges unique to this issue that have impeded progress, especially in regards to marijuana-impaired driving. Simply put, marijuana-impaired driving is a much more complex issue than alcohol-impaired driving.

The current push to legalize marijuana for both recreational and medicinal uses, the differences in the potency, metabolism, and effects of marijuana use compared to alcohol, and a general lack of awareness on the part of the public about the inherent dangers of driving under the influence (DUI) of marijuana present difficulties for policymaking. In addition, concern has been expressed among some in the traffic safety community that extending the focus of impaired driving to include drugs will somehow detract from the important work still needed to reduce drunk driving fatalities. We argue that to continue to reduce motor vehicle fatalities, the issue of impaired driving must be addressed holistically. Thus, it is imperative to develop solutions to eliminate the growing problem of marijuana-impaired driving.

In this chapter we stress the importance of taking advantage of our national success combating alcohol-impaired driving to encourage specific ways to reduce the highway safety threat created by marijuana, the most commonly detected drug among fatally injured drivers.

METABOLISM OF MARIJUANA

Given that the nature of marijuana's acute effects are relevant to driving performance, we briefly review the drug's metabolism. The metabolism of marijuana is far more complicated than the metabolism of alcohol, but it is nonetheless well understood. When a person smokes marijuana, the smoke enters the lungs, allowing Δ9-tetrahydrocannabinol (THC), the primary psychoactive component in marijuana, to be absorbed into the bloodstream. Within seconds, THC reaches the brain. Unlike alcohol, which is water-soluble, THC is fat-soluble (lipophilic) but not water soluble. The body's fatty tissues, including the brain, rapidly absorb THC out of the blood so blood concentrations fall rapidly after consumption ends. The THC then reenters the bloodstream slowly from the fatty tissues and is metabolized and excreted in the urine and feces. Within hours, 11-nor-9-carboxy-THC (THC-COOH), the primary metabolite of THC, can be detected in the user's urine and feces. After a single use, the body eliminates the remaining metabolites over a period of a few days.

When a person consumes or ingests marijuana by eating baked goods or other foods, often referred to as edibles, THC is absorbed and sent directly to the liver, where it is partially metabolized before entering the general circulation and transport to the brain. The drug next slowly reenters the bloodstream, is further metabolized to carboxy-THC, and is eliminated from the body through the urine and feces. The behavioral effects of marijuana resulting from consumption of edibles are delayed roughly an hour or so but then become pronounced and can take up to 4 hr to reach peak THC blood concentrations and longer for its full effects (Colorado Department of Public Health & Environment, 2015).

Marijuana induces psychoactive effects regardless of how it is used. The intensity of the effect is determined by many factors including the THC potency of the product; how the marijuana is smoked, inhaled, or eaten; and the presence of tolerance related to prior marijuana use. For example, the expansion of new marijuana products, including specifically marijuana concentrates sold as butane hash oil or wax that are vaporized (i.e., "dabbing") have reached new levels of THC potency, ranging to upward of 90%.

Overall, the onset of the high is much faster when it is smoked because the THC reaches the brain more quickly compared to when it is ingested. The difference between smoking and eating marijuana can be significant for highway safety. The behavioral effects of smoked marijuana typically persist anywhere from 2 to 24 hr (Couper & Logan, 2004), depending on the prior drug use experience of the marijuana user and the complexity of the task (e.g., driving vs. mopping a floor), but its effects can last much longer for chronic and frequent users. Because the slow onset of the effect from edibles may result in the consumption of higher doses of the drug, users may not feel the full effects for an hour or longer after consumption. As a result, a marijuana user who has smoked the plant may suffer from immediate impact from the drug while driving, but the user who has eaten the drug may get behind the wheel of a vehicle before the full impact of the drug has been experienced, leading to an unexpected increase in the severity of impairment.

A comprehensive discussion of testing technology is outside the scope of this chapter. Readers are referred to review various available resources that address drug testing (American Society of Addiction Medicine, 2013; Hedlund, 2015; Reisfield, Bertholf Goldberger, & DuPont, in press).

DRIVING-RELATED EFFECTS OF MARIJUANA USE AND IMPAIRMENT

Marijuana is a brain-affecting drug that can significantly impair the ability to drive a motor vehicle safely (Downey et al., 2012; Li et al., 2012; Hartman & Huestis, 2013; Mann, Brands, MacDonald, & Stoduto, 2003).

Though there remains much debate about how marijuana impairment compares to alcohol impairment, it is important to understand that no matter the substance used by a driver, there is no single measure of impairment. Driving impairment does not mean that a driver is certain to be involved in a crash, rather that impairment increases the likelihood of crash and other unsafe driving outcomes. A literature review and meta-analysis of nine studies found that acute cannabis consumption doubled the risk of a driver being involved in a crash where someone is seriously injured or killed (Asbridge, Hayden, & Cartwright, 2012). A more recent study updating and revising past meta-analyses concluded that acute cannabis intoxication is associated with a statically significant increase of low to moderate magnitude in traffic crashes (Rogeberg & Elvik, 2016).

Today there is a wealth of evidence that marijuana is an impairing substance that affects skills necessary for safe driving. However, it is relevant to note that meta-analyses compare studies that were conducted using different protocols and different measures of marijuana.

Hartman and Huestis (2013) provide an excellent summary of recent research on the effects of marijuana use. Marijuana has significant impairing psychological and physiological effects, including but not limited to disorientation, changes in perception, thought formation and mood, lack of concentration, impaired memory, drowsiness, and sedation, all of which can impair driving behaviors (Couper & Logan, 2004). Marijuana use impairs also judgment and motor coordination and slows reaction time (Hartman & Huestis, 2013). Moreover, there is a relationship between marijuana use and risky behavior in both natural settings and clinical laboratory settings (Lane, Cherek, Tcheremissine, Lieving, & Pietras, 2005).

Like alcohol and other impairing substances, the effects of marijuana are dose-related with greater effects from higher doses (Hartman & Huestis, 2013). Additionally, like alcohol, the effects of marijuana are influenced by tolerance so a given dose of marijuana will have a greater effect on a novice or occasional user than on an experienced frequent marijuana user (Desrosiers, Ramaekers, Chauchard, Gorelick & Huestis, 2015).

A recent research collaboration among the National Institute on Drug Abuse, the White House Office on National Drug Control Policy (ONDCP), and NHTSA undertook the first-ever study of the effects of marijuana on driving performance using the National Advanced Driving Simulator. This research examined the effect of marijuana on standard deviation of lateral position, commonly referred to as weaving within the lane of traffic (Hartman et al., 2015). The study also examined the effect of marijuana alone and its effect when combined with alcohol, which is the most common co-occurrence of substances among drivers. Key findings of the study were that marijuana use increases weaving within the lane, as does alcohol. Additionally, when these substances were used in combination, there was an additive effect on driving impairment.

An important aspect of this study is that the measurements of THC in the blood reflect levels at the time of driving as the researchers were able to collect samples shortly after driving ceased. In a real-world setting, measurements are not taken immediately. So while the researchers were able to determine that 13.1 ng/ml of THC produces the same effects of 0.08 g/dl BAC (as it relates to standard deviation of lateral position), those levels would be much lower in the blood by the time a sample is collected by law enforcement. This type of simulator research is ongoing and will provide more information about how marijuana affects driving performance.

Researchers have also studied the impact of marijuana on cognitive functioning likely associated with driving performance. Battistella et al. (2013) studied the impact of marijuana use on driving ability of occasional marijuana users by tracking changes in the brain network and concluded that "smoking cannabis significantly decreases psychomotor skills and globally alters the activity of the main brain networks involved in cognition" as shown in deficits in critical tracking and task performance (p. 7). Another study of recreational marijuana users showed that executive function (a general term for neurologically-based skills involving mental self-regulation) and motor control are impaired by use of high-potency marijuana (13% THC; Ramaekers et al., 2006).

Recent research shows that impairment from marijuana use can be long lasting. A study of chronic, daily marijuana users assessed over a three-week period of abstinence showed prolonged impairment of psychomotor function on critical tracking and divided attention tasks necessary for driving safely (Bosker et al., 2013). Critical tracking "assesses operator performance when the person perceives a discrepancy between a desired and actual state and aims to reduce the error by compensatory movement during a continuous closed-loop system" (Bosker et al., 2013, p. 5) while divided attention "assesses the ability to divide attention between two tasks simultaneously" (Bosker et al., 2013, p. 2). Importantly, performance on critical tracking improved over three weeks of abstinence but was never fully recovered and remained significantly worse compared to occasional drug using controls; similar results were found for divided attention.

Over the past three decades, the potency of marijuana, measured by concentration of THC, has increased by about 300% (ElSohly, 2014). As such, past

performance studies using traditionally lower doses of THC (4%) may not be reliable in identifying the effects of marijuana (Mann et al., 2003; Ramaekers et al.,
2006). Specifically, the change in potency of the drug "raises questions about
the current relevance of findings in older studies on the effects of marijuana
use" and the impact may be worse today (Volkow, Baler, Compton, & Weiss,
2014, p. 2222). Moreover, emphasizing this point with regard to current research
findings is the fact that the federally funded research studies on the effects of marijuana administer marijuana with lower THC concentrations (e.g., in Hartman
et al., 2015, 2.9%–6.7%) than the average THC concentration of marijuana sold
in Colorado, of upwards of 20%.

IMPACT OF MARIJUANA ON HIGHWAY SAFETY

Marijuana is the most frequently detected illegal drug among drivers arrested
on suspicion of DUI (Cangianelli & Walsh, 2006; Crouch, Hersch, Cook, Frank,
& Walsh, 2002). Whereas estimating rates of DUI of any substance can be
influenced by detection factors (e.g., intensity of roadside monitoring; procedures
for determining presence of substance in the driver), recent research has found
that the prevalence of DUI related to marijuana is increasing. In the 2007 NRS,
8.6% of weekend night-time drivers tested positive for THC, the psychoactive
substance in marijuana (Berning et al., 2015). The number rose significantly
during the succeeding years as several states passed laws legalizing marijuana
in various forms (i.e., recreational and medical marijuana). In 2013–2014, 12.6%
of weekend night-time drivers tested positive for THC, a disconcerting 48% increase from 2007 (Berning et al., 2015).

Not surprisingly, researchers examining data from six states found that an
increasing percentage of fatally injured drivers tested positive for marijuana,
from 4.2% in 1999 to 12.2% in 2010 (Brady & Li, 2014). National fatality data
analyzed from NHTSA's Fatality Analysis Reporting System (FARS, 2015) revealed that in 2013 nationwide, 62.6% of fatally injured drivers were tested for the
presence of drugs. Of those drivers with a known test result, a drug in the FARS
list or another drug was detected in 38%. Nearly 35% of the identified drugs were
marijuana in some form (FARS, 2015; Hedlund, 2015).

The prevalence of marijuana among both dead and injured drivers underscores
the role of this drug in highway safety. A study of seriously injured drivers
admitted to the Maryland Shock-Trauma Center over a 90-day period found that
26.9% tested positive for marijuana compared to 30.6% who tested positive for
alcohol (Walsh et al., 2005). Marijuana positives were more common in younger
ages with 50% of drivers ages 16 to 20 testing positive and only 10% positive for
THC among those 55 and older.

Two states that recently legalized marijuana, Colorado and Washington, have
reported postlegalization traffic safety data. These data suggest that marijuana-
impaired driving has increased significantly. Colorado, which established a commercial medical marijuana market beginning in 2009, first passed Amendment

64, legalizing marijuana for recreational uses in 2012 and subsequently opened recreational marijuana shops in 2014. One study showed that marijuana-related traffic deaths increased by 66% in the four-year average (2013–2016) since Colorado legalized the use of recreational marijuana compared to the four-year average (2009–2012) prior to legalization; traffic fatalities overall only increased by 16% during this same period (Rocky Mountain HIDTA Strategic Intelligence Unit, 2017).

In 2009, marijuana-related traffic deaths involving operators testing positive for marijuana represented about 9% of all traffic fatalities. As Table 7.1 shows, by 2016 that figure more than doubled to nearly 21%. Consistent with previous years, in 2016 only 44% of drivers involved in traffic deaths were tested for drug impairment. Out of those drivers tested, one in five tested positive for marijuana (Rocky Mountain HIDTA Strategic Intelligence Unit, 2017). Figure 7.1 shows how these fatalities in Colorado line up against two important eras: 2009 in which medical marijuana was commercialized and 2013 in which recreational marijuana legalization was implemented.

In Washington State, there was a significant increase in the number of drivers suspected of DUI after Initiative 502 to legalize recreational marijuana was passed in 2012. That year 18.6% of all DUI cases in the state tested for drugs were positive for THC; from January through April, 2015, 33% were positive for THC (Couper, 2015). The number of fatally injured drivers positive for marijuana in

Table 7.1 MARIJUANA-RELATED TRAFFIC DEATHS IN COLORADO WHEN A DRIVER TESTED POSITIVE FOR MARIJUANA, 2006–2016

Crash Year	Total Statewide Fatalities (n)	Fatalities with Drivers Testing Positive for Marijuana (n)	Total Marijuana-Related Fatalities (%)
2006	535	33	6.17
2007	554	32	5.78
2008	548	36	6.57
2009	465	41	8.82
2010	450	46	10.22
2011	447	58	12.98
2012	472	65	13.77
2013	481	55	11.43
2014	488	75	15.37
2015	547	98	17.92
2016	608	125	20.56%

SOURCE: National Highway Traffic Safety Administrator's Fatality Analysis Reporting System, 2006–2011, Colorado Department of Transportation 2012–2016 and Rocky Mountain HIDTA Strategic Intelligence Unit, 2017.

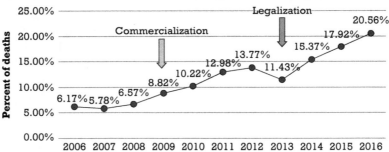

Percent of all traffic deaths that were marijuana-related when a driver tested positive for marijuana

Figure 7.1 Marijuana-related traffic deaths in Colorado by year and state marijuana policy status. Percentage of traffic fatalities where the drivers tested positive for marijuana.

NOTE: Data from National Highway Traffic Safety Administrator's Fatality Analysis Reporting System (2006–2011) and Colorado Department of Transportation (2012–2016).

SOURCE: Adapted from Rocky Mountain High Intensity Drug Trafficking Area Strategic Intelligence Unit (2017).

the state more than doubled following marijuana legalization, reaching 17% in 2014 (Tefft, Arnold, & Grabowski, 2016).

The Washington Traffic Safety Commission (WTSC) in collaboration with the State Toxicologist examined marijuana involvement in fatal crashes from 2010 to 2014 (WTSC, 2016). Among the 1,773 fatally injured drivers that were tested for both alcohol and drugs, 59.8% (*n* = 1,061) were positive for alcohol and/or drugs. This analysis not only looked at the presence of THC in drivers involved in fatal crashes, but it also differentiated between those who were positive for the presence of THC and those who were positive for the presence of the metabolite carboxy-THC. In 2014, 84.3% of the drivers who were positive for the presence of cannabinoids were positive for THC, compared to only 44.4% of cannabinoid-positive drivers in 2010.

In addition, analysts were able to determine the percentage of THC-positive drivers involved in fatal crashes who were above the state's 5 ng/ml per se limit and the percentage that was below the limit. Of the 75 drivers involved in fatal crashes in 2014 who tested positive for THC, 50.7% were above the 5 ng/ml limit (WTSC, 2016).

Self-report roadside survey data from Washington State also demonstrates that marijuana users frequently drive after using the drug. The Pacific Institute for Research and Evaluation administered a THC questionnaire in the summer of 2014 to 893 eligible participants, of which 220 identified that they had used marijuana within the past year. Of these individuals, 44% reported that they had used marijuana within two hours prior to driving. When asked about how marijuana use affected their driving ability, the majority (62%) felt that it did not have any impact. Perhaps even more alarming, 25% indicated that marijuana use improved their driving (Pacific Institute for Research and Evaluation, 2014).

A recent roadside study funded by NHTSA administered voluntary, anonymous drug tests to drivers in Washington State using oral fluid and blood tests to determine whether there were increases in the prevalence of marijuana-positive drivers postlegalization (Ramirez et al., 2016). The results of the chemical tests showed that compared to before the law (14.6% in Wave 1), more drivers were positive for THC six months (19.4% in Wave 2) and one year (21.4% in Wave 3) after implementation of the retail sales law (Ramirez et al., 2016). Although the differences were not statistically significant between waves of the study, there was a significant increase in daytime prevalence of THC between Waves 1 and 2 and Waves 1 and 3. These findings underscore the urgent need to address marijuana-impaired driving and to educate the general public about the dangers associated with this behavior. While much research has focused on states that have made policy changes to the legal status of marijuana, it is important to observe that the current and future effects of those policy changes are not limited to state boundaries.

MARIJUANA-IMPAIRED DRIVING IS NOT JUST ABOUT MARIJUANA

Combining other substances, particularly alcohol, with marijuana can have an additive or a synergistic effect, significantly increasing driving impairment (Downey et al., 2012; Griffiths, 2014; Hartman et al., 2015; Ramaekers et al., 2012). In their study utilizing driving simulator research, Hartman et al. (2015) found that using alcohol and marijuana in combination produces significantly higher blood concentrations of THC than marijuana use alone. Not only do marijuana users often simultaneously use alcohol but many also use other drugs at the same time that they use marijuana. Walsh et al. (2005) found that among seriously injured drivers, more than one third (37.9%) of drivers testing positive for marijuana also tested positive for alcohol. Additionally, of the seriously injured drivers that tested positive for marijuana, 38.7% also tested positive for another drug of abuse. Figure 7.2 shows that a large percentage of drugged drivers use multiple drugs simultaneously.

Other studies reveal this trend as well. Researchers reviewing data from drivers killed in crashes in 14 states between 2005 and 2009 found that 19.9% tested positive for two or more substances (Grady & Li, 2013). In a recent study conducted in Miami, Florida, the Miami–Dade Police Department collected samples from drivers arrested for DUI, regardless of BAC (Logan, Mohr, & Talpins, 2014). Among this sample, 79% were alcohol-positive, 41% were drug-positive, and specifically 30% tested positive for recent marijuana use. Among drivers who were alcohol-free, 78% were positive for at least one drug, most commonly marijuana (72%). Among alcohol-positive drivers with less than the illegal limit, 22% were positive for drugs, and all were positive for marijuana. Among

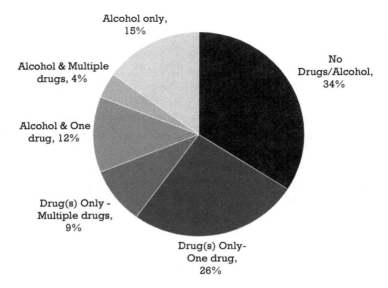

Figure 7.2 Prevalence of drugs and alcohol in a study of seriously injured drivers.
SOURCE: Adapted from Wash et al. (2005).

drivers with illegal BACs, 39% were drug-positive, and 22% were positive for marijuana. Lastly, the WTSC (2016) analysis of drivers involved in fatal crashes in Washington State reported the presence of cannabinoids in combination with other substances (alcohol and drugs). These statistics, displayed in Table 7.2, reveal that polysubstance use among fatally injured drivers in Washington State is increasing.

Table 7.2 DRIVERS INVOLVED IN FATAL CRASHES IN WASHINGTON TESTING
POSITIVE FOR ALCOHOL, THC, OR MULTIPLE SUBSTANCES, 2010–2014

	2010	2011	2012	2013	2014	Total 2010–2014	Change 2010–2014 (%)
No Drug, No Alcohol	147	151	151	147	116	712	−21.1
Alcohol Only ≥0.08	67	67	60	69	51	317	−23.9
THC Only	9	7	13	7	20	56	122.2
Carboxy-THC Only	11	10	7	3	6	37	−45.5
THC + Alcohol ≥0.08	16	16	12	16	23	83	43.8
THC + Drugs	6	3	8	5	17	39	183.3
THC + Drugs + Alcohol ≥0.08	2	5	2	3	6	18	200.0

SOURCE: Washington Traffic Safety Commission (2016).

Overall, the results of these studies clearly demonstrate the critical need for polydrug testing of all DUI suspects; unfortunately today, both legally drunk drivers (i.e., with BACs of 0.08 g/dL or greater) and those with low BACs are rarely tested for drugs other than alcohol.

PROMISING STRATEGIES FOR REDUCING MARIJUANA-IMPAIRED DRIVING

The nation has made impressive progress in reducing alcohol-impaired driving. This success can inform our strategy to reduce marijuana-impaired driving. It is illegal to drive while impaired by alcohol or other drugs in every state in the nation. That sounds simple enough, but there is no bright line standard to judge impairment, making prosecution for impaired driving difficult. In the case of alcohol, the country has evolved, over many decades, a per se standard for alcohol-impaired driving—0.08 g/dL BAC as measured in blood or breath. With alcohol, the general relationship between BAC level and impairment is supported by rigorous data (Hingson, Heeren, & Winter, 2000). The same cannot be said for other drugs. Unfortunately, reaching a nationally agreed upon illegal limit for drugs, including marijuana, is not feasible due to a lack of convergence of scientific evidence that establishes a close relationship between drug concentrations in the body and impairment.

In confronting the epidemic of drug use in the 1980s, a strategy was developed for dealing with illegal drug use based on zero tolerance, meaning that any evidence of the presence of an impairing drug in a driver's system was illegal and, thus, a violation. However, if the driver was in possession of a valid prescription for the potentially impairing drug, then this zero tolerance standard was not imposed. This means that drivers testing positive for cocaine are in violation, but if they tested positive for amphetamine and had a valid prescription, they have an affirmative defense to the charge of impaired driving.

The zero tolerance strategy was adopted in 1987 by the US Department of Transportation and imposed on commercial drivers, airline pilots, train engineers, and others in safety-sensitive jobs following a high-profile crash of a Conrail train in Chase, Maryland, on January 17, 1987. The train engineer who caused the crash tested positive for carboxy-THC, a metabolite of marijuana. No alcohol or other drugs were present in his system. Since that time, this strict standard for commercial drivers has been in existence with little controversy; however, using such a strategy for all drivers has been met with significant controversy, especially for marijuana since marijuana may be detected long after chronic use. Nonetheless, a zero tolerance standard for driving after using marijuana, despite the complications of detecting recent use, can be justified. Drivers who violate our nation's drug laws, not the general public who shares the country's roadways with them, should assume the risk of incurring adverse consequences for their criminal activities. The concerns for the use of zero tolerance can be alleviated by using testing methods with shorter windows of detection, like breath, blood, or oral fluid. Further, it makes little sense to create a legal limit for illicit drugs or the illicit use of legal drugs (i.e., taking prescriptions medications without a valid prescription).

Greater Public Education

ALCOHOL MODEL

Not every problem is best solved by changing the law or using the criminal justice system as a regulatory program. Education alters social norms and keeps many people from engaging in socially undesirable conduct. Education works even better when reinforced by legal sanctions. Consider the national effort to reduce alcohol-impaired driving. For most of the 20th century, the majority of society did not take alcohol-impaired driving seriously. That day has passed. The birth of nonprofit organizations—two in particular, Remove Intoxicated Drivers, established by Doris Aiken in 1978, and MADD, established by Candace Lightner in 1980, five days after a recidivist drunk driver killed her 13-year old daughter Cari—changed the way that Americans address alcohol-impaired driving. (For a history of these efforts, see Fell & Voas, 2006; Jacobs, 2013; Lerner, 2011). MADD humanized the problem by identifying real-life victims and revealing the devastating impact that the decision to drive drunk can have on others. This served as the catalyst for a social and political movement whose moral authority continues to grow. MADD and its many allies persuaded legislatures to adopt laws that set 21 as the minimum legal drinking age and 0.08 g/dl as the illegal per se alcohol limit, to encourage police departments to use sobriety checkpoints and saturation patrols to identify and deter drunk drivers and to persuade the nation to treat alcohol-impaired driving as a serious national health problem. MADD was so effective that it now enjoys a 94% national name recognition (Fell & Voas, 2006).

Today, MADD is joined in their work to eliminate alcohol-impaired driving by countless other individuals and nonprofit associations, including the American Automobile Association, American Association of Motor Vehicle, the Foundation for Advancing Alcohol Responsibility (Responsibility.org; formerly known as the Century Council), Governors Highway Safety Association (GHSA), International Association of Chiefs of Police (IACP), National District Attorneys Association, National Sheriffs Association, and the Society of Forensic Toxicologists, as well as government agencies, most notably the NHTSA, the National Transportation Safety Board (NTSB), the National Institute on Drug Abuse, and ONDCP.

Together, these organizations and agencies changed the way the nation views alcohol-impaired driving, "arguably the ultimate success in prevention" (El-Guebaly, 2005, p. 36). The road to success, however, has been long. It has taken more than three decades to achieve the current reductions in alcohol-impaired driving. Along the way, efforts to address the problem have spurred multiple controversies and subsequent compromises often involving legislation and court decisions. What appears now to be settled policy and consensus remains an unfinished public health and public safety priority. The good news is that these organizations and advocates alike remain steadfast in their commitment to the elimination of drunk driving. In recent years, several of these agencies and organizations have realized the need to view impaired driving as a problem that encompasses more than just alcohol. The result has been an emergence of much-needed leadership on the issue of drugged driving and an expansion of mandates and missions.

RECOGNIZING THE SEVERITY OF THE MARIJUANA HIGHWAY SAFETY THREAT

To reduce marijuana-impaired driving, it is necessary to bring the same degree of attention and commitment to reduce marijuana use by drivers that advocates and agencies brought to bear on alcohol-impaired driving. Unfortunately, these efforts face an uphill battle. In the summer of 2015, a Gallup poll revealed that only 29% of respondents view marijuana-impaired driving as a serious problem whereas 79% of respondents identified alcohol-impaired driving as a serious problem. Of note, Americans age 18 to 29 were most likely to say alcohol-impaired driving is a serious problem (88%); this age group was also least likely to consider marijuana-impaired driving to be a serious problem (22%). Not surprisingly, this young age group also holds the highest rate of approving legalization of marijuana compared to all other age groups.

It is particularly concerning that lax attitudes by youth about the dangers of marijuana-impaired driving is compounded by their lack of driving experience, which in and of itself increases their crash risk. The risk of motor vehicle crashes is higher among 16- to 19-year-olds than among any other age group. In fact, per mile driven, teen drivers ages 16 to 19 are nearly three times more likely than drivers aged 20 and older to be in a fatal crash (Insurance Institute for Highway Safety, 2013). The 2011 Monitoring the Future survey revealed that driving after using marijuana surpassed driving after drinking alcohol among 12th graders. Of those surveyed, 12.4% indicated that they had driven after using marijuana in the past two weeks whereas only 8.7% reported driving after drinking alcohol in that same time period (O'Malley & Johnston, 2013).

It is imperative that the public be educated to recognize the serious highway safety threat of marijuana use by drivers and support effective legislation to discourage it. The fact that marijuana is commonly used (and legal in some states for recreational use by those aged 21 and older), is associated with impairing effects, and is viewed by so many people as safe highlights how difficult this challenge will be. Even the National Organization for the Reform of Marijuana Laws (1996), a leading marijuana advocacy group, has long-warned users about impairment: "The responsible cannabis user does not operate a motor vehicle or other dangerous machinery while impaired by cannabis, nor (like other responsible citizens) while impaired by any other substance or condition, including some medicines and fatigue."

There are only a handful of nonprofit organizations that have consistently advocated against marijuana-impaired driving, including most notably Community Anti-Drug Coalitions of America, IACP, Institute for Behavior and

Health, National District Attorneys Association, National Sheriffs Association, and Society of Forensic Toxicologists. However, in the last two years, they have been joined by other powerful partners including GHSA, MADD, Responsibility. org, and We Save Lives.

In recent years, the federal government has gotten the message that this issue requires attention and has begun to provide leadership. Particularly noteworthy are the efforts of ONDCP that identified this issue as a high priority in 2010 following the publication of the NHTSA-funded NRS. In its 2011 National Drug Control Strategy, ONDCP set the goal of reducing the prevalence of drugged driving by 10% by the year 2015. As part of this strategy, ONDCP encouraged states to adopt per se drug laws, increase law enforcement training, and collect more and better quality data. The agency was unequivocal in stating that preventing drugged driving must become a national priority on par with preventing drunk driving. Similarly, the NTSB began prioritizing drug-impaired driving in 2012 and encouraged NHTSA to take action (NTSB, 2012). NHTSA is charged with implementing the policy and has begun the process of educating the public about its dangers as well as pursuing drugged driving research objectives.

Other agencies and groups have made important contributions to the state of knowledge, specifically the National Institute on Drug Abuse, which funded, with ONDCP, an extensive report on drugged driving research with a particular focus on marijuana in 2011 (DuPont, Logan, Shea, Talpins, & Voas, 2011). More recently, GHSA convened an expert panel and published a comprehensive report entitled *Drug-Impaired Driving—A Guide For What States Can Do*, in partnership with Responsibility.org (Hedlund, 2015). This report contains a multitude of recommendations that state officials can employ to address the problem in their jurisdictions and identifies national research and program needs.

Another promising development and step forward occurred on December 4, 2015, when the president signed the Fixing America's Surface Transportation Act, known as the FAST Act (see http://www.fhwa.dot.gov/fastact/), into law. The multiyear highway bill requires the Department of Transportation to conduct a series of research projects to examine the relationship between marijuana and driving impairment and identify methods and technology to detect marijuana-impaired drivers. NHTSA was also charged with the task of increasing public awareness about the dangerous associated with drug-impaired driving.

While all of these marijuana-highway safety efforts are helpful, the traffic safety community as a whole, including NHTSA, continues to remain primarily focused on alcohol-impaired driving (Government Accountability Office [GAO], 2015). The reluctance of some advocates to broaden their focus to include marijuana-impaired driving is an impediment to progress. Some fear that taking on drug-impaired driving will dilute their focus on and resources for reducing alcohol-impaired driving. This policy bias may be justified by government agencies from a strictly numbers perspective given the high prevalence of alcohol-impaired drivers using various transportation systems at any given time; however, advocates need not make a choice between addressing alcohol-impaired driving and drug-impaired driving.

We believe the failure to properly address drug-impaired driving is misguided and counterproductive. The research substantiates that there is an enormous overlap of alcohol use and drug use among impaired drivers. The data presented here shows that an increasing number of individuals drive after using both alcohol and marijuana. Moreover, the expanded focus on drugs, including marijuana, will enhance public support for the efforts to reduce alcohol-impaired driving and likely open additional sources of financial and public support in this area. Linking the focus on alcohol-impaired driving and drug-impaired driving is the right thing to do for the nation's health and safety and should be done, even if it is challenging.

Moving forward, federal, state, and local agencies should work collaboratively with the various relevant nonprofit organizations to bring more attention to the issue, put a face on the crime, specifically drug-impaired driving victims and families, and educate the public about the issues as they did with alcohol-impaired driving. This strategy will ultimately make our roads safer.

More Effective Laws

ALCOHOL MODEL—FEDERAL LEVEL

Congress has played an integral role in shaping state legislation for alcohol-impaired drivers by including incentives and penalties in federal appropriations bills. For example, in October 2000, Congress passed and the president signed the Department of Transportation's 2001 Appropriations Act. The law provided that states that failed to pass a 0.08 g/dl BAC law by 2004 would lose a portion of their federal highway constructions funds. At the time the law was passed, 25 states had laws prohibiting driving with a BAC of 0.08 g/dl or higher (Rodriguez-Iglesias, Wiliszowksi, & Lacey, 2001); not surprisingly the remaining 25 states passed 0.08 laws by mid-2004 (NHTSA, 2004a). Also, alcohol, which is legal for people age 21 and older, is treated differently for commercial drivers with the cut-off at 0.04 g/dl BAC, well under the legal cut-off for other drivers of 0.08 g/dl BAC for an offense. Similarly, Congress has enacted legislation encouraging states to adopt promising and effective strategies such as administrative license revocation systems, ignition interlock, DUI courts, and the 24/7 Sobriety Program (Fixing America's Surface Transportation Act, 2015).

MARIJUANA CHALLENGE—FEDERAL LEVEL

Congress can replicate the success it experienced with alcohol-impaired driving policy by encouraging states to pass effective legislation and implement evidence-based practices to combat drug-impaired driving. Unfortunately, Congress has shown little interest in passing serious legislation specifically geared toward drug-impaired driving, let alone marijuana-impaired driving, by noncommercial drivers. Congressman Jared Polis (D-Colorado) who proposed in 2015 a federal bill that would legalize marijuana (the Regulate Marijuana Like Alcohol Act; H.R. 1013), introduced H.R. 4179 (The "Lucid Act"), a bill to amend Title 23 "to establish requirements relating to marijuana-impaired driving, and for other purposes." Essentially, the bill would have prohibited a state with laws legalizing marijuana for any purpose from receiving certain federal grants unless the state had a law prohibiting people from driving or being in actual physical control of a vehicle while impaired by marijuana and (b) "enforce[d] the law using training and methods for determining cognitive or physical marijuana impairment." The bill died in the Subcommittee on Highways and Transit with good reason. Such a bill has little or no value particularly since virtually every state already prohibits drug-impaired driving (Walsh, 2009) and provides at least some basic training to its law enforcement. An example of Congress getting serious about this important issue and address it in a more effective way is the FAST Act. This act contains provisions for drugged driving research and education efforts and is a meaningful step toward making significant improvements in identifying and reducing marijuana-impaired driving.

STATE LAWS—ALCOHOL

Impaired driving, like the vast majority of crimes, is primarily a local issue. This offense is defined by state law and generally prosecuted by state and local officials. While the language varies among the states, current state laws typically prohibit:

- Anyone from driving while impaired by alcohol;
- Anyone under 21 years of age from driving with any alcohol in his or her system (i.e., zero tolerance); and
- Anyone from driving with a blood or breath alcohol level of 0.08 g/dl or higher.

The zero tolerance standard for alcohol use by those under 21 and the 0.08 g/dl illegal per se limit provisions for those aged 21 and older make it easier for officers to enforce the law and for prosecutors to prove their cases. Further, there is strong evidence suggesting that zero tolerance laws for drivers under age 21 (Goodwin et al., 2013) and the 0.08 illegal limit have significantly improved traffic safety and saved lives (NHTSA, 2004b).

STATE LAWS—MARIJUANA

As previously noted, it is illegal in every state to drive while impaired by any drug listed in the Controlled Substances Act, including marijuana. These controlled substances are drugs with abuse potential; however, only a minority of states have per se laws for drugs. These laws generally fall into two categories: (a) zero tolerance per se laws that prohibit a person from driving with any detectable amount of a drug in his or her system or (b) per se laws that establish a threshold or limit for enforcement, analogous to the 0.08 illegal limit for alcohol (DuPont et al., 2012; DuPont, Logan & Talpins, 2010; Larkin, 2015).

The federal government set the standard for drug-impaired driving in the mid-1980s when it defined any level of certain widely used illegal drugs above a specified cut-off level, including marijuana, as a violation for the estimated

10 million commercial drivers and many others in safety-sensitive occupations. This historic effort to protect highway safety treated prescribed potentially abused drugs (i.e., controlled substances) differently if the driver had a valid prescription for the drug and was using it as prescribed. This was done to avoid interfering with sound medical practice.

As previously noted, there is a distinction for alcohol—one standard for drivers who can legally consume the substance (0.08 g/dl BAC limit) and another for individuals under the minimum legal drinking age (zero tolerance). This distinction has been used for prescription drugs as previously noted. It also provides precedent for using the zero tolerance per se standard for illegal drugs.

The state-level legalization of marijuana for medical and recreational purposes has made enforcing marijuana-impaired driving more difficult because marijuana use remains illegal in all 50 states under federal law and US international treaty obligations. The US Constitution clearly states in its Supremacy Clause that federal law supersedes state law, a fact that has been reaffirmed by the Supreme Court (*Arizona v. United States*, 2012). However, the Obama administration's decision not to enforce the federal law on marijuana when it conflicts with state law enormously complicates this issue.

Regardless of the legal status of marijuana, arrest and conviction for driving under the influence of marijuana is possible. Every state has an impairment-based statute that requires law enforcement to prove impairment of the driver through the gathering and documentation of evidence. For these cases to be successfully prosecuted, linkages must be made to the documented behavioral evidence and recent drug use. While difficult, it is not impossible to prove impairment.

Two of the states where marijuana is legal for recreational uses have rejected zero tolerance laws with Washington State establishing 5 ng/ml THC per se limit and Colorado establishing a weaker 5 ng/ml THC permissible inference law. The other states that have legalized recreational marijuana (Alaska and Oregon as well as the District of Columbia) have refrained from passing their own per se statutes. Instead, these jurisdictions have opted to leave their existing impairment-based laws in effect. For states that permit marijuana for medical uses, zero tolerance per se laws should include an affirmative defense for drivers who can verify that their use of marijuana is recommended by a physician (e.g., possession of a current medical marijuana ID card). Per se laws with established illegal drug limits do not need to contain exceptions for prescription drugs or marijuana (THC) unless the thresholds are set so low that the laws essentially act as zero tolerance. An example of this might be Pennsylvania, which has a de facto 1 ng/ml THC limit.

Considering those states that have not legalized recreational marijuana, as of September 2016, eight states have zero tolerance per se laws for THC and metabolites (Arizona, Delaware, Georgia, Indiana, Oklahoma, Rhode Island, South Dakota [for drivers under 21 only], and Utah). An additional three states (Iowa, Michigan, and Wisconsin) have zero tolerance laws for THC only with no restriction on metabolites. Per se limits for THC are present in Illinois (5 ng/ml), Montana (5 ng/ml), Nevada (2 ng/ml), Ohio (2 ng/ml), Pennsylvania (1 ng/ml).

Figure 7.3 presents the current state marijuana-impaired driving laws as of September 2016 and is updated regularly by the Foundation for Advancing Alcohol Responsibility.

Some commentators on this important traffic safety issue prefer the per se illegal limit laws to the zero tolerance per se laws; however, unlike alcohol, there is no close relationship between blood concentrations of drugs (or drug metabolites)—including marijuana—and impairment (Hartman & Huestis, 2013).

Individual tolerance is an important factor that hinders the ability to set blood or other tissue limits for marijuana and other drugs. First-time and infrequent users will likely be more sensitive to the effects of marijuana than a frequent or chronic user (Desrosiers et al., 2015). An easily understood example of the

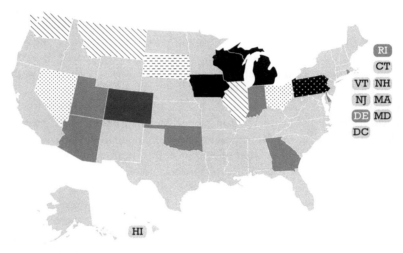

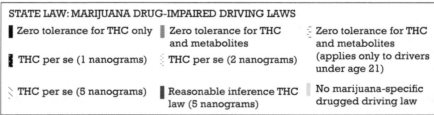

STATE LAW: MARIJUANA DRUG-IMPAIRED DRIVING LAWS		
Zero tolerance for THC only	Zero tolerance for THC and metabolites	Zero tolerance for THC and metabolites (applies only to drivers under age 21)
THC per se (1 nanograms)	THC per se (2 nanograms)	
THC per se (5 nanograms)	Reasonable inference THC law (5 nanograms)	No marijuana-specific drugged driving law

* For states without a marijuana-specific per se drugged driving law, an impairment-based statute exists that requires law enforcement to prove impairment of the driver. Successful prosecution depends on documented behavioral evidence and recent drug use.

** West Virginia's per se law applies to state-registered medical cannabis users.

To submit a law update, please contact out Director of Traffic Safety at erin.holmes@www.responsibility.org

Figure 7.3 Marijuana drug-impaired driving laws in the united states (as of December 2017).
SOURCE: Adapted from Foundation for Advancing Alcohol Responsibility (2017).

impossibility of identifying a tissue level for drugs is methadone. Methadone is typically prescribed for tolerant patients in doses of 100 mg or more a day. For most nontolerant individuals, a dose of 40 mg can be lethal, the ultimate "impairment." In addition to tolerance, impairment resulting from drug use will be related to various aspects of the individual user including age, sex, weight, and disease state of the individual (DuPont et al., 2011). The same dose of a drug will impact users differently based on these and many other factors. Furthermore, the ever-expanding number of impairing drugs and drug combinations often used with marijuana (including alcohol) that enhance the marijuana's impact prevent any single per se limit from effectively addressing all drivers (DuPont, Reisfield, Goldberger, & Gold, 2013).

The alcohol per se precedent of 0.08 g/dl BAC simply is impossible to apply for other drugs, including marijuana, because there is no stable relationship between impairment level and blood or other tissue levels. No amount of additional research can come up with blood levels above which all drivers are impaired and below which all drivers are not impaired; the pursuit of these levels for drugs, including marijuana, is a fool's errand (DuPont et al., 2011, 2013). In its recently released report on drugged driving, the GAO (2015) echoes these sentiments indicating that "identifying a link between impairment and drug concentrations in the body, similar to the 0.08 BAC threshold established for alcohol is complex and, according to officials from [the Society of Forensic Toxicologists] possibly infeasible" (p. 13). As previously described, past research has not been able to identify a quantitative correlation between impairment and THC levels (e.g., Battistella et al., 2013). We remind readers of the recently controlled driving simulator study of occasional marijuana smokers that identified while-driving THC blood levels associated with impairment related to weaving within the lane similar to that seen at 0.05 g/dl BAC and 0.08 g/dl BAC (Hartman et al., 2015). Such THC levels are not useful for any enforcement practices, however, for numerous reasons, including that (a) THC blood levels fall so rapidly that such measured levels are vastly higher than any levels that would be identified in a driver arrested for impaired driving due to the long delay in testing and (b) because THC is often used in combination with other substances by many impaired drivers.

Also complicating matters is that among some chronic heavy and frequent marijuana users, there can be a positive test for metabolites in the blood for weeks after smoking stops. This occurs because chronic marijuana use causes the fatty tissues, including the brain, to become saturated with THC. Advocates for marijuana legalization often cite this fact as an argument against drug testing and zero tolerance policies and in response some states limit zero tolerance laws for THC only rather than THC metabolites. But what is omitted from this argument is the fact that a chronic frequent marijuana user can be influenced by the drug for a long period of time after their marijuana use stops. As previously noted, research has shown that chronic marijuana use can impair a person's ability to drive for up to three weeks after stopping marijuana use (Bosker et al., 2013). Further, the marijuana lobby ignores the fact that nonchronic users who smoke one or two marijuana joints are likely to test positive for carboxy-THC at standard cut-off levels for only two or three days with many testing negative 24 hr after smoking marijuana. After three to five days, such users almost always test negative.

Some critics of urine testing for marijuana claim that no one should test for carboxy-THC because carboxy-THC is an inactive metabolite that has no impact on brain function. However, the presence of carboxy-THC means that the individual had THC in their brains when the urine sample was taken (Institute for Behavior and Health, 2015). The majority of carboxy-THC is quickly eliminated from the body, but the presence of long-term carboxy-THC is a marker that the individual has sequestered THC in his or her fatty tissues, including the brain.

Oral fluid (i.e., saliva) testing for drug use is becoming more common and is preferred by some to blood and urine testing because it requires little training for law enforcement officers, less cooperation from the subject, is minimally invasive, and does not require the officer be the same gender as the subject. Oral fluid testing is also resistant to adulteration (Private Sector Oral Fluid Testing Advisory Board, 2007). Oral fluid testing identifies THC, not carboxy-THC, and has a shorter detection window. The process of obtaining a warrant to perform a blood draw can take several hours and during this time, the THC in the suspect's body is rapidly metabolizing. Subsequently, the blood results reflect a THC level that is much lower than it was at the time the suspect was driving. The benefit of using oral fluid with impaired driving suspects is that the collection can be performed at the roadside, ensuring that the results reflect drug use that is contemporaneous with the act of driving. Using oral fluid testing to identify drugs among DUI suspects has been used successfully as a specimen for both screening and confirmation testing, although there are differences among devices in their sensitivity in screening for marijuana (Logan, Mohr, & Talpins, 2014).

LEGAL LIMITS
Setting an illegal limit for marijuana or any drug that is illicit under federal law makes little sense and sends the unintended message that driving with small amounts of illegal drugs in the system is safe or acceptable.

Some people argue that per se and zero tolerance laws violate people's rights by forcing them to choose between one activity (driving) or another (consuming drugs); however, no one has a constitutional right to drive or to consume marijuana: *Montana v. Egelhoff* (1996) ruled that a defendant does not have a right under the Due Process Clause to present an intoxication defense even to a crime requiring proof of mens rea. Further, the suggestion that use of the zero tolerance per se standard for the general public is irrational begs the question of why this standard is sensible and justified for airline pilots, flight attendants, railroad engineers, and conductors, among other groups involved in transportation, and not for drivers behind the wheel in neighborhoods and on the highway. The different standards for these groups reflect political, not scientific, decisions.

While some researchers found that the mere passage of per se and zero tolerance laws have little impact on traffic fatalities (Anderson & Rees, 2012; Holmgren, Holmgren, Kugelberg, Jones, & Ahlner, 2008), we believe that the data are more a reflection of how laws were implemented and how offenders have been treated, rather than a reflection of the laws themselves. Per se and zero tolerance laws are useful tools to address the drugged driving problem. If they are implemented properly, widely publicized, and coupled with high visibility enforcement and appropriate sanctioning, they should work well.

Overall, drug-impaired driving is an area where policy has largely outpaced research and the establishment of per se limits for THC has been done absent scientific evidence. Current research efforts are focused on determining whether the current nanogram limits are at appropriate cut-off levels for identifying impairment. Interestingly, trend data from Washington State revealed that of those fatally injured drivers who tested positive for THC between 2010 and 2014, only 56.7% were above the per se limit of 5 ng/mL (WTSC, 2015).

Analyses conducted on 302 drug recognition expert (DRE) cases where toxicology (blood tests) confirmed the presence of marijuana only found that there were no significant differences between cases where THC was above and below 5 ng/ml (Hartman, Richman, Hayes, & Huestis, 2016). The authors concluded that the 5ng/ml cut-off had limited relevance. A study conducted by Logan, Kacinko, and Beirness (2016) had similar outcomes, determining that there were minimal differences between subjects with high (>5ng/ml) and low (<5ng/ml) THC concentrations.

Some marijuana advocates are trying to take the high ground (pun intended) by establishing limits that are all but impossible to violate. For example, in 2015, in Illinois, House Bill 218 proposed a limit of 15 ng/ml of THC in the blood. Data from Sweden reporting the blood concentrations of THC among drivers arrested for driving impaired by marijuana showed that 90% of drivers had concentrations of THC lower than 5 ng/ml (Jones, Holmgren, & Kugelberg, 2008). The national limit for THC in Sweden is 0.3 ng/ml. These data support the position that setting cut-offs for highway safety at 5 ng/ml, let alone at 15 ng/ml, will be the equivalent of licenses to drive stoned. The governor of Illinois agreed that establishing such a high limit would greatly weaken the existing zero tolerance statute in the state. As a result, he opted to issue an amendatory veto of the bill. A modified version of this bill passed in the 2016 legislative session striking Illinois's existing zero tolerance law and establishing a 5 ng/ml THC per se limit. Both the 5 ng/ml limits set for Washington (per se) and Colorado (permissible inference) were political compromises rather than policy decisions rooted in science.

IMPLIED CONSENT

The vast majority of states and the District of Columbia have implied consent laws requiring drivers to provide blood, breath, and/or urine samples upon request by a law enforcement officer with probable cause to believe the person drove while impaired. Agreeing to this implied consent is a condition of obtaining a drivers permit. These provisions of the law encourage drivers to produce forensic samples, which make it easier for the prosecution to prove its case. Unfortunately, only a handful of states (Alabama, Arizona, Colorado, Georgia, Indiana, Kansas,

Louisiana, Missouri, New York, North Carolina, Ohio, Oklahoma, South Dakota, and Utah) have language in their implied consent statutes that allow for oral fluid testing in addition to traditional chemical tests. We encourage policymakers to consider including evidential oral fluid testing because of the many advantages it offers over both blood and urine testing.

TESTING RATES

One of the reasons that it is difficult to quantify the impact of drugged drivers is because so few drivers are tested for drugs. We urge testing of all drivers arrested for DUI for drugs as well as for alcohol. Despite the high prevalence rates for drug-impaired driving, officers typically do not test drivers who test above the illegal limit for alcohol for drug impairment to save time and money (GAO, 2015). This means that many drugged drivers escape detection.

In 1994, the Miami–Dade County State Attorney's Office reviewed data from 25,129 cases. It found that approximately 88% of drivers arrested for misdemeanor DUI tested at or above the alcohol illegal limit of 0.08 g/dl and that 91% tested above the limit or refused to provide breath samples for testing (Talpins & Hayes, 2004). Almost none of those individuals were tested for drugs. In the aforementioned Miami study, where police tested every driver they arrested for DUI for drugs, over 40% of the drivers had drugs in their system (Logan et al., 2014). Over half of these drivers provided breath samples above the illegal limit.

Length of time from arrest to specimen collection for drug testing is another relevant issue. A recent study determined the average length of time from arrest to blood draw among vehicular homicide and vehicular assault suspects in Colorado was over 2 hr and highlighted many of the complications that can delay testing (Wood, Brooks-Russell, & Drum, 2016).

Recent opinions released by the US Supreme Court also present challenges for testing impaired driving suspects for the presence of drugs using traditional methods. In *Missouri v. McNeely* (2013) and *Birchfield v. North Dakota* (2016), the Court held that law enforcement officers may compel breath tests without a warrant when they have probable cause to believe that a person drove while impaired as a search incident to arrest; however, they ruled that officers could not compel a blood test absent a warrant or exigent circumstances since blood testing is invasive. Consistent with that analysis, the Court opined in *Birchfield* that a state can criminalize the refusal to take a breath test but cannot criminalize the refusal to submit to a blood draw. At present, there is no breath test available to test for the presence of drugs, and states rely on either blood or urine testing. While the Court did not specifically rule on whether urine testing falls under the warrant requirement, it stands to reason that this form of testing would be treated similar to blood draws as it is more invasive than breath testing.

Oral fluid appears to provide a convenient solution. In *Maryland v. King* (2013), the Supreme Court approved the use of oral fluid DNA testing during the booking process. While one can never predict what the courts will do with 100% accuracy, we would expect the Court to treat oral fluid drug testing the same way it has treated oral fluid DNA testing. In other words, it appears that law enforcement officers may obtain oral fluid samples for drug testing without needing to obtain a warrant. Assuming this to be true, oral fluid drug testing presents a significant advantage over blood and urine drug testing.

Laboratory-based oral fluid tests can produce accurate and reliable results. On-site or so-called point of collection tests produce rapid results and can be read on-site by a law enforcement officer (DuPont et al., 2011; Bosker & Huestis, 2009; Houwing et al., 2012). Despite the significant advantages of oral fluid tests as previously discussed, there are several problems with the testing at present (Bosker & Huestis, 2009; Toennes, Steinmeyer, Maurer, Moeller, & Kauert, 2005). Some devices absorb the drug, which confounds the results. Smoking marijuana, as well as use of other drugs, can cause dry mouth, which may make oral fluid testing somewhat difficult for subjects. However, with the growing recognition of drug-impaired driving, new testing devices are being regularly developed and improved. The Integrated Project DRUID (Driving under the Influence of Drugs, Alcohol and Medicines), sponsored by the European Union, examined a number of such devices and found several promising possibilities (Schulze, Schumacher, Urmeew, & Auerbach, 2012). Research is continuing. In the meantime, on-site oral fluid devices provide a far better solution than doing nothing and are relatively inexpensive (Logan et al., 2014). All oral fluid screening test results need to be confirmed through laboratory testing before they could be introduced in criminal court.

Drug testing all DUI arrestees would greatly increase prosecution rates; however, the major impact of wider testing for drugs may be seen elsewhere. Virtually every state requires people convicted of impaired driving offenses to be evaluated for alcohol and drug problems and participate in treatment programs where indicated. Unfortunately, people convicted of DUI offenses routinely underreport their use of alcohol and drugs. In the absence of a drug test, treatment professionals are unlikely to identify or treat, or subsequently test for, concurrent drug problems. This can have significant consequences as drugged drivers appear to recidivate at far higher rates than alcohol-impaired drivers (Impinen et al., 2009; Holmgren et al., 2008; Christophersen, Skurtveit, Grung, & Morland, 2002).

Authorities also need to do a better job testing fatally injured drivers for drugs. NHTSA reported that between 56% and 65% of fatally injured drivers were tested for drugs during the years from 2005 through 2009 (NHTSA, 2010). In 2013 nationwide, only 62.3% of fatally injured drivers were tested for drugs; the percentage was considerably lower for surviving drivers with only 31.2% tested for drugs (Hedlund, 2015). Increasing the testing rate for these drivers, however, may be easier said than done.

Enforcement

BETTER TRAINED OFFICERS

An alternative option is to improve the academy and in-service training that officers receive to detect drugged drivers. A police officer can stop a motorist if the officer has a reasonable suspicion that the driver has committed or is committing any offense. Officers are trained to administer the Standardized Field Sobriety Test (SFST) to drivers they suspect are impaired. The SFST provides officers with a more objective means to determine whether a driver is impaired than the old-fashioned smell and appearance tests that officers historically used. The tests were adopted from medical science, but the standards for law enforcement officers were created by researchers who attempted to link the scoring criterion to the then-existing 0.10 g/dl BAC illegal limit. While these tests may be relatively in-sensitive when it comes to detecting many drivers who are specifically under the influence of marijuana (Moskowitz, 2007), if a driver fails the SFST, it provides further evidence of impairment and supports the officer administering alcohol and drug tests. We encourage agencies to adopt and implement programs specif-ically designed to facilitate the identification and investigation of drug-impaired drivers and at the same time to encourage the administration of drug tests for all drivers identified as impaired.

Officers who complete the Drug Evaluation and Classification Program are trained and certified as DREs. DREs rely on the SFSTs and other generally ac-cepted neurological tests as part of a standardized 12-step protocol to determine whether drivers are under the influence of drugs and, if so, what drug category or categories are most likely to be causing their impairment (Talpins & Hayes, 2004). As of December 2015, the International Association of Chiefs of Police had credentialed 7,892 DREs (International Association of Chiefs of Police, 2016). Unfortunately, DRE training is time-consuming and expensive. Officers are re-quired to complete 72 hr of classroom training as well as field certification, which takes that officer away from regular duties for several weeks. Another drawback is that even when trained, DRE officers typically conduct few investigations. This is often the result of investigations ending when a BAC above the illegal limit is detected as previously noted. Furthermore, if there are few DREs in a geographic region, it may not be possible for them to attend to every drugged driving sus-pect in a timely fashion (i.e., shortly after they are arrested). Finally, since the departments typically send their best DUI officers to DRE school, DREs often are promoted within a couple of years of completing their training.

To expand the number of officers who can identify drugged drivers, states have included blocks on drug-impaired driving in their academy training. Further, the NHTSA, IACP, and the Virginia Association of Chiefs of Police developed a mid-level training program, Advanced Roadside Impaired Driving Enforcement. This program is designed to bridge the gap between SFST and DRE examination and provides an additional 16 hr of training to educate officers on how to observe and identify signs of drug-related impairment. Advanced Roadside Impaired Driving Enforcement can be delivered in-person or online. Since 2009, in excess of 46,000 law enforcement officers have received classroom Advanced Roadside Impaired Driving Enforcement training (IACP, 2015).

HIGH VISIBILITY ENFORCEMENT

People tend to follow the law when they believe that the likelihood of being detected and apprehended for violating it is high. However, the chances of being caught driving impaired is low: In 2010, 112 million adults reported episodes of alcohol-impaired driving, but the police only arrested 1.4 million people for DUI. Thus, the police arrested a little over 1% of the people who drove while impaired. Increasing the arrest rate theoretically would improve deterrence; however, it is unlikely that we can ever increase the arrest rate sufficiently to catch enough impaired drivers to significantly impact the number of people who drive while impaired.

Fortunately, we do not need to make 10 million more annual arrests per year to make a difference. Research shows that high visibility enforcement changes the public's perception about the risks of being caught and reduces the incidence of impaired driving. Sobriety checkpoints provide the best example. While checkpoints typically do not generate a large number of arrests, their visibility sends a strong message to the community and creates a perception of heightened enforcement. Thus, they effectively reduce impaired driving trips, crashes, and fatalities (NTSB, 2013).

Administrative Remedial Measures

ALCOHOL AND ADMINISTRATIVE LICENSE REMOVAL/SUSPENSION
The wheels of justice turn slowly. Even the simplest DUI cases may take months or years to conclude. Recognizing the need for more urgent action, legislators in 42 states and the District of Columbia have adopted laws authorizing officers to immediately confiscate the licenses of motorists who drive under the influence of alcohol, who test at or above the 0.08 g/dL BAC standard, or who refuse to provide a blood or urine sample for BAC testing (NHTSA, 2008; Talpins et al., 2014; Wagenaar & Maldonado-Molina, 2007). These provide the drivers with a prompt post-revocation hearing where the drivers may contest the evidence and decision (*Mackey v. Montrym*, 1979). Administrative license removal (ALR) enforcement can be quite effective; they have reduced alcohol-related fatalities by 5-9%, or approximately 800 lives per year.

MARIJUANA AND ADMINISTRATIVE LICENSE REMOVAL/SUSPENSION
Only two states, Arizona and New Mexico, have ALR laws that apply to drugged drivers. The provisions are poorly enforced in no small part because the states historically have not had access to on-site kits to test drivers for drugs. The development of reasonably reliable oral fluid screening kits offers an opportunity to create an ALR law that works for drugged drivers. The Institute for Behavior and Health has developed a model ALR drug law that mirrors the alcohol laws (Talpins et al., 2014). The model allows officers with probable cause to believe that a driver was impaired to confiscate the driver's license if he or she tested positive for drugs at roadside using oral fluid methods. Of course, the drivers would have an opportunity to contest the officers' probable cause and the findings through an administrative process.

In the fall of 2015, GHSA published a report informed by a panel of national experts that included a recommendation that all states consider adopting ALR for drugged drivers, establishing parity with existing drunk driving revocation provisions (Hedlund, 2015).

Improved Data Collection

There remains much dispute over how serious the public safety threat is from marijuana-impaired driving; this is in part due to the available data (or lack thereof) on the marijuana-impaired driving problem. The federal government began conducting the NRS in 1973, and it has been collecting fatality data since 1975. Unfortunately, the government did not test drivers for drugs in until the 2007 NRS, and it not review the data it collected on fatally injured drivers who were tested for drugs until 2008. To this day, there remains "no national source of data on the extent of drug-impaired driving in the United States," and the sources that exist can provide only "limited" information (GAO, 2015, p. 6). Officers typically do not test drivers who test above the 0.08 illegal limit for alcohol for drug impairment. Further, "state data on impaired driving are often not centralized or complete," and there are no defined standards for drug testing (GAO, 2015, p. 12). To better appreciate the impact that drugs are having on driving, it is imperative that the states and federal government collect and analyze more data about the extent of marijuana—and other drug—use among drivers including all drivers arrested for being impaired. This amounts to an estimated 1.1 million drivers arrested for DUI each year nationally (Federal Bureau of Investigation, 2015).

The FARS data on fatally injured driver provides useful data on the role of marijuana in highway safety, but there are many improvements to the data collection, particularly related to standardization of testing and reporting, that can be made (Berning & Smither, 2014; Hedlund, 2015; Logan et al., 2013). Most important, all fatally injured drivers should be tested for alcohol as well as marijuana and other commonly used drugs of abuse. Furthermore, at present, only positive (and negative) test results for drug presence are reported to FARS; drug concentrations (i.e., nanogram levels) are not. This practice misses an opportunity to gather and analyze more robust crash data that would reveal characteristics about the drug-impaired driving problem. To make the FARS testing and reporting uniform as well as systematic will require a federal law and federal funding.

Another group of drivers to be routinely tested for drugs is seriously injured drivers. In addition to the FARS data, this would provide valuable information about the role of drugs in nonfatal injuries. The 2005 sample of seriously injured drivers in the Maryland shock-trauma centers is a landmark study in this field (Walsh et al., 2005). Ideally, a larger sample of other shock-trauma centers should be recruited to do similar studies on an ongoing, routine basis. Given the large overlap of drugs among drivers, we encourage testing all drivers who are admitted to major shock-trauma centers be tested for illicit drugs and medications as well as for alcohol.

Together, these improvements in data collection will produce valuable information about the extent of drug-impaired and polysubstance-impaired driving and provide an ongoing, comprehensive assessment of the role of marijuana and other drugs in highway safety. These changes will neither be cheap nor easy, but they are all doable, affordable, and important. Until data collection improves, it will be impossible to measure the full magnitude and characteristics of the marijuana-impaired driving problem. Readers are referred to the AAA Foundation report by Arnold and Scopatz (2016) on improving drug-impaired driving data.

More Effective Sanctions

Practitioners developed multiple programs that effectively reduce impaired driving recidivism through community corrections (DuPont, Shea, Talpins & Voas, 2010; Sabet, Talpins, Dunagan, & Holmes, 2013; Voas et al., 2011), including driving while intoxicated (DWI) courts and South Dakota's 24/7 Sobriety Program.

DWI courts are specialized, postconviction court programs that provide a structure of supervision, treatment, and accountability. These specialty courts follow the well-established drug court model and are based on the premise that repeat impaired driving can be prevented if the underlying causes of the behavior (e.g., substance abuse, mental health disorders) are identified and addressed. These programs focus on high-risk, high-need offenders who are not deterred by traditional sanctions as evidenced by multiple convictions. Traffic safety experts and other practitioners identified DWI courts as one of the 10 Promising Sentencing Practices at the 2004 NHTSA National DWI Sentencing Summit at the National Judicial College, and the program has not disappointed. The NTSB has also endorsed DWI courts as a proven strategy for addressing the repeat DWI offender problem (NTSB, 2013). A number of evaluations have found that this specialty court model reduces recidivism. Studies of DWI courts in Michigan and Georgia showed that participants recidivated at a significantly lower rate than nonparticipants (Fell, Tippetts, & Langston, 2011; Taylor, Zold-Kilbum, Carey, Fuller, & Kissick, 2008). The Georgia study reported recidivism was 63% lower for DWI court graduates after four years than that of DWI offenders who completed probation in adjacent counties (Fell, Tippetts, & Langston, 2011). As of December 2014, there were 262 stand-alone DWI courts and 407 DWI/drug (hybrid) courts established across America.

More recently, former Attorney General Larry Long developed South Dakota's 24/7 Sobriety Program for repeat DUI offenders. The 24/7 Sobriety Program does not require participants to undergo treatment initially; however, it prohibits them from drinking and using drugs. Offenders are monitored through twice-daily breath testing or continuous transdermal alcohol monitoring and random urine drug screens or drug sweat patches. Participants who test positive are subject to immediate but brief incarceration and may be ordered to participate in treatment programs (Long, Talpins, & DuPont, 2010). Researchers documented a 12% reduction of repeat DUI arrests at the county level in South Dakota communities that adopted the program (Kilmer, Nicosia, Heaton, & Midgette, 2013) and a possible 45% to 70% reduction in recidivism in Montana (Midgette & Kilmer, 2015). More recently, researchers determined that the implementation of the 24/7 Sobriety Program in South Dakota was associated with a 4.2% reduction in all-cause adult mortality with the largest reductions found among women and individuals over 40 years of age (Nicosia et al., 2016). While the 24/7 Sobriety Program initially focused on alcohol, it has been adapted for drugged drivers. The 24/7 Sobriety Program is an impressive innovation that is cost-effective. Unlike many other approaches to the problem of alcohol-impaired driving, the 24/7 Sobriety Program focuses not only on driving after drinking but also on the drinking behavior itself. This program requires drivers convicted of multiple violations of DUI laws not to drink alcohol while they are under supervision, whether or not they get behind the wheel. This is a paradigm shift that holds great promise not only to reduce alcohol and drug-impaired driving but also to promote lasting recovery from substance use disorders (DuPont & Humphreys, 2011).

The evidence that a large percentage of drivers arrested for alcohol-impaired driving also use other drugs, including marijuana, substantiates the necessity for all impaired drivers under supervision to be monitored for drug use, including marijuana use.

CONCLUSION

This chapter presents evidence that marijuana impairs driving and that marijuana use is a significant threat to highway safety. We make a series of practical and comprehensive recommendations to reduce this threat. First, greater public education using the alcohol model is needed to increase awareness of the significant highway safety threat posed by marijuana use. While public education on drugged driving in general is needed, marijuana presents the biggest threat as it is the most commonly used drug of abuse other than alcohol and because it is the primary stumbling block to better strategies to reduce drugged driving. Second, more effective laws targeting marijuana-impaired driving at the federal and state levels must be created and vigorously enforced. Third, enforcement strategies must be improved, including increased training for law enforcement officers to identify drug impairment, including marijuana impairment, among drivers. Fourth, high visibility enforcement is needed to send the message that those who drive impaired by any substance are likely to be detected and arrested and thus to deter drugged driving. Fifth, law enforcement can improve overall drugged driving detection and enforcement by testing all drivers arrested for DUI each year for marijuana and other drugs as well as for alcohol. Sixth, the use of administrative remedial measures like ALR can greatly enhance efforts to combat marijuana- and other drug-impaired driving by removing these drivers immediately from the roads. Seventh, improved data collection is needed, including standardizing testing to determine the prevalence of marijuana and other drugs among the public, fatally injured drivers, and drivers admitted to shock-trauma centers, among others. Eighth, more effective sanctions must be implemented through the development and expansion of innovative criminal justice programs including DWI courts and 24/7 Sobriety programs. Ninth, we must ensure that all drivers arrested for DUI are assessed for drug and alcohol use and referred to appropriate education and/or treatment interventions.

To conclude, there has been abundant research on marijuana-impaired driving for the past four decades not only in the United States but also in western Europe, Canada, Australia, and New Zealand (see international review by Watson and Mann, 2016). We have cited significant data demonstrating the extent of the problem and identified multiple ways to address it that are promising, if not proven. Moreover, the recent report by the National Academy of Sciences and National Academies of Science, Engineering, and Medicine (2017) contains a rigorous review of scientific research published since 1999 regarding the health impacts of cannabis/cannabis products, including an examination of marijuana's therapeutic effects and its potential for causing certain cancers, diseases, mental health disorders, and injuries. With respect to traffic safety, the National Academies of Science, Engineering, and Medicine committee explored whether there was evidence of a statistical association between cannabis use and motor vehicle crashes. The committee found "substantial evidence of a statistical association" and noted that these findings indicate a need for research to "further specify the strength of this association and to identify any mediating factors" (National Academies of Science, Engineering and Medicine, 2017, p. 237).

While we encourage additional research, today marijuana-impaired driving is a serious highway safety threat. Waiting for more research before vigorous action to reduce the problem is tragically irresponsible and results in property loss, injury, and loss of life. Strong and effective action must be taken now. Lack of research must not be an excuse for continued inaction on marijuana-impaired driving. We learned substantial lessons addressing the drunk driving problem; we can apply those lessons in the context of marijuana-impaired driving. We have a good understanding of what works to promote highway safety. We must make progress addressing marijuana-impaired driving now.

REFERENCES

American Society of Addiction Medicine. (2013). *Drug testing: A white paper of the American Society of Addiction Medicine.* Retrieved from http://www.asam.org/docs/default-source/public-policy-statements/drug-testing-a-white-paper-by-asam.pdf
Anderson, D. M., & Rees, D. I. (2012, November). Per se drugged driving laws and traffic fatalities. IZA Discussion Paper 7048. Bonn, Germany. Retrieved from http://ftp.iza.org/dp7048.pdf
Arizona v. United States, 567 U.S. 2012.

Arnold, L. S., & Scopatz, R. A. (2016). *Advancing Drugged Driving Data At The State Level: Synthesis of barriers and expert panel recommendations.* Retrieved from http://dx.www.aaafoundation.org/sites/default/files/AdvancingDruggedDrivingData.pdf

Asbridge, M., Hayden, J. A., & Cartwright, J. L. (2012). Acute cannabis consumption and motor vehicle collision risk: Systematic review of observational studies and meta-analysis. *British Medical Journal, 344,* e536. http://dx.doi.org/10.1136/bmj.e536

Battistella, B., Fornari, E., Thomas, A., Mall, J., Chtioui, H., Appenzeller, M., . . . Giroud, C. (2013). Weed or wheel! fMRI, behavioural, and toxicological investigations of how cannabis smoking affects skills necessary for driving. *PLoS ONE, 8,* e52545. http://dx.doi.org/10.1371/journal.pone.0052545

Berning, A., Compton, R., & Wochinger, K. (2015). *Results of the 2013–2014 National Roadside Survey of Alcohol and Drug Use by Drivers: Traffic safety facts research note.* Retrieved from http://www.nhtsa.gov/staticfiles/nti/pdf/812118-Roadside_Survey_2014.pdf

Berning, A., & Smither, D. D. (2014, November). *Understanding the limitations of drug test information, reporting, and testing practices in fatal crashes: Traffic safety facts research note.* Retrieved from http://www-nrd.nhtsa.dot.gov/Pubs/812072.pdf

Birchfield v. North Dakota, 579 U.S. (2016).

Bosker, W. M., & Huestis, M. A. (2009). Oral fluid testing for drugs of abuse. *Clinical Chemistry, 55,* 1910–1931. http://dx.doi.org/10.1373/clinchem.2008.108670

Bosker, W. M., Karschner, E. L., Lee, D., Goodwin, R. S., Hirvonen, J., . . . Ramaekers, J. G. (2013). Psychomotor function in chronic daily cannabis smokers during sustained abstinence. *PLoS ONE, 8,* e53127. http://dx.doi.org/10.1371/journal.pone.0053127

Brady, J. E., & Li, G. (2014). Trends in alcohol and other drugs detected in fatally injured drivers in the United States, 1999–2010. *American Journal of Epidemiology, 179,* 692–699. http://dx.doi.org/10.1093/aje/kwt327

Cangianelli, L. A., & Walsh, J. M. (2006). Evaluation of roadside oral fluid drug testing devices in Hillsborough County Florida. In A. G. Verstraete & E. Raes (Eds.), *Rosita-2 Project: Final report* (pp. 159–174). Ghent, Belgium: Ghent University.

Christophersen, A. S., Skurtveit, S., Grung, M., & Morland, J. (2002). Rearrest rates among Norwegian drugged drivers compared with drunken drivers. *Drug and Alcohol Dependence, 66,* 85–92. http://dx.doi.org/10.1016/S0376-8716(01)00187-9

Colorado Department of Public Health and Environment. (2014). Monitoring health concerns related to marijuana in Colorado: 2014: Changes in marijuana use patterns, systematic literature review, and possible marijuana-related health effects. Denver, CO: Author.

Couper, F. (2015, June 15). *Analysis of suspected impaired driving cases (DUI & DRE) received at the Washington State Toxicology Laboratory (statewide data from blood results): Preliminary data shown for 2015.* Retrieved from http://dx.learnaboutsam.org/wp-content/uploads/2015/08/THC-data-for-distribution_20150615.pdf

Couper, F. J., & Logan, B. K. (2004). *Drugs and human performance fact sheets.* Washington, DC: National Highway Traffic Safety Administration.

Crouch, D. J., Hersch, R. K., Cook, R. F., Frank, J. F., & Walsh, J. M. (2002). A field evaluation of five on-site drug-testing devices. *Journal of Analytical Toxicology, 26,* 493–499. http://dx.doi.org/10.1093/jat/26.7.493

Desrosiers, N. A., Ramaekers, J. G., Chauchard, E., Gorelick, D. A., & Huestis, M. A. (2015). Smoked cannabis' psychomotor and neurocognitive effects in occasional and frequent smokers. *Journal of Analytical Toxicology, 39*, 251–261. http://dx.doi.org/10.1093/jat/bkv012

Downey, L. A., King, R., Papafotiou, K., Swann, P., Ogden, E., Boorman, M., & Stough, C. (2012). Detecting impairment associated with cannabis with and without alcohol on the Standardized Field Sobriety Tests. *Psychopharmacology, 224*, 581–589. http://dx.doi.org/10.1007/s00213-012-2787-9

DuPont, R. L., & Humphreys, K. (2011). A new paradigm for long-term recovery. *Substance Abuse, 32*, 1–6. http://dx.doi.org/10.1080/08897077.2011.540497

DuPont, R. L. (2000). *The selfish brain: Learning from addiction.* City Center, MN: Hazelden.

DuPont, R. L., Logan, B. K., & Talpins, S. K. (2010). New strategies to curb drugged driving. *Between the Lines, 18*(4), 1–2.

DuPont, R. L., Logan, B. K., Shea, C. L., Talpins, S. K., & Voas, R. B. (2011). *Drugged driving: A white paper.* Retrieved from http://dx.www.whitehouse.gov/sites/default/files/ondcp/issues-content/drugged-driving/nida_dd_paper.pdf

DuPont, R. L., Reisfield, G. M., Goldberger, B. A., & Gold, M. S. (2013). The seductive mirage of a 0.08 g/dL BAC equivalent for drugged driving. *DATIA Focus, 6*(1), 36–43.

DuPont, R. L., Shea, C. L., Talpins, S. K., & Voas, R. B. (2010). Leveraging the criminal justice system to reduce alcohol- and drug-related crime: A review of three promising and innovative programs. *The Prosecutor, 44*, 38–42.

DuPont, R. L., Voas, R. B., Walsh, J. M., Shea, C., Talpins, S. K., & Neil, M. M. (2012). The need for drugged driving per se laws: A commentary. *Traffic Injury Prevention, 13*(1), 31–42. http://dx.doi.org/10.1080/15389588.2011.632658

El-Guebaly, N. (2005). Don't drink and drive: The successful message of Mothers Against Drunk Driving (MADD). *World Psychiatry, 4*, 35–36.

ElSohly, M.A. (2014). *Potency monitoring program quarterly report no. 123—Reporting period: 09/16/2013-12/15/2013.* Oxford, MS: University of Mississippi, National Center for Natural Products Research.

Fatality Analysis Reporting System. (2015). FARS Query System. Retrieved from http://www-fars.nhtsa.dot.gov/QueryTool/

Federal Bureau of Investigation. (2015). *Crime in the United States: 2014. Table 29, Estimated number of arrests.* Retrieved from http://dx.ucr.fbi.gov/crime-in-the-u.s/2014/crime-in-the-u.s.-2014/tables/table-29

Fell, J. C., & Voas, R. B. (2006). Mothers Against Drunk Driving (MADD): The first 25 years, *Traffic Injury Prevention, 7*(3), 195–212. http://dx.doi.org/10.1080/15389580600727705

Fell, J. C., Tippetts, A. S., & Langston, E. A. (2011). *An evaluation of the three Georgia DWI courts* (DOT HS 811 450). Washington, DC: U.S. Department of Transportation.

Fixing America's Surface Transportation Act (FAST). Pub. L. No. 114-94.

Foundation for Advancing Alcohol Responsibility. (2016). *State law: Marijuana drug-impaired driving laws.* Retrieved from http://responsibility.org/get-the-facts/state-map/issue/duid-zero-tolerance-and-per-se-laws/

Goodwin, A., Kirley, B., Sandt, L., Hall, W., Thomas, L., O'Brien, N., & Summerlin, D. (2013). Countermeasures that work: A highway safety countermeasures guide for

State Highway Safety Offices. (7th ed., Report No. DOT HS 811 727). Washington, DC: National Highway Traffic Safety Administration.

Gouvin, E. J. (1987). Drunk driving and the alcoholic offender: A new approach to an old problem. *American Journal of Law & Medicine, 12*, 99–130.

Government Accountability Office. (2015). *Drug-impaired friving: Additional support needed for public awareness initiatives* (Report to Congressional Committees, GAO-15-293). Washington, DC: Author.

Grady, J. E., & Li, G. (2013). Prevalence of alcohol and other drugs in fatally injured drivers. *Addiction, 108*, 104–114. http://dx.doi.org/10.1111/j.1360-0443.2012.03993.x

Griffiths, P. (2014). *An overview of drug-impaired driving in the EU.* Wellington: New Zealand Drug Foundation.

Hartman, R. L., & Huestis, M. A. (2013). Cannabis effects on driving skills. *Clinical Chemistry, 59*, 478–492. http://dx.doi.org/10.1373/clinchem.2012.194381

Hartman, R. L., Brown, T. L., Milavetz, G., Spurgin, A., Pierce, R. S., . . . Huestisa, M. A. (2015). Cannabis effects on driving lateral control with and without alcohol. *Drug and Alcohol Dependence, 154*, 25–37. http://dx.doi.org/10.1016/j.drugalcdep.2015.06.015

Hartman, R. L., Richman, J. E., Hayes, C. E., & Huestis, M. A. (2016). Drug Recognition Expert (DRE) examination characterisitcs of cannabis impairment. *Accident; analysis and prevention, 92*, 219–229. http://dx.doi.org/10.1016/j.aap.2016.04.012

Hedlund, J. (2015). Drug-impaired driving: A guide for what states can do. Washington, DC: Governors Highway Safety Association.

Hingson, R., Heeren, T., & Winter, M. (2000). Effects of recent 0.08% legal blood alcohol limits on fatal crash involvement. *Injury Prevention, 6*, 109–114.

Holmgren, A., Holmgren, P., Kugelberg, F. C., Jones, A. W., & Ahlner, J. (2008). High re-arrest rates among drug-impaired drivers despite zero-tolerance legislation. *Accident Analysis and Prevention, 40*, 534–540. http://dx.doi.org/10.1016/j.aap.2007.08.009

Houwing, S., Smink, B. E., Legrand, S. A., Mathijssen, R. P., Verstraete, A. G., & Brookhuis, K. A. (2012). Repeatability of oral fluid collections methods for THC measurement. *Forensic Science International, 223*, 266–272. http://dx.doi.org/10.1016/j.forsciint.2012.09.017

Impinen, A., Rahkonen, O., Karjalainen, K., Lintonen, T., Lillsunde, P., & Ostamo, A. (2009). Substance use as a predictor of driving under the influence (DUI) rearrests: A 15-year retrospective study. *Traffic Injury Prevention, 10*, 220–226. http://dx.doi.org/10.1080/15389580902822725

Institute for Behavior and Health, Inc. (2015, March). *Workplace drug testing in the era of legal marijuana.* Rockville, MD: Author.

Insurance Institute for Highway Safety. (2013). Fatality facts: Teenagers 2013. Arlington, VA: Author.

International Association of Chiefs of Police. (2016). *2015 annual report of the IACP Drug Evaluation & Classification Program.* Alexandria, VA: Author.

Jacobs, J. B. (2013). *Drunk driving: An American dilemma.* Chicago: University of Chicago Press.

Jones, A. W., Holmgren, A., & Kugelberg, F. C. (2008). Driving under the influence of cannabis: A 10-year study of age and gender differences in the concentrations of tetrahydrocannabinol in blood. *Addiction, 10*, 452–461. http://dx.doi.org/10.1111/j.1360-0443.2007.02091.x

Kilmer, B., Nicosia, N., Heaton, P., & Midgette, G. (2013). Efficacy of frequent monitoring with swift, certain, and modest sanctions for violations: Insights from

South Dakota's 24/7 Sobriety Project. *American Journal of Public Health, 103*, e37–e43. http://dx.doi.org/10.2105/AJPH.2012.300989

Lane, S. D., Cherek, D. R., Tcheremissine, O. V., Lieving, L. M., & Pietras, C. J. (2005). Acute marijuana effects on human risk taking. *Neuropsychopharmacology, 30*, 800–809. http://dx.doi.org/10.1038/sj.npp.1300620

Larkin, P. J., (2015). Medical or recreational marijuana and drugged driving. *American Criminal Law Review, 52*, 453–515.

Lerner, B. H. (2011). Drunk driving, distracted driving, moralism, and public health. *New England Journal of Medicine, 365*, 879–881. http://dx.doi.org/10.1056/NEJMp1106640

Li, M., Brady, J. E., DiMaggio, C. J., Lusardi, A. R., Tzong, K. Y., & Li, G. (2012). Marijuana use and motor vehicle crashes. *Epidemiologic Reviews, 34*, 65–72. http://dx.doi.org/10.1093/epirev/mxr017

Logan, B. K., Lowrie, K. J., Turri, J. L., Yeakel, J. K., Limoges, J. F., . . . Farrell, L. J. (2013). Recommendations for toxicological investigation of drug-impaired driving and motor vehicle fatalities. *Journal of Analytical Toxicology, 37*, 552–558. http://dx.doi.org/10.1093/jat/bkt059

Logan, B. K., Mohr, A. L., & Talpins, S. K. (2014). Detection and prevalence of drug use in arrested drivers using the Drager Drug Test 5000 and Affiniton DrugWipe oral fluid drug screening devices. *Journal of Analytical Toxicology, 38*, 444–450. http://dx.doi.org/10.1093/jat/bku050

Logan, B. K., Kacinko, S. L., & Beirness, D. J. (2016). *An evaluation of data from drivers arrested for driving under the influence in relation to per se limits for cannabis.* Washington, DC: AAA Foundation for Traffic Safety.

Long, L., Talpins, S. K., & DuPont, R. L. (2010, Spring). The South Dakota 24/7 Sobriety Project: A summary report. *Highway to Justice.* Washington, DC: ABA/National Highway Traffic Safety Administration.

Mackey v. Montrym, 443 U.S. 1 (1979).

Mann, R., Brands, B., MacDonald, S., & Stoduto, G. (2003). *Impacts of cannabis on driving: An analysis of current evidence with an emphasis on Canadian data* (Report TP 14179E). Ottawa, ON: Transport Canada.

Maryland v. King, 569 U.S. (2013).

Midgette, G., & Kilmer, B. (2015). *The effect of Montana's 24/7 Sobriety Program on DUI re-arrest: Insights from a natural experiment with limited administrative data.* Santa Monica, CA: RAND.

Missouri v. McNeely, 133 S.Ct. 1552, 185 L.Ed.2d 696 (2013).

Montana v. Egelhoff., 518 U.S. 37 (1996).

Moskowitz, A. (2007). Detecting alcohol impairment by observation of intoxication. In Transport Research Board (Ed.), *Traffic Safety and Alcohol Regulation: A Symposium* (pp. 164–168). Washington, DC: Transportation Research Board.

National Academies of Sciences, Engineering, and Medicine. (2017). *The health effects of cannabis and cannabinoids: The current state of evidence and recommendations for research.* Washington, DC: The National Academies Press.

National Highway Traffic Safety Administration. (2004a, July 2). *All U.S. states now have .08 laws, with passage of legislation in Delaware.* Retrieved from http://www.nhtsa.gov/About+NHTSA/Press+Releases/2004/All+U.S.+States+Now+Have+.08+BAC+Laws,+With+Passage+of+Legislation+in+Delaware

National Highway Traffic Safety Administration (NHTSA). (2004b, March). *.08 BAC illegal per se level* (Traffic Safety Facts, 2.1). Washington, DC: Author.

National Highway Traffic Safety Administration. (2008, January). *Administrative license revocation* (Traffic Safety Facts). Retrieved from http://www.nhtsa.gov/DOT/NHTSA/Communication%20&%20Consumer%20Information/Articles/Associated%20Files/810878.pdf

National Highway Traffic Safety Administration. (2010). *Drug involvement of fatally injured drivers* (Traffic Safety Facts). Washington, DC: NHTSA's National Center for Statistical and Analytics.

National Highway Traffic Safety Administration (2015). *Alcohol-impaired driving: 2014 data, traffic safety facts* (DOT HS 812 231). Washington, DC: US Department of Transportation.

National Transportation Safety Board. (2012, November 21). *Safety recommendation H-12-32 and H-12-33.* Washington, DC: Author.

National Transportation Safety Board. (2013). *Reaching zero: Actions to eliminate alcohol-impaired driving* (Safety Report NTSB/SR-13/01). Washington, DC: Author.

Nicosia, N., Kilmer, B., & Heaton, P. (2016). Can a criminal justice alcohol abstinence programme with swift, certain, and modest sanctions (24/7 Sobriety) reduce population morality? A retrospective observational study. *The Lancet Psychiatry, 3,* 226–232. http://dx.doi.org/10.1016/S2215-0366(15)00416-2

National Organization for the Reform of Marijuana Laws. (1996). *Principles of responsible cannabis use.* Retrieved from http://norml.org/principles/item/principles-of-responsible-cannabis-use-3#driving

Northwest High Intensity Drug Trafficking Area. (2016). *Washington State marijuana impact report.* Retrieved from http://www.mfiles.org/home/nw-hidta/marijuana-impact-report

O'Malley, P.M., & Johnston, L.D. (2013). Driving after drug or alcohol use by U.S. high school seniors, 2001–2011. *American Journal of Public Health, 103,* 2027–2034. http://dx.doi.org/10.2105/AJPH.2013.301246

Pacific Institute for Research and Evaluation. (2014). *Washington State Roadside Survey.* Retrieved from http://wtsc.wa.gov/wp-content/uploads/dlm_uploads/2014/11/Washington-State-Roadside-Survey-Wave-1-10-01-14-for-WA.pdf

Private Sector Oral Fluid Testing Advisory Board. (2007). Oral Fluid Advisory Board guidelines: Guidelines for laboratory-based oral fluid workplace drug testing. In J. Ferguson (Ed.), *The medical review officer team manual: MROCC's guide for MROs and MRO team members* (2nd ed.; pp. 289–304). Beverly Farms, MA: OEM.

Ramaekers, J. G., Kauert, G., van Ruitenbeek, P., Theunissen, E. L., Schneider, E., & Moeller, M. R. (2006). High-potency marijuana impairs executive function and inhibitory motor control. *Neuropsychopharmacology, 31,* 2296–2303. http://dx.doi.org/10.1038/sj.npp.1301068

Ramaekers, J. G., Robbe, H. W., O'Hanlon, J. F. (2000). Marijuana, alcohol and actual driving performance. *Human Psychopharmacology, 15,* 551–558. http://dx.doi.org/10.1002/1099-1077(200010)15:7<551::AID-HUP236>3.0.CO;2-P

Ramirez, A., Berning, A., Carr, K., Scherer, M., Lacey, J. H., Kelley-Baker, T., & Fisher, D. A. (2016, July). *Marijuana, other drugs, and alcohol use by drivers in Washington State* (Report No. DOT HS 812 299). Washington, DC: National Highway Traffic Safety Administration.

Reisfield, G., Bertholf, R., Goldberger, B., & DuPont, R. (in press). The science and clinical uses of drug testing. In S. C. Miller, D. A. Fiellin, R. N. Rosenthal, R. Saitz (Eds.),

The ASAM Principles of Addiction Medicine (6th ed.). Philadelphia: Lippincott Williams & Wilkins.

Robbe, H. (1998). Marijuana's impairing effects on driving are moderate when taken alone but severe when combined with alcohol. *Human Psychopharmacology, 13*(Suppl 2), S70–S78. http://dx.doi.org/10.1002/(SICI)1099-1077(1998110)13:2+<S70::AID-HUP50>3.0.CO;2-R

Rocky Mountain HIDTA Strategic Intelligence Unit. (2017). *The legalization of marijuana in Colorado: The impact* (Vol. 5). Denver: Rocky Mountain High Intensity Drug Trafficking Area.

Rodriguez-Iglesias, C., Wiliszowksi, C., & Lacey, J. H. (2001). *Legislative history of .08 per se law.* Retrieved from http://www.nhtsa.gov/people/injury/research/pub/alcohol-laws/08history

Rogeberg, O., & Elvik, R. (2016). The effects of cannabis intoxication on motor vehicle collision revisited and revised. *Addiction, 111,* 1348–1359. http://dx.doi.org/10.1111/add.13347

Sabet, K., Talpins, S. K., Dunagan, M., & Holmes, E. (2013). Smart justice: A new paradigm for dealing with offenders. *Journal of Drug Policy Analysis, 6,* 1–17. http://dx.doi.org/10.1515/jdpa-2012-0004

Schulze, H., Schumacher, M., Urmeew, R., & Auerbach, K. (2012). *DRUID final report: Work performed, main results and recommendations.* Bergisch Gladbach, Germany: Federal Highway Research Institute.

Sewell, R. A., Poling, J., & Sofuoglu, M. (2009). The effect of cannabis compared with alcohol on driving, *American Journal on Addiction, 18,* 185–193. http://dx.doi.org/10.1080/10550490902786934

Talpins, S. K., & Hayes, C. (2004, October). *The Drug Evaluation and Classification (DEC) Program.* Alexandra, VA: American Prosecutors Research Institute.

Talpins, S. K., DuPont, R. L, Voas, R. B., Holmes, E., Sabet, K. A., & Shea, C. L. (2014). License to revocation as a tool for combating drugged driving. *Impaired Driving Update, 18*(2).

Taylor, E., Zold-Kilburn, P., Carey, S. M., Fuller, B. E., & Kissick, K. (2008, March). *Michigan DUI courts outcome evaluation: Final report.* Lansing, MI: Michigan Supreme Court.

Tefft, B. C., Arnold, L. S., & Grabowski, J. G. (2016, May). *Prevalence of marijuana involvement in fatal crashes: Washington, 2010–2014.* Washington, DC: AAA Foundation for Traffic Safety.

Toennes, S. W., Steinmeyer, S., Maurer, H. J., Moeller, M. R., & Kauert, G. F. (2005). Screening for drugs of abuse in oral fluid: Correlation of analysis results with serum in forensic cases. *Journal of Analytical Toxicology, 29,* 22–27. http://dx.doi.org/10.1093/jat/29.1.22

Voas, R. B., DuPont, R. L., Talpins, S. K., & Shea, C. L. (2011). Towards a national model for managing impaired driving offenders. *Addiction, 106,* 1221–1227. http://dx.doi.org/10.1111/j.1360-0443.2010.03339.x

Volkow, N. D., Baler, R. D., Compton, W. M., & Weiss, S. R. B. (2014). Adverse health effects of marijuana use. *New England Journal of Medicine, 370,* 2219–2227. http://dx.doi.org/10.1056/NEJMra1402309

Wagenaar, A. C., & Maldonado-Molina, M. M. (2007). Effects of drivers' license suspension policies on alcohol-related crash involvement: Long-term follow-up in forty-six states. *Alcoholism, Clinical and Experimental Research, 31,* 1399–1406. http://dx.doi.org/10.1111/j.1530-0277.2007.00441.x

Walsh, J. M. (2009). *A state-by-state analysis of laws dealing with driving under the influence of drugs.* (DOT HS 811 236). Washington, DC: National Highway Traffic Safety Administration.

Walsh, J. M., Flegel, R., Atkins, R., Cangianelli, L. A., Cooper, C., Welsh, C., & Kerns, T. J. (2005). Drug and alcohol use among drivers admitted to a Level-1 trauma center. *Accident Analysis & Prevention, 37,* 894–901. http://dx.doi.org/10.1016/j.aap.2005.04.013

Washington Traffic Safety Commission. (2016). Driver toxicology testing and the involvement of marijuana in fatal crashes, 2010–2014. Olympia, WA: Author.

Watson, T. M., & Mann, R. E. (2016). International approaches to driving under the influence of cannabis: A review of evidence on impact. *Drug and Alcohol Dependence, 169,* 148–155. http://dx.doi.org/10.1016/j.drugalcdep.2016.10.023

Wood, E. Brooks-Russell, A., & Drum, P. (2016). Delays in DUI blood testing: Impact on cannabis DUI assessments. *Traffic Injury Prevention, 17,* 105–108. http://dx.doi.org/10.1080/15389588.2015.1052421

8

Risk Factors for Adolescent Marijuana Use

RICHARD F. CATALANO, ELIZABETH C. SPEAKER,
MARTIE L. SKINNER, JENNIFER A. BAILEY,
GE HONG, KEVIN P. HAGGERTY, KATARINA
GUTTMANNOVA, AND ERIN N. HARROP

INTRODUCTION

Marijuana is the third most common substance used among youth and adults in the United States, following alcohol and tobacco. Over the last two decades, marijuana has become legal for medical use in over 20 states and the District of Columbia, and several states now allow legal nonmedical use among adults but not for those under age 21. The Monitoring the Future survey and the National Survey of Drug Use and Health provide evidence of the link between lower perception of harm and higher use among youth (Johnston, O'Malley, Miech, Bachman, & Schulenberg, 2016; Substance Abuse and Mental Health Services Administration, 2013). Legalization may contribute to a decreased perception of harm related to marijuana use and, in turn, lead to increased marijuana use among youth. If these negative consequences are to be prevented, prevention efforts should be focused on children and adolescents.

Other chapters in this volume have documented a number of negative consequences associated with marijuana use for youth, including problems related to cognitive functioning and brain development, impaired driving, mental illness, pulmonary functioning, and increased risk for developing a marijuana use disorder. If these negative consequences are to be prevented, prevention efforts should be focused upstream before marijuana use is initiated or before use becomes frequent and associated with negative consequences. "Prevention science is based on a framework that identifies empirically verifiable precursors that affect the likelihood of undesired health outcomes" (Catalano et al., 2012, p. 1653). These precursors, often called risk and protective factors, have been found in longitudinal studies to predict substance use and other problematic outcomes. While there is overlap among risk and protective factors for multiple problems, given the current concerns that promarijuana laws may contribute to an increase in adolescent use, a clear detailed knowledge of risk and protective factors for marijuana involvement among youth is needed. If risk can be decreased and protection can be increased through preventive intervention, marijuana use among youth might be less likely and healthy development more likely.

RISK AND PROTECTIVE FACTORS: CONCEPTUAL ISSUES

Risk factors are person or environmental characteristics that when present increase the likelihood of later problems (Arthur, Hawkins, Pollard, Catalano, & Baglioni, 2002). The more risk factors an individual is exposed to, the higher the likelihood for problems resulting in adverse health or social consequences (Arthur et al., 2002). Protective or promotive factors are person or environmental characteristics that reduce the likelihood of problems directly or buffer the effects of risk (Hawkins, Catalano, & Miller, 1992; Stone, Becker, Huber, & Catalano, 2012). Reducing risk factors and enhancing protective factors in the individual and environment has demonstrated impact on reducing problem behaviors, including substance use (Catalano, Haggerty, Hawkins, & Elgin, 2011).

Risk and protective factors for adolescent substance use have been examined in the individual and in multiple social domains including the family, school, peer group, community, and society. This chapter examines the literature for evidence of risk and protective factors identified specifically for marijuana use among youth across these domains. Although we are examining factors for marijuana use, these identified factors may be common to other substances, or even a wide range of other problem behaviors (e.g., delinquency, school truancy, dropout).

For the purposes of this review, we have grouped risk and protective factors into six domains: society, community, school, family, peers, and individual. These domains have been studied extensively and represent a core set of factors associated with substance use. Societal factors include laws, policies, and broad social norms. Community factors include community norms and neighborhood characteristics. School factors include bonding or commitment to school and academic success or failure. Family factors focus primarily on parents' behaviors and attitudes, parenting skills, family conflict, and parent–child relationships, but also include siblings as agents of influence. Peer factors focus primarily on peer substance use and attitudes toward substance use. Individual factors include individual characteristics such as gender, race, and temperament (reflecting genetic and epigenetic influences, and other biological processes). Individual factors also include one's previous experiences and behavior.

Whereas there is considerable research on predictors of alcohol (National Research Council and Institute of Medicine, 2004) and tobacco use (Community Preventive Services Task Force, 2015), research on risk and protective factors for use of marijuana (and other illicit substances) is rarely differentiated in the literature. This chapter will focus on risk and protective factors specific to marijuana, which necessarily limits the review. The reader is referred to other more general reviews of risk and protective factors for substance use to put this review in context (Catalano et al., 2012, 2011; Hawkins et al., 1992; Stone et al., 2012).

SOCIETY

Dramatic changes have been taking place through legislation within states (and now introduced for debate in the US Congress) regarding marijuana production, distribution, and sales. The direction of influence of marijuana policy on youth marijuana use and norms is unclear. Studies from Australia, the Netherlands, and the United States indicate that the effects of legalization, decriminalization, and medical use laws on youth marijuana use are mixed, with some studies reporting small increases in youth use and others reporting no change (Anderson, Hansen, & Rees, 2012; Korf, 2002; Lynne-Landsman, Livingston, & Wagenaar, 2013; MacCoun, 2011; MacCoun & Reuter, 2001; Pacula, 2010; Pacula, Chriqui, & King, 2004; Wen, Hockenberry, & Cummings, 2014). Studies of the effects of medical use laws in the United States show higher rates of use among youth in states allowing medical use (Cerda, Wall, Keyes, Galea, & Hasin, 2012; Hasin et al., 2015; Monte, Zane, & Heard, 2015; Wall et al., 2011). However, some authors have argued that higher prevalence of use and lower perceived harm contributed to the passage of medical use laws rather than the reverse (Pacula et al., 2004; Wall et al., 2011). Although some studies have focused on broad historical trends and others have retrospectively assessed aspects of use careers (e.g., age at onset, age at regular use), few have investigated the effects of marijuana decriminalization and medical use laws on within-person or developmental patterns of use over time. No studies to date have directly examined whether legalized nonmedical use for adults constitutes a risk factor for youth marijuana use. (See chapter by Cottler and Okafor, this volume, for more details on trend data and legalization in the United States.)

COMMUNITY

Within the community domain, most of the evidence indicates community-level social norms and attitudes toward substance use in general are risk factors for marijuana use among youth (Cleveland, Feinberg, Bontempo, & Greenberg, 2008). For example, data from Monitoring the Future suggest that birth cohort norms about marijuana use predict an individual's likelihood of marijuana use independent of that individual's personal attitudes about marijuana (Keyes et al., 2011).

Studies have found that neighborhood disorder significantly predicts risk of later marijuana use among youth (Copeland-Linder, Lambert, Chen, & Ialongo, 2011; Lambert, Brown, Phillips, & Ialongo, 2004), as does lack of neighborhood cohesion (Cleveland et al., 2008), and neighborhood violence (Copeland-Linder et al., 2011; Wright, Fagan, & Pinchevsky, 2013). In another study, perceptions of neighborhood disorder, increased neighborhood general drug activity, and exposure to violence in 8th grade were associated with initiation and progression to more frequent marijuana use from 9th to 12th grade (Reboussin, Green, Milam, Furr-Holden, & Ialongo, 2014). Community cohesion, a community index composed of the following scales: Neighborhood attachment, community prosocial involvement, laws and norms favorable to drug use and firearms, perceived ability of drugs and firearms, and community disorganization, has been found to impact youth at younger ages and contributes to lifetime and recent (past-30-day) marijuana use (Cleveland et al., 2008). Conversely, the protective factor of a positive sense of community has buffered the impact of deviant peers on marijuana use (Mayberry, Espelage, & Koenig, 2009).

SCHOOL

Having a variety of problems in school, poor academic performance, and school dropout have been linked to marijuana use among youth. For example, an analysis of the 1997 and 1998 National Household Surveys on Drug Abuse data indicated that any marijuana use was positively associated with school dropout and truancy, and chronic marijuana use (weekly or more frequent) was found to be the dominant factor in these relationships (Roebuck, French, & Dennis, 2004). Also, longitudinal studies have produced evidence that school problems lead to later marijuana use. Poor grades increase the risk of later marijuana initiation (Tang & Orwin, 2009). Getting in trouble in school has been linked to initiating experimental use and the transition from initiation to regular use (van den Bree & Pickworth, 2005). Other aspects of the school experience are risk factors for youth marijuana use. School-level norms favorable to marijuana use and youth perceptions about the marijuana use of their schoolmates are related to youth marijuana use (Juvonen, Martino, Ellickson, & Longshore, 2007). Monitoring the Future data suggest that aggregate school-level norms about marijuana use were related to student use even when controlling for a student's own norms about use (Kumar, O'Malley, Johnston, Schulenberg, & Bachman, 2002).

Another important, though underresearched, area involving school risk factors is that of school policies. School policies regarding substance use not only provide behavioral guidelines for the students but may also be important signals of norms toward drug use by students. While virtually all schools in the United States have policies against substance use, there is very little literature examining the impact of school policy on substance use of any kind (Evans-Whipp et al., 2004; Evans-Whipp, Bond, Toumbourou, & Catalano, 2007). A recent study examined the impact of school substance use policy on marijuana use (Evans-Whipp, Plenty, Catalano, Herrenkohl, & Toumbourou, 2015). Results showed that perceptions of low enforcement of antidrug policies was a risk factor for later marijuana use. However, specific antidrug policies may not be effective when student perception is not in line with the policies. Evans-Whipp et al. (2015) found that schools with policies that included suspension of students from school for using illicit drugs (zero tolerance) predicted more—not less—marijuana use one year later. Finally, policies that students perceived as providing counseling for students in violation of the illicit drug policy were found to be protective against later marijuana use. These are school-wide effects, not just effects for those in violation of the policy.

School protective factors, including school commitment, positive involvement, and rewards for positive involvement are associated with reduced likelihood of future marijuana use (Cleveland et al., 2008; Kuntsche & Jordan, 2006; van den Bree & Pickworth, 2005). Students' perceptions of being respected by the adults in their school and the school providing a good education have been found to have protective effects against marijuana use as well (Mayberry et al., 2009).

FAMILY

Family factors are important predictors of youth marijuana use. Leading among these is parents' own use of substances, particularly marijuana (Fleary, Heffer, McKyer, & Newman, 2010; Griffin, Botvin, Scheier, & Nichols, 2002; Heron et al., 2013; Korhonen et al., 2008; Tang & Orwin, 2009). Evidence suggests that children with parents who use marijuana are at greater risk for initiating use themselves before adulthood. Tang and Orwin (2009) found that parental illicit drug use, including marijuana, increased the odds for marijuana initiation among 11- to 13-year-olds by 33% to 57% compared to youth with parents who did not use illicit drugs. Parental alcohol and tobacco use have also been linked to youth marijuana use (Heron et al., 2013; Korhonen et al., 2008). Parent mental health problems, particularly parental depression (Cortes, Fleming, Mason, & Catalano, 2009), also pose risk for later youth marijuana use.

Parent's norms, attitudes, or beliefs about marijuana use also significantly impact adolescent perception of risk (Fleary et al., 2010), and risk perception is closely related to marijuana initiation (Johnston, O'Malley, Miech, Bachman, & Schulenberg, 2014). In addition, family factors including parent–child bonding; family management including rule setting, monitoring, rewards, and discipline; and parental favorable attitudes toward drug use or other antisocial behaviors have all been linked to adolescent substance use (Brook, Brook, Arencibia-Mireles, Richter, & Whiteman, 2001; Cleveland et al., 2008; Fleary et al., 2010; Tang & Orwin, 2009). Brook et al. (2001) assessed several parent–child predictors together, including parent–child bonding (mutual attachment), parental control, and disciplinary style. They found that parent–child bonding acted as a protective factor, while paternal punitive discipline increased risk for marijuana engagement. Tang and Orwin found that parental monitoring was a protective factor, reducing the likelihood of later marijuana use by 38% to 54% for 12- to 13-year-olds (Tang & Orwin, 2009). Some evidence suggests that family factors, such as the ones previously noted, are stronger predictors of marijuana use for younger youth (6th to 8th grade) and become less salient in later adolescence (10th to 12th grade), when peer factors become more influential (Cleveland et al., 2008; Fleary et al., 2010; Tang & Orwin, 2009).

Consistent with the finding that harsh discipline is a risk factor for youth marijuana use, Hussey et al. (2006) examined the effects of childhood maltreatment (which happens most frequently within the family) on adverse adolescent health outcomes using the National Longitudinal Study of Adolescent Health from 2001–2002. They found adolescent marijuana use was significantly more common among victims of childhood neglect, physical assault, and contact sexual abuse. Furthermore, Wright et al. (2013) found that child abuse was significantly related to more frequent marijuana use among youth several years after the abuse occurred.

PEERS

The peer context is an important determinant of youth substance use behavior (Catalano & Hawkins, 1996; Hawkins et al., 1992). Of particular importance is perceived substance use by peers, siblings, and romantic partners. Empirical studies provide a wealth of data supporting the importance of perceptions about peer, sibling, and partner use in predicting youth substance use, including marijuana (Catalano & Hawkins, 1996; Catalano, White, Hawkins, & Pandina, 1985; Hawkins et al., 1992; Oesterle et al., 2012). Peer influences may also maintain drug use that already started in the adolescent. Drug users will tend to spend time with others who use drugs, and the group will consider drug use as normal behavior (Bauman & Ennett, 1996). Peer factors generally impact youth in adolescence (Heron et al., 2013; Hussey et al., 2006) but have been found to promote continued use as well (Cleveland et al., 2008; Fleary et al., 2010).

INDIVIDUAL

Several individual characteristics can increase marijuana use. Demographic variables are consistently related to initiation and/or self-reported use of marijuana. Not surprisingly, older adolescents are more likely to have initiated, report more frequent use, and report more problematic use (Korhonen et al., 2008; Tang & Orwin, 2009; Wright et al., 2013). As with many other types of risk-taking behaviors, marijuana use is more common among male adolescents than females (Stone et al., 2012). However, gender may moderate the relationship between individual risk factors and marijuana use. Griffin et al. (2002) examined gender differences in the impact of risk factors using a prospective study of high school marijuana use and found that girls with high self-control were at lower risk and boys with social anxiety were at higher risk. With respect to race/

ethnicity, national statistics suggest fewer racial disparities in youth marijuana use (Johnston et al., 2014), whereas, in general, White teens are at greater risk for use of other substances (alcohol, cocaine, etc.) than most ethnic minorities, especially Black youth.

An adolescent's own attitudes about marijuana use and perceptions of harmful consequences are strongly linked to youth marijuana use (Griffin et al., 2002; Simons, Neal, & Gaher, 2006). Not surprisingly, teens who perceive little or no harm associated with marijuana use are more likely to use (Guttmannova et al., in press). Also, as noted earlier, if teens believe marijuana is accepted by their parents, peers, and others, they are more likely to report using. Positive attitudes toward substance use are linked to availability and the likelihood that youth will be offered marijuana. Perceived availability of marijuana (Gillespie, Neale, & Kendler, 2009) and having been offered marijuana (Tang & Orwin, 2009) are significant risk factors for initiation of marijuana use.

Among individual risk factors for marijuana use, the teen's own history of other substance use is predictive of marijuana use. van den Bree and Pickworth (2005) looked at five stages of marijuana involvement and 21 risk factors that may impact those stages using National Longitudinal Study of Adolescent Health data from 1995 and 1996. The five stages were (a) initiation; (b) initiation to regular use; (c) progression to regular use; (d) failure to discontinue experimental use; and (e) failure to discontinue regular use. Individual involvement with other substances, particularly tobacco and alcohol, was one of the strongest predictors for all stages of marijuana involvement. Also, regular and occasional use of cannabis as an adolescent is linked with a greater risk of other illicit drug consumption in early adulthood (Taylor et al., 2017). Similarly, individual alcohol and tobacco use were among the strongest risk factors for marijuana engagement (Tang & Orwin, 2009).

Other individual constitutional or temperament factors have been identified as risk factors for marijuana use. Heron et al. (2013) examined the relationship between conduct disorder trajectories between the ages of 4 and 13 and marijuana use by age 16 in a birth cohort study in England. They found that early-onset conduct problems led to a sixfold increase in risk for problem marijuana use, with early onset conduct problems explaining 25% of the variance in problem marijuana use. Although some exceptions exist, there are several studies that support the view that childhood attention problems, including the presence of an attention deficit/hyperactivity disorder, have also been linked to a greater likelihood to use marijuana during adolescence (August et al., 2006; Disney, Elkins, McGue, & Iacono, 1999; Elkins, McGue, & Iacono, 2007). Fleary et al. (2010) examined marijuana use from the bio-ecological model. They found that being older and having lower impulse control were the two strongest predictors of adolescent marijuana use. Sensation seeking can also increase the likelihood for marijuana engagement throughout adolescence (Cleveland et al., 2008; Fleary et al., 2010; Heron et al., 2013; Hussey et al., 2006). Creemers, Verhulst, and Huizink (2009) examined temperament factors related to marijuana use and found high levels of intensity seeking and low levels of shyness were associated with early onset marijuana use.

Perhaps underlying these individual constitutional factors are potential genetic or epigenetic influences. In a meta-analysis of twin studies that reported genetic and shared and unshared environmental influences, the heritability of marijuana initiation was estimated to be between 40% and 48%, and between 51% and 59% for problematic use (Verweij et al., 2010). Kendler et al. (2003) examined data from male twin pairs and found that illicit drugs (including marijuana, cocaine, hallucinogens, sedatives, stimulants, and opiates) share a single inherited factor for vulnerability to dependence. However, when examining early substance use (including marijuana), family environmental factors were more influential at early ages, and genetic factors did not become the most influential until the mid-20s (Kendler, Myers, & Prescott, 2007; McGue, Elkins, & Iacono, 2000). Recent results in a study of female twin pairs suggest heritability influences are low for ever using marijuana but high for heavy use, abuse, and dependence (Kendler & Prescott, 1998). This finding fits with genetic influences being stronger for more severe marijuana use and marijuana use disorder, rather than for patterns that reflect experimental or less frequent use.

SUMMARY AND FUTURE DIRECTIONS

There is considerable research on predictors of alcohol (National Research Council and Institute of Medicine, 2004) and tobacco use (Community Preventive Services Task Force, 2015). In contrast, less research is available on predictors of illicit substances, and this research rarely differentiates between drug types. Given the changing legal landscape related to marijuana, understanding the specific predictors of marijuana use and abuse is necessary for marijuana-specific prevention efforts. As is clear from the epidemiology of substance use, the most used and abused substances are legal substances, whether the user is an adolescent or adult. States that have passed legislation decriminalizing or legalizing marijuana use for adults may face unique challenges for youth under the minimum legal age. More states may join those currently adopting legal use of marijuana for those age 21 and older, and it will be increasingly important for researchers to understand the marijuana-specific risk and protective factors. Even though marijuana use is still illegal for youth in states with legal marijuana use for adults, the availability, norms, and marketing of marijuana may be important predictors of youth uptake, as has been the case for alcohol and tobacco.

Identifying the longitudinal predictors of youth marijuana use, heavy or regular use, and marijuana use disorder is critical for the development of marijuana prevention programs and, specifically, important if marijuana use increases with legalization. Research on prevention programs' effects on youth marijuana use has been sparse. Many studies have combined marijuana use with other illegal drug use, making it difficult to distinguish whether there are specific marijuana use reductions. Further, there are no known studies examining the effects of prevention programs in the normative context of legal marijuana use for adults. A recent search of evidence-based programs identified 13 programs with demonstrated effectiveness in preventing marijuana use in youth and young adults, and only 9 of these 13 programs were judged to have a positive return on investment (Washington State Institute for Public Policy, 2015). This chapter has identified specific relationships between adolescent marijuana use and risk and protective factors in the societal, community, school, family, peer, and individual domains. Prevention science is based on the premise that effective prevention programs address predictors of behavior problems. The risk and protective factors for marijuana use and abuse identified in this chapter are targets for prevention programs seeking to affect marijuana use among children, adolescents, and young adults. As the environment changes with more states legalizing marijuana use for adults, the levels of several risk factors may change, including not only norms, attitudes, early use, and peer use, but also parent and community favorable attitudes toward use. It will be important for federal, state, and community monitoring systems to track the levels of these and other risk and protective factors as marijuana policy changes take place so prevention efforts can target the most elevated risk factors and most depressed protective factors for youth marijuana use.

Further, new research efforts are needed to understand the impact that legalization of adult marijuana use has on youth marijuana engagement. This effort should attempt to delineate the mechanisms through which legalization (for medical and/or nonmedical use) influences patterns of marijuana use among youth. For example, does the legalization of adult marijuana use (which is itself a reflection of favorable societal norms toward marijuana use) reduce perceptions of harm among adults first, which leads to shifts in attitudes among children and youth? Do parents change their guidelines and consequences for marijuana use in response to legal use for adults? Under conditions of legal use, are parents more likely to use marijuana when their children are present, providing both a message about norms and a model of behavior? Does medical use versus legal use by a parent differentially influence marijuana use by the child? Also, given that adult attitudes may change as a function of the monitoring of local health data, how do such changes affect their child's attitudes? Disentangling these pathways will require a variety of research approaches, including population-based longitudinal studies, analyzing big data from social media, conducting focus groups with youth and parents to describe emerging trends and practices, and using observational and qualitative studies to understand the emerging environment in which marijuana use occurs in states where marijuana is legal.

Research priorities should also focus on the impact of school policies on youth marijuana use and their impact on later substance use in young adulthood. While zero-tolerance school policies are in place across the United States, in some cases the implementation of elements of these policies may have an iatrogenic impact on marijuana use (Evans-Whipp et al., 2015). Research on alcohol and tobacco has demonstrated the usefulness of different policies, including access, cost, and compliance checks, on use. It is critical that we learn lessons from this research and investigate the impact of aspects of state, community, and school policies regarding marijuana use on underage as well as adult marijuana use.

Despite a few studies establishing the causal ordering of risk and protective factors and later marijuana use, further longitudinal research that describes the causal process, including directionality, that links risk and protective factors to the trajectory of marijuana use and problems associated with use is warranted. The connection between marijuana use and school is an example. Understanding the impact of school factors on marijuana initiation and patterns of use, as well as the consequences of marijuana use on dropout and grades, requires carefully conducted longitudinal studies to disentangle potential bidirectional effects or sequencing of effects between school factors and marijuana use (McCaffrey, Liccardo Pacula, Han, & Ellickson, 2010). Further, more research that focuses on the interplay between school factors (e.g., policies, other qualities of the school environment), and risk and protective factors in family, peer, and individual domains is needed.

An area that has been understudied pertains to protective factors. Despite growing awareness of the impact of peer risk factors on later adolescent substance use, less research has investigated their role as a protective factor. For example, peer-to-peer mentoring is an important component of many school-based approaches to substance abuse prevention, yet little is known about the influence of positive peers or close age mentors on preventing marijuana use uptake or progression. Family variables (e.g., favorable family climate, strong antidrug attitudes by parents) can also serve as a protective influence.

Research priorities for family predictors of youth marijuana use include understanding the changing nature of family relationships and parenting practices across development. Do the effects of family factors become less predictive as the influence of peers increases over the course of adolescence, or do parenting protective and risk factors endure from an early age like the effects of early physical and sexual abuse? As noted earlier, the behavioral genetics literature suggests that environmental factors, such as family variables, likely exert more influence than genetic factors during adolescence, compared to young adulthood. Also, we have noted the changing context of legal marijuana use and its potential impact on parent's marijuana use, marijuana-specific parenting practices, and attitudes toward use on their children's marijuana use. With regard to alcohol and tobacco use, lax parental norms and parentally provided access to alcohol and tobacco were found to be important risk factors for use. Many alcohol and tobacco prevention and control interventions in the late 1970s and 1980s focused on these risks, as well as substance-specific parenting practices around cigarettes and alcohol, including parent–child discussion of rules and expectations around substance use, which are in part responsible for reducing the use of these substances from historically peak levels (Chassin et al., 2005; Hill, Hawkins, Catalano, Abbott, & Guo, 2005; van der Vorst, Engels, Meeus, & Deković, 2006). Given these findings, it seems likely that marijuana-specific parenting practices also would be important targets for preventing adolescent marijuana use.

Research has demonstrated the importance of individual temperament-related factors on a variety of risk-taking behaviors including marijuana use during adolescence. These temperament factors have been linked to genetic factors (Kreek,

Nielsen, Butelman, & LaForge, 2005) and vulnerability to addiction. Although twin studies have found significant variance explained by inherited characteristics, the search for genes for marijuana use has yet to bear fruit (e.g., Samek et al., 2016). New ways of examining and understanding molecular genetic influences on youth marijuana use may be in order (e.g., epigenetic strategies). However, the search of the interaction between preventive interventions and specific genetic risk profiles is promising and may lead to useful prevention approaches given a person's genetic risk (e.g., Howe, Beach, Brody, & Wyman, 2015). Another emerging avenue related to individual biology is research on stress-responsive physiology and how it influences substance use behavior (Sinha, 2008). With regard to marijuana use, most of the research on stress-responsive physiology has focused on the health consequences of early or heavy marijuana use (Huizink, Ferdinand, Ormel, & Verhulst, 2006; Moss, Vanyukov, Yao, & Kirillova, 1999; van Leeuwen et al., 2011; Volkow, Baler, Comptom & Weiss, 2014). Very little is known about the possible relationship between stress-responsive physiology during childhood and adolescence and the risk for future marijuana involvement. Thus, future research should examine whether aspects of individual stress responsivity operate as risk or protective factors for youth marijuana use.

This chapter has identified a number of societal, community, family, school, peer, and individual risk and protective factors. The current interest in marijuana medicalization and legalization often focuses on the reduction of harm and expense involved in arrest and incarceration of marijuana users. Countering this interest is the concern that legalization of marijuana may increase other harms at the population level related to use and consequences of use detailed in this volume. This may particularly be true for underage marijuana use given the possible impact of marijuana on the developing brain's cognitive control regions and other health risks associated with early onset use (Compton, Weiss, & Wargo, this volume). While the risk and protective factors identified here will be important targets for preventing underage uptake and preventing youth harm from marijuana use, further research identified here will also be important to prevention efforts given the numerous signs that we are experiencing a growing promarijuana era.

REFERENCES

Anderson, D. M., Hansen, B., & Rees, D. I. (2012). *Medical marijuana laws and teen marijuana use.* IZA Discussion Paper No. 6592 2012. Bonn: IZA.

Arthur, M. W., Hawkins, J. D., Pollard, J. A., Catalano, R. F., & Baglioni, A. J., Jr. (2002). Measuring risk and protective factors for substance use, delinquency, and other adolescent problem behaviors: The Communities That Care Youth Survey. *Evaluation Review, 26,* 575–601. http://dx.doi.org/10.1177/0193841X0202600601

August, G. J., Winters, K. C., Realmuto, G. M., Fahnhorst, T., Botzet, A., & Lee, S. (2006). Prospective study of adolescent drug use among community samples of ADHD and non-ADHD participants. *Journal of the American Academy of Child & Adolescent Psychiatry, 45,* 824–832. http://dx.doi.org/10.1097/01.chi.0000219831.16226.f8

Bauman, K. E., & Ennett, S. T. (1996). On the importance of peer influence for adolescent drug use: Commonly neglected considerations. *Addiction, 91*, 185–198. http://dx.doi.org/10.1111/j.1360-0443.1996.tb03175.x

Brook, J. S., Brook, D. W., Arencibia-Mireles, O., Richter, L., & Whiteman, M. (2001). Risk factors for adolescent marijuana use across cultures and across time. *Journal of Genetic Psychology, 162*, 357–374. http://dx.doi.org/10.1080/00221320109597489

Catalano, R. F., Fagan, A. A., Gavin, L. E., Greenberg, M. T., Irwin, C. E., Ross, D. A., & Shek, D. T. L. (2012). Worldwide application of the prevention science research base in adolescent health. *The Lancet, 379*(9826), 1653–1664. http://dx.doi.org/10.1016/S0140-6736(12)60238-4

Catalano, R. F., Haggerty, K. P., Hawkins, J. D., & Elgin, J. (2011). Prevention of substance use and substance use disorders: The role of risk and protective factors. In Y. Kaminer & K. C. Winters (Eds.), *Clinical manual of adolescent substance abuse treatment* (pp. 25–63). Washington, DC: American Psychiatric Publishing.

Catalano, R. F., & Hawkins, J. D. (1996). The social development model: A theory of antisocial behavior. In J. D. Hawkins (Ed.), *Delinquency and crime: Current theories* (pp. 149–197). New York: Cambridge University Press.

Catalano, R. F., White, H. R., Hawkins, J. D., & Pandina, R. J. (1985, November). *Predicting delinquency and marijuana use among adolescents*. Paper presented at the annual meeting of the American Society of Criminology, San Diego, CA.

Cerda, M., Wall, M., Keyes, K. M., Galea, S., & Hasin, D. (2012). Medical marijuana laws in 50 states: Investigating the relationship between state legalization of medical marijuana and marijuana use, abuse and dependence. *Drug and Alcohol Dependence, 120*, 22–27. http://dx.doi.org/10.1016/j.drugalcdep.2011.06.011

Chassin, L., Presson, C. C., Rose, J., Sherman, S. J., Davis, M. J., & Gonzalez, J. L. (2005). Parenting style and smoking-specific parenting practices as predictors of adolescent smoking onset. *Journal of Pediatric Psychology, 30*, 333–344. http://dx.doi.org/10.1093/jpepsy/jsi028

Cleveland, M. J., Feinberg, M. E., Bontempo, D. E., & Greenberg, M. T. (2008). The role of risk and protective factors in substance use across adolescence. *Journal of Adolescent Health, 43*, 157–164. http://dx.doi.org/10.1016/j.jadohealth.2008.01.015

Community Preventive Services Task Force. (2015, May 15). *The guide to community preventive services*. Retrieved from http://www.thecommunityguide.org/index.html

Copeland-Linder, N., Lambert, S., Chen, Y.-F., & Ialongo, N. (2011). Contextual stress and health risk behaviors among African American adolescents. *Journal of Youth and Adolescence, 40*, 158–173. http://dx.doi.org/10.1007/s10964-010-9520-y

Cortes, R. C., Fleming, C. B., Mason, W. A., & Catalano, R. F. (2009). Risk factors linking maternal depressed mood to growth in adolescent substance use. *Journal of Emotional and Behavioral Disorders, 17*, 49–64. http://dx.doi.org/10.1177/1063426608321690

Creemers, H. E., Verhulst, F. C., & Huizink, A. C. (2009). Temperamental risk factors for adolescent cannabis use: A systematic review of prospective general population studies. *Substance Use & Misuse, 44*, 1833–1854. http://dx.doi.org/10.3109/10826080802494933

Disney, E. R., Elkins, I. J., McGue, M., & Iacono, W. G. (1999). Effects of ADHD, conduct disorder, and gender on substance use and abuse in adolescence. *American Journal of Psychiatry, 156*, 1515–1521. http://dx.doi.org/10.1176/ajp.156.10.1515

Elkins, I. J., McGue, M., & Iacono, W. G. (2007). Prospective effects of attention-deficit/ hyperactivity disorder, conduct disorder, and sex on adolescent substance use and abuse. *Archives of General Psychiatry, 64,* 1145–1152. http://dx.doi.org/10.1001/ archpsyc.64.10.1145

Evans-Whipp, T., Beyers, J. M., Lloyd, S., Lafazia, A. N., Toumbourou, J. W., Arthur, M. W., & Catalano, R. F. (2004). A review of school drug policies and their impact on youth substance use. *Health Promotion International, 19*(2), 227–234. http://dx.doi. org/10.1093/heapro/dah210

Evans-Whipp, T. J., Bond, L., Toumbourou, J. W., & Catalano, R. F. (2007). School, parent, and student perspectives of school drug policies. *Journal of School Health, 77,* 138–146. http://dx.doi.org/10.1111/j.1746-1561.2007.00183.x

Evans-Whipp, T. J., Plenty, S. M., Catalano, R. F., Herrenkohl, T. I., & Toumbourou, J. W. (2015). Longitudinal effects of school drug policies on student marijuana use in Washington State, US and Victoria, Australia. *American Journal of Public Health, 105,* 994–1000. http://dx.doi.org/10.2105/AJPH.2014.302421

Fleary, S. A., Heffer, R. W., McKyer, E. L. J., & Newman, D. A. (2010). Using the bioecological model to predict risk perception of marijuana use and reported marijuana use in adolescence. *Addictive Behaviors, 35,* 795–798. http://dx.doi.org/ 10.1016/j.addbeh.2010.03.016

Gillespie, N. A., Neale, M. C., & Kendler, K. S. (2009). Pathways to cannabis abuse: A multi-stage model from cannabis availability, cannabis initiation and progression to abuse. *Addiction, 104,* 430–438. http://dx.doi.org/10.1111/ j.1360-0443.2008.02456.x

Griffin, K. W., Botvin, G. J., Scheier, L. M., & Nichols, T. R. (2002). Factors associated with regular marijuana use among high school students: A long-term follow-up study. *Substance Use and Misuse, 37,* 225–238. http://dx.doi.org/10.1081/JA-120001979

Guttmannova, K., Skinner, M. L., Oesterle, S., White, H. R., Catalano, R. F., & Hawkins, J. D. (in press). The interplay between marijuana-specific risk factors and marijuana use over the course of adolescence. *Prevention Science.*

Hasin, D. S., Wall, M., Keyes, K. M., Cerdá, M., Schulenberg, J., O'Malley, P. M., . . . Feng, T. (2015). Medical marijuana laws and adolescent marijuana use in the USA from 1991 to 2014: Results from annual, repeated cross-sectional surveys. *The Lancet Psychiatry, 2,* 601–608. http://dx.doi.org/10.1016/S2215-0366(15)00217-5

Hawkins, J. D., Catalano, R. F., & Miller, J. Y. (1992). Risk and protective factors for alcohol and other drug problems in adolescence and early adulthood: Implications for substance abuse prevention. *Psychological Bulletin, 112,* 64–105. http://dx.doi.org/ 10.1037/0033-2909.112.1.64

Heron, J., Barker, E. D., Joinson, C., Lewis, G., Hickman, M., Munafò, M., & Macleod, J. (2013). Childhood conduct disorder trajectories, prior risk factors and cannabis use at age 16: Birth cohort study. *Addiction, 108,* 2129–2138. http://dx.doi.org/ 10.1111/add.12268

Hill, K. G., Hawkins, J. D., Catalano, R. F., Abbott, R. D., & Guo, J. (2005). Family influences on the risk of daily smoking initiation. *Journal of Adolescent Health, 37,* 202–210. http://dx.doi.org/10.1016/j.jadohealth.2004.08.014

Howe, G. W., Beach, S. R. H., Brody, G. H., & Wyman, P. A. (2015). Translating genetic research into preventive intervention: The baseline target moderated mediator design. *Frontiers in Psychology, 6: 1911.* http://dx.doi.org10.3389/fpsyg.2015.01911

Huizink, A. C., Ferdinand, R. F., Ormel, J., & Verhulst, F. C. (2006). Hypothalamic–pituitary–adrenal axis activity and early onset of cannabis use. *Addiction, 101*, 1581–1588. http://dx.doi.org/10.1111/j.1360-0443.2006.01570.x

Hussey, J. M., Chang, J. J., & Kotch, J. B. (2006). Child maltreatment in the United States: Prevalence, risk factors, and adolescent health consequences. *Pediatrics, 118*, 933–942. http://dx.doi.org/10.1542/peds.2005-2452

Johnston, L. D., O'Malley, P. M., Miech, R. A., Bachman, J. G., & Schulenberg, J. E. (2014). *Monitoring the Future national results on drug use, 1975–2013: Overview, key findings on adolescent drug use.* Ann Arbor: Institute for Social Research, University of Michigan.

Johnston, L. D., O'Malley, P. M., Miech, R. A.,Bachman, J. G., & Schulenberg, J. E. (2016). *Monitoring the Future national survey results on drug use, 1975–2015: Overview, key findings on adolescent drug use.* Ann Arbor: Institute for Social Research, University of Michigan.

Juvonen, J., Martino, S. C., Ellickson, P. L., & Longshore, D. (2007). "But others do it!": Do misperceptions of schoolmate alcohol and marijuana use predict subsequent drug use among young adolescents? *Journal of Applied Social Psychology, 37*, 740–758. http://dx.doi.org/10.1111/j.1559-1816.2007.00183.x

Kendler, K. S., Jacobson, K. C., Prescott, C. A., & Neale, M. C. (2003). Specificity of genetic and environmental risk factors for use and abuse/dependence of cannabis, cocaine, hallucinogens, sedatives, stimulants, and opiates in male twins. *American Journal of Psychiatry, 160*, 687–695. http://dx.doi.org/10.1176/appi.ajp.160.4.687

Kendler, K. S., Myers, J., & Prescott, C. A. (2007). Specificity of genetic and environmental risk factors for symptoms of cannabis, cocaine, alcohol, caffeine, and nicotine dependence. *Archives of General Psychiatry, 64*, 1313–1320. http://dx.doi.org/10.1001/archpsyc.64.11.1313

Kendler, K. S., & Prescott, C. A. (1998). Cannabis use, abuse, and dependence in a population-based sample of female twins. *American Journal of Psychiatry, 155*, 1016–1022. http://dx.doi.org/10.1176/ajp.155.8.1016

Keyes, K. M., Schulenberg, J. E., O'Malley, P. M., Johnston, L. D., Bachman, J. G., Li, G., & Hasin, D. (2011). The social norms of birth cohorts and adolescent marijuana use in the United States, 1976–2007. *Addiction, 106*, 1790–1800. http://dx.doi.org/10.1111/j.1360-0443.2011.03485.x

Korf, D. J. (2002). Dutch coffee shops and trends in cannabis use. *Addictive Behaviors, 27*, 851–866. http://dx.doi.org/10.1016/S0306-4603(02)00291-5

Korhonen, T., Huizink, A. C., Dick, D. M., Pulkkinen, L., Rose, R. J., & Kaprio, J. (2008). Role of individual, peer and family factors in the use of cannabis and other illicit drugs: A longitudinal analysis among Finnish adolescent twins. *Drug and Alcohol Dependence, 97*, 33–43. http://dx.doi.org/10.1016/j.drugalcdep.2008.03.015

Kreek, M. J., Nielsen, D. A., Butelman, E. R., & LaForge, K. S. (2005). Genetic influences on impulsivity, risk taking, stress responsivity and vulnerability to drug abuse and addiction. *Nature Neuroscience, 8*, 1450–1457. http://dx.doi.org/10.1038/nn1583

Kumar, R., O'Malley, P. M., Johnston, L. D., Schulenberg, J. E., & Bachman, J. G. (2002). Effects of school-level norms on student substance use. *Prevention Science, 3*, 105–124. http://dx.doi.org/10.1023/A:1015431300471

Kuntsche, E., & Jordan, M. D. (2006). Adolescent alcohol and cannabis use in relation to peer and school factors: Results of multilevel analyses. *Drug and Alcohol Dependence, 84,* 167–174. http://dx.doi.org/10.1016/j.drugalcdep.2006.01.014

Lambert, S., Brown, T., Phillips, C., & Ialongo, N. (2004). The relationship between perceptions of neighborhood characteristics and substance use among urban African American adolescents. *American Journal of Community Psychology, 34,* 205–218. http://dx.doi.org/10.1007/s10464-004-7415-3

Lynne-Landsman, S., Livingston, M. D., & Wagenaar, A. C. (2013). Effects of state medical marijuana laws on adolescent marijuana use. *American Journal of Public Health, 103,* 1500–1506. http://dx.doi.org/10.2105/AJPH.2012.301117

MacCoun, R. J. (2011). What can we learn from the Dutch cannabis coffeeshop system? *Addiction, 106,* 1899–1910. http://dx.doi.org/10.1111/j.1360-0443.2011.03572.x

MacCoun, R., & Reuter, P. (2001). Evaluating alternative cannabis regimes. *British Journal of Psychiatry, 178,* 123–128. http://dx.doi.org/10.1192/bjp.178.2.123

Mayberry, M., Espelage, D., & Koenig, B. (2009). Multilevel modeling of direct effects and interactions of peers, parents, school, and community influences on adolescent substance use. *Journal of Youth and Adolescence, 38,* 1038–1049. http://dx.doi.org/10.1007/s10964-009-9425-9

McCaffrey, D. F., Liccardo Pacula, R., Han, B., & Ellickson, P. (2010). Marijuana use and high school dropout: The influence of unobservables. *Health Economics, 19,* 1281–1299. http://dx.doi.org/1002/hec.1561

McGue, M., Elkins, I., & Iacono, W. G. (2000). Genetic and environmental influences on adolescent substance use and abuse. *American Journal of Medical Genetics, 96,* 671–677. http://dx.doi.org/10.1002/1096-8628(20001009)96:5<671::AID-AJMG14>3.0.CO;2-W

Monte, A. A., Zane, R. D., & Heard, K. J. (2015). The implications of marijuana legalization in Colorado. *JAMA, 313,* 241–242. http://dx.doi.org/10.1001/jama.2014.17057

Moss, H. B., Vanyukov, M., Yao, J. K., & Kirillova, G. P. (1999). Salivary cortisol responses in prepubertal boys: The effects of parental substance abuse and association with drug use behavior during adolescence. *Biological Psychiatry, 45,* 1293–1299. http://dx.doi.org/10.1016/S0006-3223(98)00216-9

National Research Council and Institute of Medicine. (2004). *Reducing underage drinking: A collective responsibility.* Washington, DC: National Academies Press.

Oesterle, S., Hawkins, J. D., Steketee, M., Jonkman, H., Brown, E. C., Moll, M., & Haggerty, K. P. (2012). A cross-national comparison of risk and protective factors for adolescent drug use and delinquency in the United States and the Netherlands. *Journal of Drug Issues, 42,* 337–357. http://dx.doi.org/10.1177/0022042612461769

Pacula, R. L. (2010). *Examining the impact of marijuana legalization on marijuana consumption: Insights from the economics literature.* RAND Working Papers. Santa Monica, CA: RAND.

Pacula, R. L., Chriqui, J. F., & King, J. (2004). *Marijuana decriminalization: What does it mean in the United States?* NBER Working Paper No. 9609. Cambridge, MA: National Bureau of Economic Research.

Reboussin, B., Green, K., Milam, A., Furr-Holden, C. D., & Ialongo, N. (2014). Neighborhood environment and urban African American marijuana use during high school. *Journal of Urban Health, 91,* 1189–1201. http://dx.doi.org/10.1007/s11524-014-9909-0

Roebuck, M. C., French, M. T., & Dennis, M. L. (2004) Adolescent marijuana use and school attendance. *Economics of Education Review, 23*, 133–141. http://dx.doi.org/10.1016/S0272-7757(03)00079-7

Samek, D. R., Bailey, J. A., Hill, K. G., Wilson, S., Lee, S., Keyes, M. A., McGue, M. (2016). A test-replicate approach to candidate gene research on addiction and externalizing disorders: A collaboration across five longitudinal studies. *Behavior Genetics, 46*, 608–626. http://dx.doi.org/10.1007/s10519-016-9800-8

Simons, J. S., Neal, D. J., & Gaher, R. M. (2006). Risk for marijuana-related problems among college students: An application of zero-inflated negative binomial regression. *American Journal of Drug and Alcohol Abuse, 32*, 41–53. http://dx.doi.org/10.1080/00952990500328539

Sinha, R. (2008). Chronic stress, drug use, and vulnerability to addiction. *Annals of the New York Academy of Sciences, 1141*, 105–130. http://dx.doi.org/10.1196/annals.1441.030

Stone, A. L., Becker, L. G., Huber, A. M., & Catalano, R. F. (2012). Risk and protective factors of substance use and problem use in emerging adulthood. *Addictive Behaviors, 37*, 747–775. http://dx.doi.org/10.1016/j.addbeh.2012.02.014

Substance Abuse and Mental Health Services Administration. (2013). *Report to Congress on the nation's substance abuse and mental health workforce issues.* Retrieved from http://calswec.berkeley.edu/sites/default/files/uploads/samhsa-bh_workforce.pdf

Tang, Z., & Orwin, R. G. (2009). Marijuana Initiation among American youth and its risks as dynamic processes: Prospective findings from a national longitudinal study. *Substance Use & Misuse, 44*, 195–211. http://dx.doi.org/10.1080/10826080802347636

Taylor, M., Collin, S. M., Munafò, M. R., MacLeod, J., Hickman, M., & Heron, J. (2017). Patterns of cannabis use during adolescence and their association with harmful substance use behaviour: Findings from a UK birth cohort. *Journal of Epidemiology and Community Health, 71*, 764–770. http://dx.doi.org/10.1136/jech-2016-208503

van den Bree, M. M., & Pickworth, W. B. (2005). Risk factors predicting changes in marijuana involvement in teenagers. *Archives of General Psychiatry, 62*(3), 311–319. http://dx.doi.org/10.1001/archpsyc.62.3.311

van der Vorst, H., Engels, R. C. M. E., Meeus, W., & Deković, M. (2006). The impact of alcohol-specific rules, parental norms about early drinking and parental alcohol use on adolescents' drinking behavior. *Journal of Child Psychology and Psychiatry, 47*, 1299–1306. http://dx.doi.org/10.1111/j.1469-7610.2006.01680.x

van Leeuwen, A. P., Creemers, H. E., Greaves-Lord, K., Verhulst, F. C., Ormel, J., & Huizink, A. C. (2011). Hypothalamic–pituitary–adrenal axis reactivity to social stress and adolescent cannabis use: The TRAILS study. *Addiction, 106*, 1484–1492. http://dx.doi.org/10.1111/j.1360-0443.2011.03448.x

Verweij, K. J. H., Zietsch, B. P., Lynskey, M. T., Medland, S. E., Neale, M. C., Martin, N. G., . . . Vink, J. M. (2010). Genetic and environmental influences on cannabis use initiation and problematic use: A meta-analysis of twin studies. *Addiction, 105*, 417–430. http://dx.doi.org/10.1111/j.1360-0443.2009.02831.x

Volkow, N. D., Baler, R. D., Compton, W. M., & Weiss, S. R. (2014). Adverse health effects of marijuana use. *New England Journal of Medicine, 370*, 2219–2227. http://dx.doi.org/10.1056/NEJMra1402309

Wall, M. M., Poh, E., Cerda, M., Keyes, K. M., Galea, S., & Hasin, D. S. (2011). Adolescent marijuana use from 2002 to 2008: Higher in states with medical marijuana laws, cause still unclear. *Annals of Epidemiology, 21,* 714–716. http://dx.doi.org/10.1016/j.annepidem.2011.06.001

Washington State Institute for Public Policy. (2015). Substance abuse benefit-cost results. Olympia, WA: Author.

Wen, H., Hockenberry, J., & Cummings, J. R. (2014). *The effect of medical marijuana laws on marijuana, alcohol, and hard drug use.* NBER Working Paper No. 20085. Cambridge, MA: National Bureau of Economic Research.

Wright, E. M., Fagan, A. A., & Pinchevsky, G. M. (2013). The effects of exposure to violence and victimization across life domains on adolescent substance use. *Child Abuse & Neglect, 37,* 899–909. http://dx.doi.org/10.1016/j.chiabu.2013.04.010

9

Status Update on the Treatment of Cannabis Use Disorder

ALAN J. BUDNEY, CATHERINE STANGER,
ASHLEY A. KNAPP, AND DENISE D. WALKER

"When I wanted to quit smoking cannabis a few years ago and found that I couldn't do it under my own steam I went in search of a self-help book to show me the way. Annoyingly all I could find were books on how to cultivate the damn stuff."

CHRIS SULLIVAN, *The Joy of Quitting Cannabis: Freedom From Marijuana*

INTRODUCTION

The neuropharmacology, behavioral pharmacology, phenomenology, and clinical epidemiology of cannabis use and cannabis use disorder (CUD) closely parallel most other psychoactive substances that are used recreationally. That is, cannabis ingestion activates specific receptors in the brain that stimulate increases in dopamine; cannabis functions as a positive reinforcer, meaning that it produces effects that increase the probability that it will be used again; tolerance to its effects can develop and a withdrawal syndrome can occur following abstinence from regular, heavy use; intoxication adversely impacts cognitive and behavioral processes, increasing the probability of poor decision-making and acute adverse consequences; it is "enjoyed" in solitude or social settings; frequency and amount of use escalate over time in some users; some users maintain a nonproblematic pattern of use, while others develop a CUD that ranges from mild to severe; those who develop a use disorder experience a broad array of associated problems related to school/employment, family, finances, exacerbation of emotional disorders, low self-esteem, guilt, procrastination, memory, and related problems; a significant number of those who develop a problematic pattern of use wish to cut down or quit but are not successful; a substantial proportion of those who develop a CUD have at least one other co-occurring mental disorder; and, last, some individuals with CUD seek treatment, although as observed with those who have other types of substance use disorders (SUDs), the great majority do not seek or receive treatment.

This last point merits additional attention. The number of persons that might benefit from treatment and who seek treatment for CUD is not inconsequential. The National Survey on Drug Use and Health estimates that about 4.2 million people in the United States had a CUD in 2014, with a slight decreasing trend observed over the past couple years among youth less than 26 years old (Center for Behavioral Health Statistics and Quality, 2015). Treatment seeking at state-funded substance use treatment facilities for cases that report cannabis use as their primary substance problem ranks third behind alcohol and opioids among those 12 years and older, and among those younger than 20, cannabis remains by far the most common primary substance reported for treatment admissions. Of note, however, among adults with a CUD in the past year, only 7.2% received any type of service for cannabis problems, with rates of receiving services for mild, moderate, and severe CUD being 4.1%, 6.0%, and 15.7%, respectively (Hasin et al., 2016).

In the United States and elsewhere, we are in the midst of an unprecedented shift in cannabis laws and regulations. This change in legal status should not be perceived as a sign that cannabis suddenly has been deemed harmless with little potential for development of addictive-type problems. On the contrary, rates of heavy cannabis use and the development of CUDs have increased over the past 10 years, and as just discussed, relatively stable rates of treatment seeking have been observed. Indeed, the proliferation of new higher potency cannabis products, novel ways to use it, and increased access and promotion of use have raised concerns about possible increases in the potential for problem development among those that use cannabis (Budney, Sargent, & Lee, 2015). Alcohol, tobacco, and, to some extent, opioids are examples of legal drugs that have addictive potential yet can be devastating to those who develop problems (although, like with cannabis, most users of those substances do not experience substantial problems), and, importantly, regulations that influence products, sales, access, and marketing of substances can impact rates of problem development, exacerbation, and maintenance.

Given the parallels with other SUDs, it is not surprising that the treatment research literature focused on interventions for CUD has investigated similar approaches to those studied for other substances. Of the psychosocial interventions, behavioral approaches such as motivational enhancement, cognitive-behavioral therapy (CBT), and contingency management (CM) have received the most study. With adolescents, multiple types of family-based interventions have been developed and tested, in addition to similar evidence-based behavioral approaches used with adults. Increased understanding of the neuropharmacology of cannabis, in particular, its interaction with the endogenous cannabinoid system and the identification and characterization of a clinically relevant cannabis withdrawal syndrome, has also led to a proliferation of laboratory and clinical investigations of medications that might assist in cannabis reduction or cessation.

In this chapter, we will provide a brief overview of the scientific clinical literature evaluating the efficacy and effectiveness of interventions for those with CUD. This will primarily comprise a summary of recently published review articles that have synthesized controlled studies on psychosocial and pharmacological interventions for adults and adolescents. We will then discuss select recent findings of note, particularly focusing on promising approaches such as the use of technological-delivered interventions and providing brief interventions in nonspecialty community settings. Last, we will provide thoughts about future directions that may further enhance our efforts to assist those experiencing problems related to their cannabis use.

ADULT PSYCHOSOCIAL TREATMENT LITERATURE

At least eight reviews of controlled trials evaluating psychosocial treatments for CUD focused on adults have been published in the last 10 years (Budney, Roffman, Stephens, & Walker, 2007; Budney, Vandrey, & Fearer, 2011; Budney, Vandrey, & Stanger, 2010; Cooper, Chatters, Kaltenthaler, & Wong, 2015; Danovitch & Gorelick, 2012; Davis et al., 2015; Gates, Sabioni, Copeland, Le Foll, & Gowing, 2016; Halah, Zochniak, Barr, & George, 2016; Sherman & McRae-Clark, 2016). In the following discussion, we briefly describe the psychosocial treatment approaches for adults that have been most studied. We then review primary outcomes from three of the most recent reviews, highlighting common observations and issues relevant to their known efficacy and limitations.

Treatment Approaches

Motivational enhancement therapy (MET), CBT, and CM approaches to CUD have received the most study. The goal of MET is to address ambivalence about quitting cannabis as well as increase motivation and commitment to change. The clinician strategically employs counseling skills, such as empathy, reflective listening, summarizing, and affirmation to engender motivation and action toward change. Both the number of MET sessions (one to four) and the duration of sessions (45–90 min) have varied across trials evaluating its efficacy.

CBT targets the reduction or cessation of cannabis through psychoeducation and development of coping and relapse prevention skills. Psychoeducation typically focuses on analysis of factors relevant to use. Skills training focuses on a broad range of general coping skills (e.g., stress and mood management, problem-solving) and cannabis-specific cessation or reduction skills (e.g., functional analysis of use patterns and consequences, cannabis refusal skills, coping with withdrawal symptoms), which are taught and practiced in session and assigned for practice between sessions. CBT has been evaluated in both group and individual delivery formats, varying in session time (e.g., 45–60 min) and number (e.g., 6–14 sessions).

CM approaches systematically use reinforcement and sometimes punishment to engender change in a targeted behavior. Typically with treatment of CUD and other forms of SUDs, the target behavior is abstinence from the drug and/or attendance at therapy sessions. Documented achievement of these targets (e.g., provision of cannabis-negative urine specimens) are reinforced or rewarded with monetary-based incentives. Such incentives can then be used to obtain or establish prosocial reinforcers (e.g., clothing, activities, hobbies) that can replace or compete with cannabis use.

Reviews

Gates et al. (2016) conducted a narrative review of 23 randomized trials for adults with either CUD or daily cannabis use. Cooper et al. (2015) conducted a narrative review of 33 randomized trials for CUD or regular cannabis use comparing psychosocial interventions administered in community and out-patient settings across several nations. Davis et al. (2015) conducted a meta-analysis on 10 randomized control trials, only including studies that compared behavioral therapies with active and nonactive control comparison conditions. Across reviews, psychosocial treatments compared to no treatment consistently produced significant reductions in quantity, frequency, and severity of cannabis use as well as severity of dependence symptoms (Davis et al., 2015; Gates et al., 2016). There was little to no evidence, however, to suggest psychosocial treatments produced significantly more change in motivation to quit, personal and social problems related to cannabis use, and additional substance use compared to no-treatment controls (Gates et al., 2016). Also, inconsistent conclusions across reviews were offered regarding effects on improvements in psychosocial functioning (e.g., employment, mental health), with the smaller meta-analytic review finding support for a positive impact on psychosocial functioning (Davis et al., 2015), but the larger narrative review not finding evidence for this effect (Gates et al., 2016). This discrepant finding could be related to definition and measurement of psychosocial functioning as the studies in the smaller meta-analysis were primarily based on indicators from the Addiction Severity Index, whereas the larger narrative review relied on more heterogeneous measures of psychopathology and psychosocial functioning.

Regarding specific types of treatment, the reviews concluded that CBT, MET, combined MET/CBT, and combined MET/CBT/CM were the most effective therapies for reducing frequency of cannabis use and cannabis dependence severity in the short term (up to nine months posttreatment). Mixed support was found for CBT outperforming the more brief MET interventions, although the bulk of the evidence suggested CBT tended to engender greater effects on cannabis use. Combining CM (abstinence-based incentives) with the other interventions

BOX 9.1

ADULT CUD PSYCHOSOCIAL TREATMENT: SUMMARY AND FUTURE DIRECTIONS

- Approaches that are efficacious with other SUDs are also efficacious for CUD.
- Support for the efficacy of CBT, MET, and abstinence-based CM as first-line interventions is strong.
- Longer duration CBT produces more robust effects than more brief CBT or MET.
- Abstinence-based CM can substantially increase achievement of abstinence, and a combination of MET/CBT/CM appears to engender superior outcomes to any of the individual interventions delivered alone.
- Even with MET/CBT/CM, less than 50% of participants achieve abstinence, and fewer maintain abstinence six months posttreatment.
- Effectiveness of all interventions wane such that most studies show only weak signs, if any, of efficacy one-year following the start of treatment.
- Nonabstinence, cannabis reduction targets and measures are needed to explore potentially important change engendered in treatment interventions.
- More research is needed on psychosocial approaches to CUD with co-occurring psychopathology.
- More research is needed to identify specific mechanisms of change activated by the efficacious psychosocial treatments for CUD.

was observed to optimize short-term treatment outcomes. Specifically, frequency of cannabis use, abstinence, and severity of dependence were enhanced when CM was integrated with other approaches, and these combinations optimize abstinence outcomes out to 12 months posttreatment.

Generally, this literature suggests that more intense psychosocial treatments over longer intervals (i.e., four or more sessions) appear more robust than the briefer motivational approaches, but future studies are necessary to better determine adequate or optimal durations of treatment. Also important is the observation that the great majority of those receiving treatment do not achieve cannabis abstinence for substantial durations of time, and many of those who do, relapse within a month posttreatment. Box 9.1 provides a summary of and possible future directions for adult psychosocial treatment.

ADOLESCENT PSYCHOSOCIAL TREATMENT LITERATURE

Most evaluations of treatment for adolescents with SUDs have included youth who use and misuse various substances and, as such, have not isolated effects on

CUD. However, in most studies, cannabis is the primary substance used by the adolescents and CUD the primary SUD diagnosis. At least eight reviews of this literature have appeared in the last 10 years (Hogue, Henderson, Ozechowski, & Robbins, 2014; Simpson & Magid, 2016; Stanger, Lansing, & Budney, 2016; Tanner-Smith, Wilson, & Lipsey, 2013; Waldron & Turner, 2008; Winters, Botzet, & Fahnhorst, 2011; Winters, Tanner-Smith, Bresani, & Meyers, 2014). In the following section, we first describe one of the very few clinical trials focused specifically on CUD in adolescents, which also happens to be the largest trial published to date. We then discuss the findings from three of the reviews, highlighting cannabis-related outcomes when possible.

The Cannabis Youth Treatment (CYT) study is the largest trial conducted to date among adolescent cannabis users (Dennis et al., 2004). This multisite study ($N = 600$) utilized five treatment approaches that included individual (MET, adolescent community reinforcement approach), group (CBT), and family-based (family support network, multidimensional family therapy) interventions in several combinations (MET + CBT, MET/CBT + Family support network), and of different durations (5, 12, and 14 weeks). All treatments were equally effective and no one treatment outperformed another. That is, adolescents across conditions and trials evidenced significant improvement in days of abstinence and recovery rates at the one-year follow-up (all in reference to substances in general, including cannabis, alcohol, and other drugs). While significant treatment gains were achieved, it is important to note that most adolescents did not achieve abstinence, well over half experienced periods of relapse across the study period, and the great majority evidenced substance-related problems or use at the one-year assessment.

Hogue et al. (2014) evaluated 19 well-controlled studies of outpatient psychosocial therapies for adolescent substance use published from 2007 to 2013 to identify those meeting criteria as well-established or probably efficacious. Tanner-Smith et al. (2013) conducted a meta-analysis of 45 adolescent outpatient treatment studies published since 1980. Across both reviews, several family-based therapies (i.e., functional family therapy and multidimensional family therapy) had strong support. In addition, CBT, whether delivered both individually and in group settings, showed positive effects. Tanner-Smith et al. reported direct comparisons between evidence-based interventions and found that family-based approaches showed significantly larger effects on substance use than MET/CBT interventions. They also indicated that, across studies, cannabis use evidenced the largest change compared with other substances being used by these youth.

Several stand-alone interventions delivered in integrated packages (e.g., CBT + Family therapy, MET + CBT, CM + Family therapy) have also received strong support. As Hogue et al. (2014) note, the support for these integrated models suggests that increasing the scope and intensity of adolescent substance use treatments by combining evidence-based interventions can enhance outcomes. More research is needed to identify the mechanisms of individual components and their optimal dose and timing. Hogue et al. also noted that these evidence-based interventions showed particularly strong effects among more impaired

BOX 9.2

ADOLESCENT SUD PSYCHOSOCIAL TREATMENT: SUMMARY AND FUTURE DIRECTIONS

- As in the adult literature, MET/CBT and CM have demonstrated efficacy for adolescent substance use disorders.
- In addition, several specific types of family therapies are highly efficacious for adolescent substance use.
- Although helpful to many, as in the adult studies, the majority of youth that receive these interventions typically do not show a clinically meaningful reduction in substance use, and posttreatment assessments indicate substantial relapse among those who do respond.
- Adolescent studies have not focused specifically on cannabis and often do not report cannabis outcomes separate from other substances, making comparison with the adult literature challenging.
- There have been few studies testing mechanisms of change in adolescent interventions, yet identification of mechanisms holds promise as a means to enhance the efficacy of existing interventions, and the development of new more effective interventions.
- Similarly, little is known about moderators of treatment outcomes, including the possible role individual and family characteristics, as well as what indicators predict early response across key mechanisms. Such markers could be tested in prospective designs to test approaches to tailoring treatment (e.g., delivering intensive interventions to those who need them, and briefer, less expensive interventions to those who do not).

youth, particularly those with more severe substance use and comorbid conduct problems.

Stanger et al. (2016) reviewed the latest research on CM approaches for SUD among youth, examining the six most recent controlled trials. As in the adult studies previously reviewed, CM was combined with various evidence-based psychosocial interventions (e.g., MET, CBT). The majority of trials reviewed provided support for the use of CM to optimize treatment outcomes. The maintenance of treatment effects, however, did not endure posttreatment. Stanger et al. called for future work to carefully examine the most optimal CM parameters (e.g., incentive magnitude and schedule, intervention target, monitoring strategy, etc.) that lead to the best treatment outcomes. Box 9.2 provides a summary of and possible future directions for adolescent psychosocial treatment.

BRIEF INTERVENTIONS IN NONCLINICAL SETTINGS

The majority of individuals who might benefit from some intervention related to their use of cannabis do not access treatment services of any kind; fewer than 10% with SUD symptoms in the past year have ever received treatment (Dennis, Clark, & Huang, 2014). Moreover, the barriers of youth and young adults enrolling in treatment for SUDs are heightened because young people almost never self-refer but, instead, are referred by parents, the juvenile justice system, or schools, and when they do enter treatment for cannabis, few (20%) believe their use is problematic (Diamond, Leckrone, Dennis, & Godley, 2006), suggesting that novel approaches to reach people directly and motivate regular users to reduce their use or abstain are needed.

Opportunistic settings such as schools or medical settings offer the ability to identify and reach more persons experiencing problems related to their use of cannabis. Several brief interventions aimed at youth have been developed to facilitate intervention efforts in these settings, with most of this work involving the adaptation or evaluation of motivational interviewing (MI) interventions. Two brief interventions for youth were developed for use in primary care or the emergency department with either a focus on substance abuse generally, of which most participants used cannabis (D'Amico, Miles, Stern, & Meredith, 2008), or cannabis specifically (Bernstein et al., 2009). Both were adaptations of MI and consisted of a 15 to 20 min session plus a 10-min booster phone call. Findings from both trials showed significant reductions in cannabis use compared to assessment control and suggest that both primary care and emergency room settings may be effective intervention settings. Offering the session at the time of the visit appeared to increase session completion.

School settings are also a compelling environment for delivery of services. Brief interventions delivered in schools have been conducted in the United States and England. One large trial identified students suspected of misusing alcohol or drugs (Winters, Fahnhorst, Botzet, Lee, & Lalone, 2012; Winters, Lee, Botzet, Fahnhorst, & Nicholson, 2014). Two sessions of an MI-based intervention reduced cannabis use and CUD symptoms more than assessment only at a one-year follow-up. Two studies conducted in the United Kingdom offered a one session MI discussing alcohol, tobacco, and illicit drug use to further education college students (age 16–20 years). One trial showed significant reductions in cigarettes, alcohol, and cannabis (McCambridge & Strang, 2004) but not in a second trial in which intervention delivery fidelity varied (McCambridge, Slym, & Strang, 2008). Overall, these studies also suggest that interventions targeting drug and alcohol use more generally among adolescents can prompt reductions in cannabis use (see recent meta-analysis; Carney & Myers, 2012).

An alternative school-based approach, offering interventions that are voluntary and not labeled as treatment can attract, engage, and effectively intervene with students with substantial cannabis and other substance use. Walker et al. (2006, 2011, 2016) recruited large numbers of nontreatment-seeking high school students to participate in a brief intervention called the Teen Marijuana Checkup (TMCU). This approach attracts those not interested or not willing to go to treatment, those who have questions or concerns about their cannabis use but do not identify as having a problem, and those who are currently not thinking about changing their use. Across three controlled trials, students with cannabis use levels comparable to levels observed in published outpatient treatment studies volunteered in response to in-school posters and classroom presentations. Students exposed to TMCU reliably show greater decreases in cannabis use relative to those in control conditions.

The TMCU has been adapted and evaluated in Australia (Martin & Copeland, 2008; Martin, Copeland, & Swift, 2005) and the Netherlands (de Gee, Verdurmen, Bransen, de Jonge, & Schippers, 2014), although neither of these adapted versions offered the service in school or directly focused recruitment on self-referred adolescents. Rather, most of the participants in these trials were recruited through more traditional routes such as advertising at potential referral sources such as juvenile justice offices and substance abuse treatment facilities or through concerned parents. Results were mixed from these trials, with the Australian Adolescent Cannabis Check-Up showing greater reductions in use compared to a delayed control. The Dutch study failed to find significant differences between the check-up and an informational control session except among heavier users. Similar types of brief interventions are being tested with college students. For example, an intervention similar to the TMCU was compared to assessment only in college students from two institutions who regularly used marijuana (Lee et al., 2013). Significant but very weak effects were observed on marijuana use. Box 9.3 provides a summary of and possible future directions for brief interventions.

BOX 9.3

BRIEF INTERVENTIONS: SUMMARY AND FUTURE DIRECTIONS

- MI approaches have been by far the most researched brief interventions for adolescents.
- Effects on reduction in cannabis use are small to moderate; research to develop more potent brief models is needed.
- Various settings, such as schools and healthcare clinics, can facilitate interventions for youth who would not typically access treatment in traditional SUD clinics.
- Reducing barriers to participation (providing interventions where adolescents already are, not requiring parental consent) increases engagement and completion.
- Studies that utilized practitioners in community settings rather than research staff reported worse outcomes.
- More research needs to focus on dissemination and implementation of these interventions—specifically if these small to moderate effect sizes are maintained when delivered under real-world conditions or by existing community program staff.

TECHNOLOGY-DELIVERED INTERVENTIONS

As previously mentioned, the great majority of youth and adults with CUD do not seek or receive treatment, the availability of evidence-based services at community clinics or other settings is low, and outcomes among those who do receive treatment is not optimal. These observations suggest that novel approaches to reach those who might benefit and to more effectively motivate reduction in use or abstinence are needed. Technology-delivered interventions (TDIs) hold substantial promise to extend reach and enhance outcomes of efforts to prevent escalation of cannabis use and to treat CUD. TDIs offer alternative strategies for providing evidence-based treatments and have fewer requirements for trained personnel and, in turn, lower costs.

TDIs for adult CUD have been tested in multiple, controlled clinical trials. These interventions, which utilized effective learning methodologies and adapted face-to-face evidence-based interventions for delivery via computer or mobile devices, have demonstrated positive impact on treatment outcomes comparable to or exceeding therapist-delivered interventions (Budney, Fearer, et al., 2011; Budney, Stanger, et al., 2015; Kay-Lambkin, Baker, Kelly, & Lewin, 2011; Kay-Lambkin, Baker, Lewin, & Carr, 2009; Marsch, Carroll, & Kiluk, 2014; Schaub et al., 2015). One TDI model, tested in two trials, involved a nine-session, office-based, computer-delivered MET/CBT program integrated with abstinence-based CM and three brief, in-person supportive sessions with a therapist (Budney, Fearer, et al., 2011; Budney, Stanger, et al., 2015). Cannabis use and abstinence outcomes observed during treatment in both studies did not differ between computer-assisted and therapist-delivered MET/CBT/CM, and no differences were observed on other secondary outcomes. The second trial demonstrated that computer-assisted MET/CBT/CM produced comparable outcomes throughout a 12-month follow-up period. Of additional importance, initial cost analyses showed substantial savings associated with the computer-assisted intervention.

An Australian group developed and tested a similar computer-delivered MET/CBT program to treat cannabis or alcohol problems and depression in adults (Kay-Lambkin et al., 2009, 2011). Again, results from two randomized trials supported the efficacy of this TDI that involved 10 MET/CBT sessions and 10 to 15 min check-ins with a therapist each session. In the initial study, treatment retention and therapeutic alliance did not differ between completely therapist-delivered MET/CBT and the computer-delivered MET/CBT intervention, and both produced better cannabis, alcohol, and depression outcomes than a brief intervention alone. A large replication trial produced similar findings, again showing that therapist- and computer-delivered interventions engendered comparable outcomes with both outperforming a 10-session person-centered therapy (Kay-Lambkin et al., 2011). A subsequent implementation study showed that community clinicians were open to using this computer-assisted intervention, but only 34% chose to do so, suggesting the importance of providing ongoing support and encouragement to clinicians to facilitate the adoption of innovative technologies into practice (Kay-Lambkin, Simpson, Bowman, & Childs, 2014).

Surprisingly, TDIs have been underdeveloped and tested for use with adolescents (Marsch & Borodovsky, 2016). Two studies have tested a brief intervention delivered on a mobile tablet with youth who did or did not screen positive for cannabis use across seven health clinics (Walton et al., 2013, 2014). Compared to assessment only, the TDI reduced self-reported cannabis-related problems but had minimal impact on cannabis use frequency among those using cannabis at baseline; however, it prevented cannabis use over the subsequent 12 months in those who were not using cannabis at baseline. Some innovative studies have used ecological momentary assessments as an intervention tool. One pilot study used ecological momentary assessment to intervene with cannabis-using youth (Shrier, Rhoads, Burke, Walls, & Blood, 2014). After two in-person MET sessions, youth were instructed to report triggers, cravings, and cannabis use with their mobile phone for two weeks. Youth received text messages to help them cope with the identified triggers. Preliminary data suggested that use of this program reduced frequency of cannabis use and was acceptable to youth. Last, a Web-based, computer-delivered TDI similar to that previously described for adults in outpatient setting was tested in a small controlled trial. Youth entering a SUD treatment program who were assigned to the TDI condition, which replaced in-person sessions, achieved similar reductions in substance use and mental health outcomes compared with the therapist-delivered intervention and rated the TDI as highly acceptable (Acosta et al., 2016).

Of note, completely Web-based interventions are being developed and beginning to undergo testing. A few of these have focused on marijuana use among college students. For example, a one-session Web-based intervention for at-risk, marijuana-using students transitioning to college that provided personalized feedback similar to that previously described for the TMCU was compared to assessment only (Lee, Neighbors, Kilmer, & Larimer, 2010). No overall treatment effects were observed, but there was suggestion of a positive effect among more motivated students and those with family histories of substance use problems. Another study tested a similar type of Web-based screening and brief intervention in students attending the on-campus health clinic but found no robust effects on marijuana use (Palfai et al., 2014). A Swiss group developed a Web-based, eight module MET/CBT self-help program for the general population and tested it with and without one to two "chat" counseling sessions delivered by a therapist over the Internet (Schaub et al., 2015). Program retention and completion were not high, but those who received the program with the "chat" counseling reported greater cannabis reduction outcomes than those who were assigned to receive only the Web-based program or to a wait list control group. Box 9.4 provides a summary of and possible future directions for technology-delivered interventions.

PHARMACOTHERAPY FOR CUD

As with treatment approaches to all SUDs, the need to develop more potent and effective interventions has led to the development and evaluation of potential

BOX 9.4

TECHNOLOGY-DELIVERED INTERVENTIONS SUMMARY AND FUTURE DIRECTIONS

- TDIs offer alternative methods for delivering evidence based treatment with high fidelity and integrity and reduced provider training requirements.
- TDIs can be cost effective and increase access to services.
- TDIs offer the possibility of enhancing outcomes by increasing access to interventions when needed in real time or when convenient, prompting use of coping strategies, and tailoring interventions for the individual.
- A number of TDIs for CUD have demonstrated efficacy in controlled studies, most of these involve at least minimal contact with a therapist.
- Brief TDIs may be of great value in nonclinical settings when cannabis use or problems are identified.
- Integration of TDIs into community systems will require careful study of optimal implementation strategies to promote acceptance and engagement by providers.

pharmacotherapies for CUD. Advances in the understanding of the neurobiology of cannabis and the complex functions of the endocannabinoid systems, together with the characterization of a clinically important withdrawal syndrome, have guided these efforts. Paralleling efforts from other SUDs, the pharmacotherapies tested have included (a) agonist-like medications targeting the CB1 receptor that could reduce withdrawal or substitute for cannabis; (b) antagonist-like or inverse agonist medications that block the CB1 receptor, reducing the reinforcing effects of cannabis; (c) medications targeting specific withdrawal symptoms; (d) medications that target craving or decrease desire for cannabis; (e) most recently, medications that block opioid receptors that interact with the cannabinoid system; and (f) medications that target co-morbid psychiatric conditions.

Multiple reviews of this CUD pharmacotherapy literature have appeared over the past few years. Much of the research to date has been limited to human laboratory studies, open-label trial, or relatively small placebo-controlled clinical trials. No medications have yet to receive sufficient empirical research support for approval by the Food and Drug Administration in the United States or to justify clear clinical recommendations. In the following discussion, we briefly summarize findings from two of the most recent reviews of this literature (Copeland & Pokorski, 2016; Mason, Mustafa, Filbey, & Brown, 2016) and provide a status update on progress being made and future directions.

Laboratory studies have demonstrated that potential agonist therapies, such as dronabinol (an oral formulation of delta-9-tetrahydrocannabinol [THC]) and nabilone (oral synthetic CB1 receptor agonist), can reduce withdrawal symptoms, subjective and physiological effects of smoked cannabis, and cannabis self-administration; however, two outpatient clinical trials failed to demonstrate the efficacy of dronabinol or a combination of lofexidine (an alpha-2 agonist) and dronabinol for CUD (Levin et al., 2011, 2016). A recent inpatient clinical trial of a nabiximols, an oramucosal medication that combines a delta-9-THC with cannabidiol (a compound in the cannabis plant with unclear neurobiological action), showed a positive effect on reducing withdrawal symptoms compared to placebo but did not engender greater cannabis abstinence postdischarge (Allsop et al., 2014). Antagonist therapies have received much less study in humans. A large laboratory study showed that Rimonabant, a CB1 receptor inverse agonist, effectively decreased (blocked) the intoxicating effects of smoked cannabis (Huestis et al., 2001); however, rimonabant has since been withdrawn from the European market because of serious psychiatric side effects. To date, no other antagonists or inverse agonists have been systematically tested in humans.

A host of medications targeting mood or stress have undergone tests in the laboratory and research clinics (e.g., baclofen, buspirone, bupropion, divalproex, fluoxetine, lithium, mirtazapine, nefazadone, quitiepine, topirimate, venlafaxine; Copeland & Pokorski, 2016; Mason et al., 2016), but none of these have produced results that offer substantial promise for use by community providers. One small clinical trial of a GABA-ergic medication (i.e., gabapentin) showed reductions in withdrawal symptoms, days and amount of cannabis use, and improved sleep compared to a placebo condition (Mason et al., 2012); a larger replication trial is ongoing. A controlled trial of N-acetylcysteine (NAC), a naturally occurring amino acid that putatively modulates glutamate, also showed positive effects in treatment-seeking youth (Gray et al., 2012). A greater percentage of those who received NAC compared to placebo achieved cannabis abstinence. A subsequent multisite trial of NAC versus placebo with adults seeking treatment for CUD did not support its efficacy for reducing cannabis use or achievement of abstinence (Gray, 2016).

The opiate antagonist, naltrexone, has been tested in the laboratory as a potential medication for CUD because of the bidirectional modulatory effects of the endogenous cannabinoid and opioid systems and the potential for opioid receptor blockade to decrease the positive effects of cannabis. A recent study showed that chronic dosing decreased the reinforcing effects of cannabis smoking in lab sessions and appeared to influence cannabis use patterns in the natural environment (Haney et al., 2015). No clinical trials of naltrexone for CUD have been conducted.

A few medications have been tested for the treatment of CUD and co-morbid psychiatric conditions. For example, a large multisite trial tested an attention deficit hyperactivity disorder (ADHD) medication, methylphenidate, in teens with both ADHD and a SUD, which included over 90% with CUD (Riggs et al., 2011). The impact of the medication on ADHD symptoms was minimal compared to placebo, no difference was observed on self-reported days of substance use (the primary outcome), and a minimal, yet significant difference in substance abstinence (number of negative urine tests) favored the medication group. Other studies testing atomoxetine for CUD patients with ADHD, and vanalfexine or fluoxetine for CUD and depression also did not produce robust findings. A number of studies have focused on the impact of antipsychotic

BOX 9.5

PHARMACOTHERAPY: TAKE HOME POINTS AND LOOKING TO THE FUTURE

- No medications are currently approved by the FDA for treating CUD.
- CB1 receptor agonist and antagonist approaches show promise, but testing of alternative doses and dosing schedules, and new compounds with fewer side effects is needed.
- Approaches that test opiate receptor blockade warrant additional study.
- Replication of effects observed with gabapentin and NAC are needed to further evaluate their clinical potential.
- More testing of medications within subgroups of persons with CUD who exhibit specific co-occurring psychiatric symptoms or disorders is needed, rather than testing psychiatric medications on the general population of CUD patients.
- Development of novel medications that directly target the endogenous cannabinoid system (e.g., directly manipulate brain levels of specific endocannabinoids; i.e., FAAH inhibitors) may prove valuable in the future.
- Testing of medications needs to be conducted in combination with various psychosocial treatments and in isolation to best determine their impact and potential for dissemination.

medications on cannabis use in persons with diagnoses of schizophrenia and CUD. Observational studies show that cannabis use may be reduced with clozapine compared to other antipsychotics, and a small, randomized trial reported a small effect of clozapine on reductions in cannabis use (Brunette et al., 2011). Box 9.5 provides an overview of the future of pharmacotherapy.

CONCLUSIONS AND FUTURE DIRECTIONS

The relatively large number of persons in need of and seeking treat for CUD relative to other types of SUDs clearly indicates the public health significance of ensuring adequate access to effective interventions for those experiencing the negative consequences of this disorder. Although a changing cannabis regulatory environment and the proliferation of US state-sanctioned medical use of cannabis may provide the perception that cannabis is relatively harmless, many youth and adults struggle with the consequences of their use and have difficulty quitting or substantially reducing their use. During the last 20 years, clinical research on the development and testing of interventions for those with CUD has progressed such that we have accumulated a wealth of information on the efficacy of psychosocial treatments and, to a lesser extent, pharmacotherapies. For psychosocial interventions, the extant outcome literature points to the view that the same types of approaches used for other SUDs appear to produce comparable outcomes for CUD. Observed outcomes clearly indicate that CUD is not easily treated as the majority of those who enter treatment struggle to make enduring significant changes in their cannabis use. Continued efforts to produce more effective intervention approaches are sorely needed, which might involve the development of more potent interventions, better strategies for matching individuals with interventions that best meet their needs, or offering of stepped care or adaptive approaches that address high levels of nonresponding to initial treatment episodes. Parallel to what is transpiring across health care research of all types, innovative applications of technology, including the use of mobile devices, to enhance access to and efficacy of evidence-based interventions offer great promise for the treatment and perhaps prevention of CUD. Moreover, TDIs would appear optimal for reaching the 80% to 90% of youth and adults that might benefit from addressing problematic cannabis use but who do not receive treatment. Brief interventions designed for delivery in nontraditional healthcare setting also have shown promise for extending the reach of psychosocial interventions.

The more nascent efforts to develop pharmacotherapies for CUD have yet to produce strong support for the efficacy of any one class of medications or a specific medication. Nonetheless, findings from the human laboratory suggest that CB1 agonists hold promise, but a clearly efficacious protocol (dose or duration) or specific agonist medication has yet to be identified. Similarly, agonist medications, both that block the CB1 receptor and opioid receptors show promise in the laboratory, but much more work is needed to identify and test optimal dose and dosing schedules and identifying CB1 antagonists with low risk-adverse effect profiles. Much more basic and clinical science is necessary if we are to expect major breakthroughs in our efforts to more effectively prevent and treat SUDs, including CUD. Efforts to increase knowledge related to cannabis use and its consequences, good or bad, will likely increase in importance as more and more states and countries move toward legalizing its use. Fortunately, many alternatives for effective assistance have already been identified, and ongoing research promises to provide the information needed to offer even more potent options for helping those in need.

REFERENCES

Acosta, M. C., Marsch, L. A., Xie, H., Kim, S. J., Grabinski, M., Kaminer, Y., et al. (2016). The Step Up Program: development and evaluation of a Web-based psychosocial treatment for adolescents with substance use disorders. Manuscript under review.

Allsop, D. J., Copeland, J., Lintzeris, N., Dunlop, A. J., Montebello, M., Sadler, C., . . . McGregor, I. S. (2014). Nabiximols as an agonist replacement therapy during cannabis withdrawal: a randomized clinical trial. *JAMA Psychiatry, 71,* 281–291. http://dx.doi.org/10.1001/jamapsychiatry.2013.3947

Bernstein, E., Edwards, E., Dorfman, D., Heeren, T., Bliss, C., & Bernstein, J. (2009). Screening and brief intervention to reduce marijuana use among youth and young adults in a pediatric emergency department. *Academy of Emergency Medicine, 16,* 1174–1185. http://dx.doi.org/10.1111/j.1553-2712.2009.00490.x

Brunette, M. F., Dawson, R., O'Keefe, C. D., Narasimhan, M., Noordsy, D. L., Wojcik, J., . . . Green, A. I. (2011). A randomized trial of clozapine vs. other antipsychotics for cannabis use disorder in patients with schizophrenia. *Journal of Dual Diagnosis, 7,* 50–63. http://dx.doi.org/10.1080/15504263.2011.570118

Budney, A. J., Fearer, S. A., Walker, D. D., Stanger, C., Thostensen, J., Grabinski, M. J., & Bickel, W. K. (2011). An initial trial of a computerized behavioral intervention for cannabis use disorder. *Drug Alcohol Dependence, 115,* 74–79. http://dx.doi.org/10.1016/j.drugalcdep.2010.10.014

Budney, A. J., Roffman, R., Stephens, R. S., & Walker, D. (2007). Marijuana dependence and its treatment. *Addictive Science and Clinical Practice, 4,* 4–16.

Budney, A. J., Sargent, J. D., & Lee, D. C. (2015). Vaping cannabis (marijuana): Parallel concerns to e-cigs? *Addiction, 110,* 1699–1704. http://dx.doi.org/10.1111/add.13036

Budney, A. J., Stanger, C., Tilford, J. M., Scherer, E. B., Brown, P. C., Li, Z., . . . Walker, D. (2015). Computer-assisted behavioral therapy and contingency management for cannabis use disorder. *Psychology of Addictive Behaviors, 29,* 501–511. http://dx.doi.org/10.1037/adb0000078

Budney, A. J., Vandrey, R., & Fearer, S. A. (2011). Cannabis (marijuana). In P. Ruiz & E. Strain (Eds.), *Lowenson & Ruiz's Substance Abuse: A Comprehensive Textbook* (5th ed., pp. 214–237). Baltimore, MD: Lippincott Williams & Wilkins.

Budney, A. J., Vandrey, R. G., & Stanger, C. (2010). Pharmacological and psychosocial interventions for cannabis use disorders. *Revista Brasileira de Psiquiatria, 3*(Suppl 1), S46–S55. http://dx.doi.org/10.1590/S1516-44462010000500008

Carney, T., & Myers, B. (2012). Effectiveness of early interventions for substance-using adolescents: Findings from a systematic review and meta-analysis. *Substance Abuse Treatment and Prevention Policy, 7,* 25. http://dx.doi.org/10.1186/1747-597X-7-25

Center for Behavioral Health Statistics and Quality. (2015). Behavioral health trends in the United States: Results from the 2014 National Survey on Drug Use and Health (HHS Publication No. SMA 15-4927, NSDUH Series H-50). Washington, DC: Substance Abuse and Mental Health Services Administration.

Cooper, K., Chatters, R., Kaltenthaler, E., & Wong, R. (2015). Psychological and psychosocial interventions for cannabis cessation in adults: A systematic review short report. *Health Technology Assessment, 19*(56), 1–130. http://dx.doi.org/10.3310/hta19560

Copeland, J., & Pokorski, I. (2016). Progress toward pharmacotherapies for cannabis-use disorder: An evidence-based review. *Substance Abuse Rehabilitation, 7,* 41–53. http://dx.doi.org/10.2147/SAR.S89857

D'Amico, E. J., Miles, J. N., Stern, S. A., & Meredith, L. S. (2008). Brief motivational interviewing for teens at risk of substance use consequences: A randomized pilot study in a primary care clinic. *Journal of Substance Abuse Treatment, 35,* 53–61. http://dx.doi.org/10.1016/j.jsat.2007.08.008

Danovitch, I., & Gorelick, D. A. (2012). State of the art treatments for cannabis dependence. *Psychiatric Clinics of North America, 35,* 309–326. http://dx.doi.org/10.1016/j.psc.2012.03.003

Davis, M. L., Powers, M. B., Handelsman, P., Medina, J. L., Zvolensky, M., & Smits, J. A. (2015). Behavioral therapies for treatment-seeking cannabis users: a meta-analysis of randomized controlled trials. *Evaluation of Health Professions*, 38, 94–114. http://dx.doi.org/10.1177/0163278714529970

de Gee, E. A., Verdurmen, J. E., Bransen, E., de Jonge, J. M., & Schippers, G. M. (2014). A randomized controlled trial of a brief motivational enhancement for non-treatment-seeking adolescent cannabis users. *Journal of Substance Abuse Treatment*, 47, 181–188. http://dx.doi.org/10.1016/j.jsat.2014.05.001

Dennis, M. L., Clark, H. W., & Huang, L. N. (2014). The need and opportunity to expand substance use disorder treatment in school-based settings. *Advances in School Mental Health Promotion*, 7, 75–87. http://dx.doi.org/10.1080/1754730X.2014.888221

Dennis, M. L., Godley, S. H., Diamond, G., Tims, F. M., Babor, T., Donaldson, J., . . . Funk, R. (2004). The cannabis youth treatment (CYT) study: Main findings from two randomized trials. *Journal of Substance Abuse Treatment*, 27, 197–213. http://dx.doi.org/10.1016/j.jsat.2003.09.005

Diamond, G., Leckrone, J., Dennis, M., & Godley, S. H. (2006). The cannabis youth treatment study: The treatment models and preliminary findings. In R.A. Roffman & R.S. Stephens (Eds.), *Cannabis Dependence: Its Nature, Consequences, and Treatment* (pp. 247–269). Cambridge: Cambridge University Press.

Gates, P. J., Sabioni, P., Copeland, J., Le Foll, B., & Gowing, L. (2016). Psychosocial interventions for cannabis use disorder. *Cochrane Database System Reviev*, 5, CD005336. http://dx.doi.org/10.1002/14651858.CD005336.pub4

Gray, K. M. (2016). Adolescent considerations in cannabis use disorder pharmacotherapy. *Child and Adolescent Psychiatry*, 55(Suppl), S67. http://dx.doi.org/10.1016/j.jaac.2016.07.698

Gray, K. M., Carpenter, M. J., Baker, N. L., DeSantis, S. M., Kryway, E., Hartwell, K. J., . . . Brady, K. T. (2012). A double-blind randomized controlled trial of N-acetylcysteine in cannabis-dependent adolescents. *American Journal of Psychiatry*, 169, 805–812. http://dx.doi.org/10.1176/appi.ajp.2012.12010055

Halah, M. P., Zochniak, M. P., Barr, M. S., & George, T. P. (2016). Cannabis use and psychiatric disorders: Implications for mental health and addiction treatment. *Current Addiction Reports*, 3, 450–462. http://dx.doi.org/10.1007/s40429-016-0128-5

Haney, M., Ramesh, D., Glass, A., Pavlicova, M., Bedi, G., & Cooper, Z. D. (2015). Naltrexone maintenance decreases cannabis self-administration and subjective effects in daily cannabis smokers. *Neuropsychopharmacology*, 40, 2489–2498. http://dx.doi.org/10.1038/npp.2015.108

Hasin, D. S., Kerridge, B. T., Saha, T. D., Huang, B., Pickering, R., Smith, S. M., . . . Grant, B. F. (2016). Prevalence and correlates of DSM–5 cannabis use disorder, 2012–2013: Findings from the National Epidemiologic Survey on Alcohol and Related Conditions–III. *American Journal of Psychiatry*, 173, 588–599. http://dx.doi.org/10.1176/appi.ajp.2015.15070907

Hogue, A., Henderson, C. E., Ozechowski, T. J., & Robbins, M. S. (2014). Evidence base on outpatient behavioral treatments for adolescent substance use: updates and recommendations 2007–2013. *Journal of Clinical Child & Adolescent Psychology*, 43, 695–720. http://dx.doi.org/10.1080/15374416.2014.915550

Huestis, M. A., Gorelick, D. A., Heishman, S. J., Preston, K. L., Nelson, R. A., Moolchan, E. T., & Frank, R. A. (2001). Blockade of effects of smoked marijuana by the CB1-sective cannabinoid recptor antagonist SR141716. *Archives of General Psychiatry, 58*, 322–328. http://dx.doi.org/10.1001/archpsyc.58.4.322

Kay-Lambkin, F. J., Baker, A. L., Kelly, B., & Lewin, T. J. (2011). Clinician-assisted computerised versus therapist-delivered treatment for depressive and addictive disorders: a randomised controlled trial. *Medical Jouranl of Australia, 195*(Suppl), S44–S50.

Kay-Lambkin, F. J., Baker, A. L., Lewin, T. J., & Carr, V. J. (2009). Computer-based psychological treatment for comorbid depression and problematic alcohol and/or cannabis use: a randomized controlled trial of clinical efficacy. *Addiction, 104*, 378–388. http://dx.doi.org/10.1111/j.1360-0443.2008.02444.x

Kay-Lambkin, F. J., Simpson, A. L., Bowman, J., & Childs, S. (2014). Dissemination of a computer-based psychological treatment in a drug and alcohol clinical service: An observational study. *Addiction Science and Clinical Practice, 9*, 15. http://dx.doi.org/10.1186/1940-0640-9-15

Lee, C. M., Kilmer, J. R., Neighbors, C., Atkins, D. C., Zheng, C., Walker, D. D., & Larimer, M. E. (2013). Indicated prevention for college student marijuana use: A randomized controlled trial. *Journal of Consulting and Clinical Psychology, 81*, 702–709. http://dx.doi.org/10.1037/a0033285

Lee, C. M., Neighbors, C., Kilmer, J. R., & Larimer, M. E. (2010). A brief, web-based personalized feedback selective intervention for college student marijuana use: a randomized clinical trial. *Psychology of Addictive Behaviors, 24*, 265–273. http://dx.doi.org/10.1037/a0018859

Levin, F. R., Mariani, J. J., Brooks, D. J., Pavlicova, M., Cheng, W., & Nunes, E. V. (2011). Dronabinol for the treatment of cannabis dependence: A randomized, double-blind, placebo-controlled trial. *Drug and Alcohol Dependence, 116*, 142–150. http://dx.doi.org/10.1016/j.drugalcdep.2010.12.010

Levin, F. R., Mariani, J. J., Pavlicova, M., Brooks, D., Glass, A., Mahony, A., . . . Choi, J. C. (2016). Dronabinol and lofexidine for cannabis use disorder: A randomized, double-blind, placebo-controlled trial. *Drug and Alcohol Dependence, 159*, 53–60. http://dx.doi.org/10.1016/j.drugalcdep.2015.11.025

Marsch, L. A., & Borodovsky, J. T. (2016). Technology-based interventions for preventing and treating substance use among youth. *Child and Adolescent Psychiatric Clinics of North America, 25*, 755–768. http://dx.doi.org/10.1016/j.chc.2016.06.005

Marsch, L. A., Carroll, K. M., & Kiluk, B. D. (2014). Technology-based interventions for the treatment and recovery management of substance use disorders: A JSAT special issue. *Journal of Substance Abuse Treatment, 46*, 1–4. http://dx.doi.org/10.1016/j.jsat.2013.08.010

Martin, G., & Copeland, J. (2008). The adolescent cannabis check-up: Randomized trial of a brief intervention for young cannabis users. *Journal of Substance Abuse Treatment, 34*, 407–414. http://dx.doi.org/10.1016/j.jsat.2007.07.004

Martin, G., Copeland, J., & Swift, W. (2005). The Adolescent Cannabis Check-Up: Feasibility of a brief intervention for young cannabis users. *Journal of Substance Abuse Treatment, 29*, 207–213. http://dx.doi.org/10.1016/j.jsat.2005.06.005

Mason, B. J., Crean, R., Goodell, V., Light, J. M., Quello, S., Shadan, F., . . . Rao, S. (2012). A proof-of-concept randomized controlled study of gabapentin: Effects on cannabis use, withdrawal and executive function deficits in cannabis-dependent adults. *Neuropsychopharmacology, 37*, 1689–1698. http://dx.doi.org/10.1038/npp.2012.14

Mason, B. J., Mustafa, A., Filbey, F., & Brown, E. S. (2016). Novel pharmacotherapeutic interventions for cannabis use disorder. *Current Addiction Reports, 3*, 214–220. https://doi.org/10.1007/s40429-016-0094-y

McCambridge, J., Slym, R. L., & Strang, J. (2008). Randomized controlled trial of motivational interviewing compared with drug information and advice for early intervention among young cannabis users. *Addiction, 103*, 1809–1818. http://dx.doi.org/10.1111/j.1360-0443.2008.02331.x

McCambridge, J., & Strang, J. (2004). The efficacy of single-session motivational interviewing in reducing drug consumption and perceptions of drug-related risk and harm among young people: results from a multi-site cluster randomized trial. *Addiction, 99*, 39–52. http://dx.doi.org/10.1111/j.1360-0443.2004.00564.x

Palfai, T. P., Saitz, R., Winter, M., Brown, T. A., Kypri, K., Goodness, T. M., . . . Lu, J. (2014). Web-based screening and brief intervention for student marijuana use in a university health center: Pilot study to examine the implementation of eCHECKUP TO GO in different contexts. *Addictive Behaviors, 39*, 1346–1352. http://dx.doi.org/10.1016/j.addbeh.2014.04.025

Riggs, P. D., Winhusen, T., Davies, R. D., Leimberger, J. D., Mikulich-Gilbertson, S., Klein, C., . . . Lui, D. (2011). Randomized controlled trial of osmotic-release methylphenidate with cognitive-behavioral therapy in adolescents with attention-deficit/hyperactivity disorder and substance use disorders. *Journal of the American Academy of Child and Adolescent Psychiatry, 50*, 903–914. http://dx.doi.org/10.1016/j.jaac.2011.06.010

Schaub, M. P., Wenger, A., Berg, O., Beck, T., Stark, L., Buehler, E., & Haug, S. (2015). A Web-based self-help intervention with and without chat counseling to reduce cannabis use in problematic cannabis users: Three-arm randomized controlled trial. *Journal of Medical International Research, 17*, e232. http://dx.doi.org/10.2196/jmir.4860

Sherman, B. J., & McRae-Clark, A. L. (2016). Treatment of cannabis use disorder: Current science and future outlook. *Pharmacotherapy, 36*, 511–535. http://dx.doi.org/10.1002/phar.1747

Shrier, L. A., Rhoads, A., Burke, P., Walls, C., & Blood, E. A. (2014). Real-time, contextual intervention using mobile technology to reduce marijuana use among youth: a pilot study. *Addictive Behaviors, 39*, 173–180. http://dx.doi.org/10.1016/j.addbeh.2013.09.028

Simpson, A. K., & Magid, V. (2016). Cannabis use disorder in adolescence. *Child and Adolescent Psychiatic Clinics of North America, 25*, 431–443. http://dx.doi.org/10.1016/j.chc.2016.03.003

Stanger, C., Lansing, A. H., & Budney, A. J. (2016). Advances in research on contingency management for adolescent substance use. *Child and Adolescent Psychiatic Clinics of North America, 25*, 645–659. http://dx.doi.org/10.1016/j.chc.2016.05.002

Tanner-Smith, E. E., Wilson, S. J., & Lipsey, M. W. (2013). The comparative effectiveness of outpatient treatment for adolescent substance abuse: A meta-analysis. *Journal of Substance Abuse Treatment, 44*, 145–158. http://dx.doi.org/10.1016/j.jsat.2012.05.006

Waldron, H. B., & Turner, C. W. (2008). Evidence-based psychosocial treatments for adolescent substance abuse. *Journal of Clinical Child and Adolescent Psychology, 37*, 238–261. http://dx.doi.org/10.1080/15374410701820133

Walker, D. D., Roffman, R. A., Stephens, R. S., Wakana, K., Berghuis, J., & Kim, W. (2006). Motivational enhancement therapy for adolescent marijuana users: A preliminary randomized controlled trial. *Journal of Consulting and Clinical Psychology, 74*, 628–632. http://dx.doi.org/10.1037/0022-006X.74.3.628

Walker, D. D., Stephens, R., Roffman, R., Demarce, J., Lozano, B., Towe, S., & Berg, B. (2011). Randomized controlled trial of motivational enhancement therapy with nontreatment-seeking adolescent cannabis users: A further test of the teen marijuana check-up. *Psychology of Addictive Behaviors, 25*, 474–484. http://dx.doi.org/10.1037/a0024076

Walker, D. D., Stephens, R. S., Blevins, C. E., Banes, K. E., Matthews, L., & Roffman, R. A. (2016). Augmenting brief interventions for adolescent marijuana users: The impact of motivational check-ins. *Journal of Consulting and Clinical Psychology, 84*, 983–992. http://dx.doi.org/10.1037/ccp0000094

Walton, M. A., Bohnert, K., Resko, S., Barry, K. L., Chermack, S. T., Zucker, R. A., . . . Blow, F. C. (2013). Computer and therapist based brief interventions among cannabis-using adolescents presenting to primary care: one year outcomes. *Drug and Alcohol Dependence, 132*, 646–653. http://dx.doi.org/10.1016/j.drugalcdep.2013.04.02

Walton, M. A., Resko, S., Barry, K. L., Chermack, S. T., Zucker, R. A., Zimmerman, M. A., . . . Blow, F. C. (2014). A randomized controlled trial testing the efficacy of a brief cannabis universal prevention program among adolescents in primary care. *Addiction, 109*, 786–797. http://dx.doi.org/10.1111/add.12469

Winters, K. C., Botzet, A. M., & Fahnhorst, T. (2011). Advances in adolescent substance abuse treatment. *Current Psychiatry Reports, 13*, 416–421. http://dx.doi.org/10.1007/s11920-011-0214-2

Winters, K. C., Fahnhorst, T., Botzet, A., Lee, S., & Lalone, B. (2012). Brief intervention for drug-abusing adolescents in a school setting: Outcomes and mediating factors. *Journal of Substance Abuse Treatment, 42*, 279–288. http://dx.doi.org/10.1016/j.jsat.2011.08.005

Winters, K. C., Lee, S., Botzet, A., Fahnhorst, T., & Nicholson, A. (2014). One-year outcomes and mediators of a brief intervention for drug abusing adolescents. *Psychology of Addictive Behaviors, 28*, 464–474. http://dx.doi.org/10.1037/a0035041

Winters, K. C., Tanner-Smith, E. E., Bresani, E., & Meyers, K. (2014). Current advances in the treatment of adolescent drug use. *Adolescent Health, Medicine and Therapeutics, 5*, 199–210. http://dx.doi.org/10.2147/AHMT.S48053

10

What Is the Evidence of Marijuana
as Medicine?

KEVIN A. SABET, DAVID ATKINSON,
AND SHAYDA M. SABET

INTRODUCTION

Since research on marijuana's potential medicinal properties does not have a long history in Western civilization—as opposed to research on the opium poppy, for instance—the underdeveloped concept of marijuana as medicine today is controversial and often distorted. Medical marijuana in the United States has bypassed the usual process of scientific rigor that is required to make medicine available and has created a political controversy among the American public. The controversy lays, in part, in the question of whether marijuana's potential benefits outweigh its potential harms. Though some research suggests that components in marijuana can treat nausea from cancer chemotherapy, reduce seizures in epileptic children, assist with muscle spasticity, and may offer pain relief, studies also find (as described in many chapters in this book) that regular and heavy use of whole-plant marijuana is linked to a variety of adverse effects, including mental illness, poor cognitive development, lack of motivation and productivity, and poor academic performance.

Given the potential harmfulness of marijuana, opinion on its use as medicine is strongly divided between the scientific community and the public. According to most opinion polls, the public agrees with medical marijuana when asked (Nelson, 2016). However, virtually every single medical organization stands strongly against state-based medical marijuana programs that permit widespread use.

About half of US states as of 2017 have legalized the use of marijuana for medicinal purposes, in particular, to treat illnesses such as HIV/AIDS, cancer, and glaucoma. Yet, a growing body of literature shows that a very small percentage of medical marijuana patients suffer from serious, life-threatening illnesses. As will be discussed in more detail later in the chapter, over 90% of patients in most medical marijuana states cite chronic pain as the primary purpose for their use (Sabet & Grossman, 2014).

This chapter delineates the history of marijuana's development as a medicine, gathering the early evidence of its harms and effectiveness. It provides an overview of its medicinal components and the pharmaceutically developed medicines based on such components. The chapter further attempts to analyze the impacts of medical marijuana laws in the United States and the challenges associated with doing so.

HISTORY OF MEDICAL MARIJUANA

Though the history of marijuana's use for therapeutic purposes traces back thousands of years, it was not introduced to Western medicine until the mid-19th century. In 1839, Irish physician William B. O'Shaughnessy introduced the European world to the therapeutic properties of cannabis, which he discovered during his nine years at the Medical College of Calcutta in India. Following his discovery, early applications of various components of marijuana were used to treat ailments such as melancholia and migraines and to act as sleeping aids and anticonvulsants.

An early pharmacopoeia, written by Wood and Bache in 1854 and referenced in Leslie Iversen's (2007) *The Science of Marijuana*, offers an insightful view of the perceived medical benefits of marijuana in the 19th century:

Extract of hemp is a powerful narcotic, causing exhilaration, intoxication, delirious hallucinations, and, in its subsequent action drowsiness and stupor, with little effect upon the circulation. It is asserted also to act as a decided aphrodisiac, to increase the appetite, and occasionally to induce the cataleptic state. In morbid states of the system, it has been found to produce sleep, to allay spasm, to compose nervous inquietude, and to relieve pain. In these respects it resembles opium in its operation; but it differs from that narcotic in not diminishing the appetite, checking the secretions, or constipating the bowels. It is much less certain in its effects; but may sometimes be preferably employed, when opium is contraindicated by its nauseating or constipating effects, or its disposition to cause headache, and to check the bronchial secretion. The complaints to which it has been specially recommended are neuralgia, gout, tetanus, hydrophobia, epidemic cholera, convulsions, chorea, hysteria, mental depression, insanity, and uterine hemorrhage. (p. 121)

During this time, Western medicine also witnessed the advent of new synthetic drugs. For example, the active ingredient in the opium poppy, morphine, was identified and isolated, and its salts could be readily formulated for oral use or for injection by hypodermic needle. Soon after, other opioids and oral synthetic medicines, such as aspirin—with defined composition and potency—were also developed. Yet throughout its medical history, individuals never smoked opium for medicinal purposes.

Despite considerable research spanning many decades, the active ingredient in cannabis remained unknown for decades. Because cannabinoids are not water soluble, it was extremely difficult to produce medical products of reliable composition and predictable effect. Patient response was uncertain, and marijuana products gradually fell out of favor with the medical profession. In 1937, the Marijuana Tax Act, which placed a tax on physicians prescribing cannabis, on retail pharmacists selling cannabis, and on the cultivation or manufacturing of medical cannabis, made cannabis-based medicines a much less attractive treatment option. Following the enactment of the tax, Robert Walton, a professor of pharmacology at the University of Mississippi, documented the drug's decline in popularity, maintaining:

> The popularity of the hemp drugs can be attributed partly to the fact that they were introduced before the synthetic hypnotics and analgesics. Chloral hydrate was not introduced until 1869 and was followed in the next 30 years by paraldehyde, sulfonal and the barbitals. Antipyrine and acetanilide, the first of their particular group of analgesics [aspirin-like drugs], were introduced about 1884 [aspirin, not until 1899]. For general sedative and analgesic purposes, the only drugs commonly used at this time were the morphine derivatives and their disadvantages were very well known. In fact, the most attractive feature of the hemp narcotics was probably the fact that they did not exhibit certain of the notorious disadvantages of the opiates. The hemp narcotics do not constipate at all, they more often increase rather than decrease appetite, they do not particularly depress the respiratory center even in large doses, they rarely or never cause pruritus or cutaneous eruption and, most importantly, the liability of developing addiction is very much less than with the opiates. These features were responsible for the rapid rise in popularity of the drug. Several features can be recognised as contributing to the gradual decline of popularity. Cannabis does not usually produce analgesia or relax spastic conditions without producing cortical effects and, in fact, these cortical effects usually predominate. The actual degree of analgesia produced is much less than with the opiates. Most important, the effects are irregular due to marked variations in individual susceptibility and probably also to variable absorption of the gummy resin. (Walton 1938, as quoted in Iversen, 2007, pp. 121–122)

By the 1960s, technology enabled chemists to identify (and synthesize) tetrahydrocannabinol (THC) as the primary psychoactive ingredient of marijuana. At the same time, anecdotal reports of therapeutic benefits from recreational users of marijuana emerged in the 1960s and 1970s. These developments led to increased research interest in developing a medication for cancer chemotherapy-induced nausea and vomiting.

More recently, new techniques have identified other cannabinoids in the plant, allowing for the production of a wide range of medicines with varying cannabinoids or cannabinoid ratios, and different therapeutic synergies and effects. Modern drug delivery methods now permit researchers to develop bioavailable formulations in appropriate dosage forms like oral or oromucosal (e.g., absorbed in the mouth). Had technology been more advanced in the early 1900s, cannabinoid medicines may have developed as opiates did, and there might be a much different medical marijuana controversy – or none at all – today.

THE POLITICAL CONTROVERSY

The case of opium is instructive when discussing marijuana and its possible medical benefit. In the 1800s, a clear path for medicalizing the opium poppy plant was established. That is, opium was processed into purified forms to produce medicines like morphine, but it was also frequently abused, particularly with hypodermic needles. Though some derivatives were promising, a diacetyl derivative called heroin created more benefits for pain relief than possibly imagined from its marketed role as a cough suppressant. However, cannabis did not follow these paths—medical research on the drug did not start in earnest until the mid-20th century—and thus, today we are left with a political controversy.

Today the issue seems to be distorted, with *medical marijuana* earning a place in the modern lexicon. The all too narrow references to smoking the marijuana plant versus the more scientifically accurate medical *cannabinoids* further reinforce this distortion. Marijuana legalization proponents have taken advantage of this misleading view of medicine. For years, proponents of legalization have attempted to use medical marijuana as a stepping-stone to broader liberalization of the drug. Keith Stroup, the founder of the National Organization for the Reform of Marijuana Laws (NORML), said in 1979, "We [NORML] are trying to get marijuana reclassified medically. If we do that (we'll do it in at least 20 states this year for chemotherapy patients) we'll be using the issue as a red herring to give marijuana a good name. That's our way of getting to them." ("NORML Chairman Keith Stroup Talks on Pot Issues," 1979).

Though NORML would not succeed in legalizing marijuana for medical purposes for another 15 years, the long-term messaging strategy seems to have paid off. In 1996, the Compassionate Use Act passed in California, allowing people with qualifying medical conditions to legally obtain and grow marijuana. In time, the director of NORML, Allen St. Pierre flatly stated, "In California, marijuana has also been *de facto* legalized under the guise of medical marijuana" (St. Pierre, 2009).

Since 1996, about two dozen additional states and the District of Columbia have also legalized the use of marijuana for medical purposes, and there is considerable variability among them in terms of regulation and eligible ailments or disorders (Bestrashniy & Winters, 2015). Table 10.1 provides a summary of all medical marijuana laws in the United States (National Council of State

Table 10.1 State Medical Marijuana/Cannabis Program Laws

State	Statutory Language (Year)	Patient Registry or ID cards	Allows Dispensaries	Specifies Conditions	Recognizes Patients from Other States	State Allows for Retail Sales/Adult Use
Alaska	Measure 8 (1998) SB 94 (1899) Statute Title 17, Chapter 37	Yes	No	Yes	Yes, for AZ; approved conditions, but not for dispensary purchases	Ballot Measure 2 (2014) Not yet fully operational/ regulated production or sales
Arizona	Proposition 203 (2010)	Yes	Yes	Yes	Yes	
Arkansas	Issue 6 (2016) Details pending	Pending	Pending	Pending	Pending	
California	Proposition 215 (1996) SB 420 (2003)	Yes	Yes (cooperatives and collectives)	No	No	Proposition 64 (2016)
Colorado Medical program info Adult- use info	Amendment 20 (2000)	Yes	Yes	Yes	No	Amendment 64 (2012) Task Force Implementation Recommendations (2013) Analysis of CO Amendment 64 (2013) Colorado Marijuana Sales and Tax Reports 2014 "Edibles" regulation measure FAQ about CO cannabis laws by the *Denver Post*
Connecticut	HB 5389 (2012)	Yes	Yes	Yes		
Delaware	SB 17 (2011)	Yes	Yes	Yes	Yes, for DE; approved conditions.	

District of Columbia	Initiative 59 (1998) L18-2010 (2010)	Yes	Yes	Yes		Initiative 71 (2014)
Florida	Amendment 2 (2016) Details pending	Pending	Pending	Pending	Pending	
Guam	Proposal 14A Approved in Nov. 2014, not yet operational. Draft rules released in July 2015	Yes	Yes	Yes	No	
Hawaii	SB 862 (2000)	Yes	No	Yes	No	
Illinois	HB 1 (2013) Eff. 1/1/2014 Rules	Yes	Yes	Yes	No	
Maine	Question 2 (1999) LD 611 (2002) Question 5 (2009) LD 1811 (2010) LD 1296 (2011)	Yes	Yes	Yes	Yes, but not for dispensary purchases	Question 1 (2016)
Maryland	HB 702 (2003) SB 308 (2011) HB 180/ SB 580 (2013) HB 1101-Chapter 403 (2013) SB 923 (signed 4/14/14) HB 881-similar to SB 923	Yes	Yes	Yes	No	
Massachusetts	Question 3 (2012) Regulations (2013)	Yes	Yes	Yes	No	Question 4 (2016)

(continued)

Table 10.1 Continued

State	Statutory Language (Year)	Patient Registry or ID cards	Allows Dispensaries	Specifies Conditions	Recognizes Patients from Other States	State Allows for Retail Sales/Adult Use
Michigan	Proposal 1 (2008)	Yes	Not in state law, but localities may create ordinances to allow them and regulate them	Yes	Yes, for legal protection of posession, but not for dispensary purchases	
Minnesota	SF 2471, Chapter 311 (2014)	Yes	Yes, limited, liquid extract products only	Yes	No	
Montana	Initiative 148 (2004) SB 423 (2011) Initiative 182 (2016)	Yes New details pending	No** New details pending	Yes New details pending	No New details pending	
Nevada	Question 9 (2000) NRS 453A NAC 453A	Yes	No	Yes	Yes, if the other state's program are "substantially similar"; patients must fill out Nevada paperwork	Question 2 (2016)
New Hampshire	HB 573 (2013)	Yes	Yes	Yes	Yes, with a note from their home state, but they cannot purchase through dispensaries	

New Jersey	SB 119 (2009) Program information	Yes	Yes	Yes	No	
New Mexico	SB 523 (2007) Medical Cannabis Program	Yes	Yes	Yes	No	
New York	A6357 (2014) Signed by governor 7/15/14	Yes	Ingested doses may not contain more than 10 mg of THC, Product may not be combusted (smoked)	Yes	No	
North Dakota	Measure 5 (2016) Final details pending	Pending	Pending	Pending	Pending	
Ohio	HB 523 (2010) Approved by legislature, signed by governor 6/8/16, not yet operational			Yes		
Oregon	Oregon Medical Marijuana Act (1998) SB 161 (2007)	Yes	No	Yes	No	Measure 91 (2014)

(continued)

Table 10.1 Continued

State	Statutory Language (Year)	Patient Registry or ID cards	Allows Dispensaries	Specifies Conditions	Recognizes Patients from Other States	State Allows for Retail Sales/Adult Use
Pennsylvania	SB 3 (2016) Signed by governor 4/17/16, not yet operational	Yes	Yes	Yes		
Puerto Rico	Public Health Department Regulation 155 (2016), not yet operational		Cannot be smoked			
Rhode Island	SB 791(2007) SB 185(2009)	Yes	Yes	Yes	Yes	
Vermont	SB 76 (2004) SB 7 (2007) SB 17 (2011)	Yes	Yes	Yes	No	
Washington	Initiative 692 (1998) SB 5798 (2010) SB 5073 (2011)	No	Yes, approved as of Nov. 2012, stores opened in July, 2014	Yes	No	Initiative 502 (2012) WAC marijuana rules: Chapter 314-55 WAC FAQ about WA cannabis laws by the Seattle Times

Legislatures, 2017). Seven of the 23 states allow for-profit medical marijuana dispensaries to operate, 3 states place qualifying conditions under the discretion of physicians, and 13 states delineate 10 or more qualifying conditions.

WHO USES MEDICAL MARIJUANA AND WHY?

As noted in Table 10.1, the medical use of unrefined marijuana is currently legalized in nearly half of the American states and the District of Columbia; also, there are a number of countries across the globe, including Canada and Australia, that permit medical marijuana. Today, there are thousands of medical marijuana dispensaries across the United States and hundreds of thousands of medical marijuana cardholders. Though the initial campaigns to pass medical marijuana laws in the United States have typically been associated with cancer, HIV/AIDS, and glaucoma patients, today, relatively little is known about the real conditions afflicting medical marijuana cardholders. Still, the few studies that exist find that only a small minority of medical marijuana users report serious, life-threatening illnesses.

Most previous research on who uses medical marijuana and why is limited to California, where legislation passed in 1996 permitting the use of marijuana for "cancer, anorexia, AIDS, chronic pain, spasticity, glaucoma, arthritis, migraine, *or any other illness for which marijuana provides relief*" (Compassionate Use Act of 1996; emphasis added). In 2007, the *Harm Reduction Journal* published a study that examined of 4,117 medical marijuana users in California between 2001 and mid-2007 (O'Connell & Bou-Matar, 2007). The authors found that during this period, 77% of medical marijuana users were male with a median age of 31 years, and nearly 70% of all users were White—not representative of the American adult population. Moreover, 88% of all users first used marijuana before the age of 19 and almost 90% report near daily use (O'Connell & Bou-Matar, 2007). In a study of a series of 623 psychiatric patients, Nussbaum, Thurstone, McGarry, Walker, and Sabel (2015) found that possession of medical marijuana cards was associated with being more likely to use marijuana over 20 times in the past month. Furthermore, the study identified 282 individuals who report using marijuana, and 133 who have bought or received medical marijuana from a cardholder. Forty-one percent of cardholders in this population reported ever having shared or sold their medical marijuana (Nussbaum et al., 2015).

A recent study by Lankenau et al. (2017) reveals that in the past 90 days medical marijuana patients were using the drug during an average of 76.4 days and spent an average of $565 on marijuana during that 90-day period; 22.6% reported reselling the dispensary products to someone else during the past 90 days.

Another study analyzed a sample of 1,746 medical marijuana users within nine medical marijuana assessment clinics (i.e., clinics that charged $100 to $125 for an assessment of eligibility for medical marijuana but did not dispense marijuana) in California in mid-2006 (Reinarman, Nunberg, Lanthier, & Heddleston, 2011). Similar to the findings from O'Connell and Bou-Matar (2007), Reinarman et al. reported that nearly three fourths of all patients were male and 62% were White. Sixty-seven percent of patients reported using marijuana daily, and 53% reported use at least twice a day. The study also found that nearly 83% of patients self-report that pain relief is the primary reason for using medical marijuana. Nunberg, Kilmer, Pacula, and Burgdorf's (2011) further analysis of the data found that the most frequently diagnosed conditions were musculoskeletal and neuropathic chronic pain such as back pain and arthritis, while HIV/AIDS, cancer, and glaucoma combined comprised of only 4.4% of diagnoses.

A problem inherent in these reports is that there is an overabundance of illnesses that can only be demonstrated by subjective report. Without objective criteria, it is difficult to assess which individuals are using marijuana for their stated medical conditions, since incentive exists to report a medical need in states where the drug is illegal for recreational use or taxed at different rates for medical and recreational use.

Oregon passed medical marijuana legislation in 1998 for patients diagnosed with qualifying conditions such as cancer, glaucoma, Alzheimer's disease, HIV/AIDS, and posttraumatic stress disorder (PTSD). As of 2015, there were over 72,000 medical marijuana patients in Oregon. State records have found that 92.8% of patients reported using medical marijuana to treat severe pain, while only 8.1% are diagnosed with the original qualifying conditions: cancer, glaucoma, HIV/AIDS, or Alzheimer's disease (Oregon Health Authority, 2015). According to the Oregon Health Authority's 2015 report on Oregon's Medical Marijuana Program, 23 physicians (1.4% of all physicians associated with Oregon's Medical Marijuana Program) were responsible for 78% of all patient registrations (Oregon Health Authority, 2015). In Colorado, there are 113,585 active medical marijuana patients, signed for by only 226 physicians (Colorado Department of Health and Environment, 2015). Of these patients, 99.8% reported severe pain as the primary condition for seeking medical marijuana, while less than 5% also reported having cancer, glaucoma, or HIV/AIDS (Colorado Department of Health and Environment, 2015).

An analysis of over 200,000 medical marijuana patients from seven different states found that 91% of users report using marijuana primarily to alleviate severe or chronic pain (Sabet & Grossman, 2014). Consistent with Nunberg et al. (2011), Reinarman et al. (2011), and O'Connell and Bou-Matar (2007), Sabet and Grossman found that a very small percentage of their sample are cancer, glaucoma, or HIV/AIDS patients (3.2, 1.3, and 1.4%, respectively).

TREATING CHRONIC PAIN

As previously noted, the majority of medical marijuana users cite pain as the main reason for its use. When examining this literature, there are issues of whether cannabis is inhaled to treat the pain, the potency of the product, and whether acute or chronic pain was treated. The clinical trials reviewed in the recent report by the National Academies of Sciences, Engineering, and Medicine

(2017) all had a fairly short follow-up, and the clinical laboratory studies showed simply the short-term relief of pain, rather than a sustained reduction in pain, which limits the ability to determine whether cannabis is efficacious for chronic pain. The report, and press related to it, often confused whole-plant cannabis with components within cannabis, frustrating the head of the National Institute on Drug Abuse in a remarkably candid blogpost (Volkow, 2017). It should be noted that the long-term efficacy data supporting the use of opioids for pain in these conditions are also lacking, and efficacy for chronic pain is limited by the practical difficulties in continuing placebo-controlled studies for a long period of time.

Of note regarding the debate of smoked versus non-smoked cannabis is the recent publication by Andreae et al. (2015), in which the authors pooled patient data from multiple randomized controlled trials. Their main conclusion was a significant effect for smoked cannabis. Yet this method differs from a conventional meta-analysis, which examines the effect sizes of each individual study. The decision by Andreae et al. to pool individual patient data increases the statistical power to determine whether the treatment is effective, but, by doing so, it adds potential confounds as studies with varying parameters are combined. The authors noted that the studies in the review varied with respect to the duration of marijuana use (it varied from a few days to a few weeks), the length of follow-up assessments, and difficulties determining whether subjects knew which treatment they had been allocated to (i.e., unblinding; when an experienced marijuana user would likely know if he or she were in a placebo condition, even if the design were double-blind) and thus could be susceptible to the placebo effect.

To ensure validity of the studies showing that cannabis may be an effective and sufficiently safe treatment option for chronic pain, the treatment should not just be for acute pain, and if inhaled cannabis is used, the safer, noninhaled cannabinoid preparations should be tested as a comparison. If studies show efficacy, it would be important for state medical marijuana programs to approximate the controls used in the studies to ensure that users are in accordance with what the science may show to be effective. Unfortunately, the robust controls in these studies are typically very different from those afforded by medical marijuana programs, including limits on frequency, quantity, and using a known concentration of THC in the marijuana. In addition, findings from clinical laboratory studies may not generalize in the face of rigorous clinical trials. For example, Wilsey et al. (2016) demonstrated in a laboratory experiment that marijuana was associated with pain reduction in the lab, an effect that is well-known for cannabis. But the study does not add to our knowledge of whether this is an effective medical treatment for chronic pain in the clinical setting requiring day-to-day pain relief. Frequently, substances lose their effect when used over days and weeks as the body adapts to the "new normal" of having the drug in its system.

Clinical studies should also address whether there are any benefits to inhaled cannabis as opposed to orally administered purified forms, because the additional addiction risk incurred through the oral route of administration along with other intoxication effects and variabilities in dosing are significant concerns for the patient using medical marijuana. Moreover, there is the issue of side effects. For example, as noted by Wallace, Marcotte, Umlauf, Gouaux, and Atkinson (2015) impairment in neuropsychological task performance was associated with marijuana dosage levels.

Furthermore, whereas authors report that medical marijuana has reduced opioid use, there is a difficulty in determining whether this effect is directly due to cannabis or simultaneous increasingly strict laws against opioids that happened to coincide with medical cannabis. The Michigan study (Boehnke et al., 2016) did not look at the changes in opioid use of a control group and used only one marijuana dispensary in that state, leaving questions of generalizability. Bradford and Bradford (2016) used all prescriptions filled by Medicare Part D enrollees from 2010 to 2013 and found that use of prescription drugs for which cannabis could serve as a therapeutic alternative dropped significantly subsequent to the implementation of medical marijuana laws. This finding is most interesting and could signal a means by which patients eschew opioid abuse. But these findings would have been strengthened if the authors had also examined whether possible changes in opioid access laws and standards had been considered in the analysis.

MARIJUANA'S ADVERSE EFFECTS

The first rule of all physicians is *primum non nocer.* That is, whatever treatment a doctor prescribes to a patient, first and foremost, that treatment must not do anything that the doctor has good reason to believe will cause a net increase of harm to the patient. This principle is at the heart of the medical marijuana debate on the political, health and social fronts, the most contentious aspect of which regards the degree of potential harm associated with the drug's use.

Marijuana's adverse mood reactions may include anxiety and paranoia, panic, depression, dysphoria, and hallucination. These reactions are more likely to be observed in new or heavy marijuana users. For example, a 2015 article published in the *Lancet* suggests that regular use of high-potency THC (often referred to as "skunk-like" and containing 14 to 15% THC) is associated with 24% of new cases of psychotic disorder in South London (Di Forti et al., 2015).

The Institute of Medicine's report (Joy, Watson & Benson, 1999), as well as the follow-up report by the National Academies of Sciences, Engineering, and Medicine (2017), thoroughly examined both the psychological and physiological risks of marijuana. Like that of many other drugs, the regular use of marijuana produces chronic adverse effects such as tolerance, physical dependence, and withdrawal symptoms (Budney, Hughs, Moore, & Vandrey, 2004; Chung & Winters, this volume). With respect to its other health effects, at the time of the IOM report in 1999, the effects of marijuana were mainly evidenced by statistical associations; yet subsequent research, which is presented in numerous chapters in this volume, provides more evidence of marijuana playing a causal role.

For the purposes of this chapter, we discuss a health issue pertinent to the medical marijuana issue: childhood exposure. Perhaps due to a media-driven enthusiasm for high-cannabidiol [CBD]/low-THC oil, many parents are turning to CBD-oil for their epileptic children. One difficulty with outcomes of observational studies done in the context of media hype is the potential of the placebo effect to bias open-label research. The question was raised in an open-label study (Press, Knupp & Chapman, 2015) finding that parents who came to Colorado from out-of-state were more likely to report response to marijuana preparations. Of the eight responders who had EEG data, none showed improvement in electroencephalogram. Porter and Jacobson (2013) reported that some children treated with high CBD oil were getting up to 0.8 mg/kg of THC. Since a "typical" joint contains 29 mg of THC (Hunault et al., 2008), this means that even 36 kg (79 pound) kids would be getting one joint's worth of THC every day. Given the substantial harms that have been linked to daily, or near-daily, marijuana use, it seems that this is a very important consideration when maintaining CBD purity. Furthermore, the addition of THC to CBD could lead to the untrained eye mistaking improvements in spasticity or locomotor activity after THC administration for a genuine reduction in epileptic seizures. There is also potential concern that THC would be used for the amelioration of behavior problems, because exhausted parents might see the reductions in locomotor activity as therapeutic benefits—while the action raises an ethical concern regarding tranquilizing a disruptive child instead of using behavioral modifications.

Groups such as MAMMA (Mothers Advocating Medical Marijuana for Autism) have made striking claims of efficacy, but it remains to be seen how the drug affects these youth in the short and long-terms. Given the drug's adverse effects on reinforcement learning (Oleson & Cheer, 2012) and social functioning (Platt, Kamboj, Morgan, & Curran, 2010), extreme caution is needed prior to giving the drug to individuals with autism, who rely on the evidence-based treatment with behavioral modifications and social skills training for their psychotherapeutic treatment. The sedating effects of cannabis also raise the danger that the drug could be simply used to reduce these children's undesirable behaviors rather than improve their developmental growth.

MEDICINAL PROPERTIES OF CANNABIS: WHAT DOES THE SCIENCE SAY?

The marijuana plant constitutes approximately ten groups of closely related cannabinoids, which have a variety of effects on the brain. Recent advances in science have identified two cannabinoid receptors in the brain, CB1 and CB2. CB1 receptors mediate the psychoactive effects of THC, while the CB2 receptors are expressed mainly in the immune system and other areas outside the brain (Felder & Glass, 1998; Munro, Thomas & Abu-Shaar, 1993; Pertwee, 1999, 2006), but they are also present in special cells that nourish and promote neuronal function, called microglial cells. These cells are thought to have some potential role in substance use disorders and other psychiatric disorders (Cutando et al., 2013). While the role of CB2 receptors remains somewhat mysterious, the role of the type 1 receptors is much clearer.

CB1 receptors are abundantly located throughout the brain and regulate numerous functions such as brain development, memory and cognition, motivational systems, appetite, immunological functions, reproduction, movement coordination, and pain regulation, though the extent and direction of each effect depends on the dosage of marijuana administered (Joy, Watson, & Benson, 1999). The original function of these receptors was, of course, not to be acted upon by THC but to respond to chemical messages in the brain. The natural activators of these receptors are called endocannabinoids, and they activate the cannabinoid receptors much less potently than THC or synthetic cannabinoids do. Chemicals that activate receptors are frequently called agonists, and those that block the receptors are called antagonists.

The modulation of the endocannabinoid system in ways that are more sophisticated than simple CB1 agonist action represents an enormous therapeutic opportunity (Picone & Kendall, 2015). There is hope in the future to affect regulators of the endocannabinoid system such as fatty acid amyl hydrolase, monoacylglycerol lipase (Tuo et al., 2017) for a more targeted improvement in therapeutic symptoms that does not disrupt endocannabinoid signaling. Certain drugs that act at sites related to the CB1 receptor, termed allosteric modulators, that do not fully agonize the CB1 receptor, also hold significant promise (Nguyen, Li, Thomas, Wiley, & Kenakin, 2016).

There are a number of marijuana-based medicines legally available that do not require smoking or inhaling the raw plant, and most current research on the efficacy of cannabinoids is not focused on crude marijuana extract but on the individual components of the plant that may have medical value. It should go without saying that smoking would not be an accepted therapeutic delivery system for reasons of dosage control, cognitive side effects, enhanced reinforcement leading to increased medicine self-administration, cardiac effects, and the acute and chronic respiratory effects on the lungs. Most drug delivery systems, with the exceptions of drugs like bronchodilators and nitroglycerine, are designed to deliver steady blood levels over many hours, whereas smoking produces rapid peaks.

Whole Plant Marijuana

Advocates of using the entire marijuana plant or whole-plant extracts frequently invoke the concept of entourage effects, whereby the mixture of all of the cannabinoid chemicals together would produce new therapeutic effects not seen with the components alone. Combining other components judiciously with CBD may add to clinical benefits. Also, additional cannabinoid compounds contributing to therapeutic benefits of medical marijuana is biologically plausible, but they have not been proven to contribute in a clinically meaningful way. Potential downsides to adding these chemicals exist, such as a lack of therapeutic specificity and a multiplication of potential side effects with different compounds. As to whether the whole plant is superior to the individual components, there is limited research. One study compared purified components to whole-plant extract, and it showed that THC actually outperformed the whole plant extract (Zajicek et al., 2005), and another study showed no benefit of the whole plant extract over purified components, but neither treatment had stronger effects than the placebo in that study (Strasser et al., 2006).

Though many maintain that marijuana's whole plant extract is superior to its individual chemicals, use of the former is associated with potential risks. First, the inherent inconsistency of a plant will vary with the genetic endowment of its parents and varies greatly with the conditions of growth. Unlike purified extracts of THC and cannabidiol that are negative in the Ames test, whole plant extract has been shown to be carcinogenic (Wehner, van Rensburg, & Thiel, 1980), and there is great incertitude regarding the long-term toxicity of each of the many additional chemicals in the plant. Two studies point to the effects of smoke condensate in animals, one in female rats (Murthy et al., 1985), and one in Swiss Albino mice (Hoffman, Brunneman, Gori, & Wynder, 1975).

Matching the dose of THC in whole-plant extract with a purified pharmaceutical extract is difficult due to plant variability, and matching doses with the smoked plant is especially difficult due to the different concentrations (varying 24–462 µg/L with the same dose of the drug smoked by a dozen different individuals) that individual users achieve (Hunault et al., 2008).

Several studies have tested whole plant marijuana for pain relief, but these studies have not used an active comparator of oral THC to demonstrate that the therapeutic benefits are superior when inhaled, which would be necessary to justify the increased risk of smoked plant. Studies of inhaled THC have also not shown superiority to the higher doses (Wilsey et al., 2016), The well-controlled conditions of these studies are also not analogous to the way in which ad lib cannabis is being recommended in American medical marijuana programs, and the benefits relatives to harms are much more difficult to maximize without these controls.

THC

Dronabinol (also known as Marinol˚ and Syndros) is a laboratory-synthesized THC capsule approved in 1985 in the United States for treatment of nausea and vomiting associated with cancer chemotherapy. By 1992, the Food and Drug Administration (FDA) also approved it for appetite stimulation for AIDS patients. Currently, it is the only cannabis-based drug approved for distribution in the United States. Its most common side effects include anxiety, confusion, depersonalization, dizziness, euphoria, dysphoria, and somnolence, though clinical trials suggest that lowering its dosage can significantly alleviate these effects (Joy et al., 1999).

Nabilone (also known as Cesamet), also based on THC, is used for nausea and vomiting related to cancer chemotherapy, but it has significant side effects such as dizziness and vertigo (Ward & Holmes, 1985) that have limited its use. Recently, nabilone has risen in popularity as a potential treatment for PTSD after benefits were suggested by an open-label trial (Fraser, 2009) and a preliminary randomized double-blind trial (Jetley, Heber, Fraser, & Boisvert, 2015). More data are sure to arrive regarding the use and effects of nabilone, and it will be important to investigate its relative efficacy and side effect frequency compared to other cannabinoids and standard treatments for PTSD.

CBD

CBD is one of the main components of marijuana that has been investigated for medical use and has been investigated for FDA approval. In the mid-2000s, researchers and activists began to educate interested patients and others about the therapeutic potential of CBD, which had been selectively bred-out of high-THC marijuana in the United States. Indeed, not long ago many individuals in the United States believed that CBD was an inert compound. There were also anecdotal reports of some adults with epilepsy who discovered that inhaled marijuana seemed to prevent or reduce their seizures. As more and more scientific research demonstrated that CBD had a variety of therapeutic effects, interest in the use of CBD in epilepsy grew.

Cannabidiol has been widely held to be the component of marijuana with better anti-seizure efficacy and certainly has evidenced a much better safety profile (Devinsky et al., 2014), since THC is a toxin to the developing child. For this reason, proper medical management would involve the maximization of the therapeutic potential of cannabidiol. Some have reported that the addition of THC to a CBD treatment could further improve the treatment of seizures, but it would seem advantageous to maintain independent dosing of CBD and THC to minimize potential harms of THC administration by keeping the dose as low as possible. Assuming an actual benefit to the addition of THC, slowly titrating THC would allow the physician to optimize the risk/benefit ratio in the partially protective presence of cannabidiol.

Since the mid-2000s, several pharmaceutical companies have been intensively researching CBD as treatment for medical conditions, including epilepsy. Several companies are currently developing CBD-based medications. One such product is the highly-purified CBD product, Epidiolex. Pediatric neurologists around the country, concerned that the desperate families of their pediatric patients were seeking access to artisanal CBD preparations of unknown quality and potency, began to seek FDA and US Drug Enforcement Agency (DEA) approval of expanded access or compassionate access investigational new drug programs to treat their patients with intractable epilepsy with Epidiolex. Approximately 20 such investigational new drug programs, covering over 400 children, have been approved by the FDA as of 2015 and many have secured DEA research registrations. One open-label study was reported by Devinsky et al. (2016) at the American Academy of Neurology, and it showed that in 137 out of 213 study completers, cannabidiol led to a mean reduction of seizures by 54%. GW Pharmaceuticals is also conducting four placebo-controlled clinical trials in children with two types of intractable epilepsy. Phase three studies released in 2016 found that Epidiolex achieved a median reduction in monthly convulsive seizures of 39% compared with a reduction on placebo of 13%, which was highly statistically significant ($p = 0.01$). Sativex (nabiximols), an orally administered 1:1 CBD–THC marijuana extract is currently in use in Canada and across Europe to treat neuropathic pain, as well as spasticity and other symptoms of multiple sclerosis (MS). Sativex is now approved for MS spasticity in 27 countries and is completing Phase 3 trials in almost 60 research sites in the United States in advanced cancer patients with significant pain.

The CNN program hosted by Dr. Sanjay Gupta in August 2013 (Gupta, 2013) reported the case of a toddler with horrible, life-threatening, intractable epilepsy. According to Dr. Gupta, her condition was greatly improved by a CBD-rich preparation produced by purveyors in Colorado. Though many were dismayed at how Dr. Gupta's program interchangeably used THC and CBD and further confused the issue of recreational and medical marijuana (especially since the program was called "Weed"), the program resulted in enormous interest in CBD from families of children with epilepsy.

As desperate parents sought high CBD products wherever they could purchase them, a number of dispensaries and other opportunistic vendors began to sell these products. However, the labeled potency and composition of these products are often inaccurate and uneven, depending on the marijuana strain from which they come, the methods of manufacture used to prepare them, and the quality of the testing facility/procedures—leading the FDA to issue its first-ever warnings against medical marijuana companies ("2016 Warning Letters and Test Results for Cannabidiol-Related Products," n.d.). At many stages in the cultivation and manufacturing process, lack of standardization can result in higher levels of THC and lower levels of CBD—as well as the varying levels of dangerous microbes or pesticides—in the final preparation. For example, growing from seed rather than clones; differences in the cultivation, harvesting, and drying conditions; uneven decarboxylation; and use of toxic extraction chemicals, such as butane or non-pharmaceutical ethanol.

Manufacturers and other purveyors of CBD products make many therapeutic claims that bring those products within the scope of the Food, Drug, and Cosmetic Act. For manufacturers of other products such as pharmaceutical products, dietary supplements, and even foods, the FDA reviews all sources of promotional statements (including websites, Facebook, Twitter, and other online media sources) that could be interpreted as making improper therapeutic claims. Claims are often made for a wide variety of medical conditions and risks are rarely mentioned. In a survey administered by the journal *Epilepsia*, a minority of epileptologists and general neurologists said that there were sufficient safety (34%) and efficacy (28%) data, and 48%

would advise using medical marijuana in severe cases of epilepsy (Mathern, Beninsig, & Nehlig, 2014). By comparison, nearly all patients and the public said there were sufficient safety (96%) and efficacy (95%) data, and 98% would recommend medical marijuana in cases of severe epilepsy. General physicians, basic researchers, nurses, and allied health professions sided more with patients, agreeing that there are sufficient safety (70%) and efficacy (71%) data, and 83% would advise using marijuana in severe cases. A majority (78%) said there should be pharmacologic-grade compounds containing CBD, and there were no differences between specialists, general medical personal, and patients and the public. The huge gap between what the public thinks and what medical doctors believe is emblematic of the medical marijuana debate generally. Despite not producing euphoria or addiction, use of cannabidiol with a developing brain still carries concerns. The development of axons and proper synapses is dependent upon the growth of small projections termed filopodia, whose growth can be inhibited by cannabidiol's disruption of G protein-coupled receptor 55 signaling (Cherif et al., 2015), and the practical consequences of this on brain development are unknown.

Some studies find that CBD can counteract some of the adverse effects of THC (Morgan, Freeman, Schafer, & Curran, 2010). However, research finds that it does not do so by blocking the CB1 receptors, but rather by modifying these receptors and acting at a different site (Laprairie, Bagher, Kelly, & Denovan-Wright, 2015). The interactions between CBD and THC are very complex, and involve actions of CBD at other sites.

Dosage Issues of THC and CBD

An urgent and critically important concern regarding the combined use of THC and CBD is the fact that the dosing ranges for therapeutic benefits are quite different, and the THC: CBD ratios found in the plants do not approximate the difference in the drugs therapeutic doses. The therapeutic doses of THC for FDA-approved indications range from 2 to 20 mg of THC per day, while the dose of cannabidiol that is theorized to be effective for treating seizures is between 200 and 600 mg/day, and perhaps higher, making the therapeutic dosing of THC and CBD at a minimum to be a 1:10 THC:CBD ratio (max of 20 mg of THC/ day, and a minimum of 200 mg of CBD/day). Because the ratio of THC:CBD is at least 1:1 in most plants, and can be as high as 20:1, it makes it very difficult to find a strain of C. indica or C. sativa that would meet these requirements. Also, it makes sense to give clinicians the ability to individually titrate doses of THC and CBD, rather than be at the mercy of whatever the plan produces. As it stands now, clinicians who do not have access to pure, or near-pure, cannabidiol are locked into giving a much higher dose of THC than is medically indicated if they are titrating cannabidiol up to its therapeutic dose.

Also, it is very important to disentangle the effects of high-dose CBD from the effects of high-dose THC. THC has more developmentally neurotoxic effects and can acutely produce a good deal of sedation and euphoria that might color subjective reports of efficacy, as well as measures of seizure efficacy based on motor activity, as is the case of parental-reported seizure frequency. Limiting the amount of THC is also important when considering the 1938 statements of Walton (p. 152) who reported that medical use was practically limited due to "cortical" effects often predominating over the other physical effects at typical marijuana doses, which is echoed in the modern MS literature, reporting significant cognitive impairment among individuals with MS who use cannabis (Honarmand, Tierney, O'Connor, & Feinstein, 2011).

Other Cannabinoids

While considerably less researched, tetrahydrocannabivarin (THCV) is another component of marijuana with potentially important effects. THCV is an antagonist of the CB1 and receptor (Pertwee et al., 2007; Thomas et al., 2005), which means that it is highly unlikely that co-administering it would add to the therapeutic benefit of THC, but would probably counteract it. However, there is a possibility that this drug would have therapeutic potential for other indications, because it is a neutral antagonist of the CB1 receptor. This is opposed to rimonabant, which is an inverse agonist, meaning rimonabant destabilizes the endocannabinoid system by doing the opposite of what THC does. The neutral antagonist could be potentially therapeutic. It is also likely to be a partial agonist of CB2 (Pertwee, 2008), which could have therapeutic potential to affect that system, which is thought to be more important to diseases outside the central nervous system.

Another chemical component of marijuana with possible antiepileptic pharmacologic effect is cannabidivarin (Hill et al., 2012, 2013). Though it has not demonstrated a unique mechanism of action compared to CBD and THC on TRPV3 and TRPV4 channels (De Petrocellis et al., 2012), it's antiepileptic effect is not CB1 dependent (Hill et al., 2013). It remains to be researched more extensively before its potential medical role is elucidated.

EVIDENCE OF MARIJUANA AND ITS COMPONENTS' EFFECTIVENESS AS MEDICINE

The *Journal of the American Medical Association* recently published a meta-analysis that reviewed the medicinal benefits and adverse effects of using different cannabinoid drugs (Whiting et al., 2015). The authors' analysis of 79 randomized medical trials examines the impact of using cannabinoids on nausea or vomiting from chemotherapy, appetite stimulation for HIV/AIDS patients, chronic pain, spasticity or paraplegia due to MS, anxiety disorder, sleep disorder, glaucoma, and psychosis, as well as any adverse effects such as dizziness, dry mouth, nausea, fatigue, somnolence, euphoria, vomiting, disorientation, drowsiness, confusion, loss of balance, and hallucination.

Though the study's findings suggest that the use of cannabinoids is associated with certain improved benefits compared with placebos or comparators, few of its results are statistically significant. Specifically, treatment of nausea/vomiting, appetite stimulation, treatment of chronic pain or spasticity, glaucoma, or psychosis all yielded no improvements or statistically insignificant ones (Whiting et al., 2015). For marijuana to be effective for glaucoma, the person would need to smoke every three hours (Tomida et al., 2006), something not practical and highly dangerous if the user neglected to follow the regimen because glaucoma treatment requires continuous reduction of intraocular pressure. The positive benefits were limited to anxiety and sleep disorders; the meta-analysis finds that cannabidiol, compared to placebo, is associated with a greater improvement in anxiety symptoms as well as sleep disorders. However, the researchers judged many of the trials included in the analysis are at high risk of bias and thus should be interpreted with caution (Whiting et al., 2015).

Regarding adverse effects of marijuana use in these therapeutic studies, an analysis of 62 trials finds that there is a statistically significant increased risk of short-term adverse effects such as balance problems, confusion, disorientation, euphoria, and hallucination associated with the drug's use (Whiting et al., 2015, p. 2466).

Sallan, Cronin, Zelen, and Zinberg (1980) compared prochlorperazine and THC for nausea and found that among these patients, there was a subjective preference for THC in the users, when both reduced nausea to seemingly equal levels. However, there are now many medications that are preferred to prochlorperazine for nausea, and these may outperform THC with greater breadth of treatment acceptance and fewer cognitive side effects. When a group of oncologists listed their preferred medications for nausea, they listed THC in ninth place among treatments and sixth out nine as a potential treatment for severe nausea (Schwartz & Beveridge, 1994). The emergence of cannabis-induced hyperemesis syndrome (Kim, Anderson, Saghafi, Heard, & Monte, 2015) suggests that it is very important to talk to patients who are using cannabis for nausea and vomiting about whether the drug is actually causing the problem, rather than relieving it.

A study of oral cannabis extract by Strasser et al. (2006) found that oral cannabis extract for cancer-related cachexia and wasting does not have any improvements in symptoms or quality of life compared with a placebo or THC extract. In fact, there were no differences in any outcome measure of the groups at any of the time measures.

In the unending quest to obtain a greater THC potency, plants are being bred and grown in conditions that maximize the conversion of the precursor material CBD to THC. While many medical marijuana strains show a lower THC:CBD ratio, some scientific evidence suggests the importance of giving THC and CBD together. A study comparing THC:CBD extract to THC alone showed that the combined treatment was associated with better improvement in pain, although it produced more nausea (Johnson et al., 2010). Whereas it is associated with a reduction in the intensity of the high (Morgan et al., 2010), this difference is not observed in all laboratory measures (Hindocha et al., 2015; Karschner et al., 2011).

Wade, Collin, Stott, and Duncombe (2010) and Novotna et al. (2011) demonstrated that Sativex (nabiximols) led to reduction in spasticity, and more recent open-label observational studies have supported the findings of efficacy and tolerability of nabiximols (Serpell, Notcutt, & Collin, 2013; Trojano & Vila, 2015). Corey-Bloom et al. (2012) showed efficacy of smoked marijuana for spasticity, but there was danger of unblinding, as it would be easy for the individual to know which treatment arm they had been allocated to based on the rather noticeable effects cannabis has on the user. This study also showed adverse cognitive effects, as have been found in other studies (Honarmand et al., 2011). Not all studies have seen cognitive problems, but there have been other correlations observed, such as a correlation between THC concentration and psychopathologic symptoms (Aragona et al., 2009).

The promise of cannabinoids in neuropathic pain is somewhat dampened by the mixed results of Langford et al. (2013), showing equivocal results. A very high placebo response in the first phase of the study was possibly responsible for hiding the positive benefits of nabiximols, but in the second phase of the study, which was a study following to discontinuation/treatment failure, the group given nabiximols performed better than placebo. An earlier study in diabetic peripheral neuropathy showed that cannabis was ineffective, but the authors suggested that depression was a confounding variable in their sample (Selvarajah, Gandhi, Emery, & Tesfaye, 2010).

Abrams showed some reduction of neuropathic pain in the short term with smoked cannabis, but the treatment also induced hyperalgesia (Abrams et al., 2007), a condition of increased pain sensitivity, as has been shown in other studies (Kraft et al., 2008). Opioids have been well-established to cause hyperalgesia and is a major limiting factor in their long-term therapeutic use (Yi & Pryzbylkowski, 2015), and this is a potentially important under-investigated parameter of long-term cannabinoid use (Kraft et al., 2008). A dose-dependent effect of THC on capsaicin-induced hyperalgesia has been suggested in the literature, with low doses of THC (2% THC joints) improving hyperalgesia, and high doses (8% THC joints) worsening it (Wallace et al., 2007). The smoked form of the medication also presents other problems.

Moore (2005) showed that long-term use of marijuana was associated with lung functioning; beyond the chronic cough, the study also found persistent bronchitis. Although as Tashkin (this volume) notes, the link between marijuana use and lung health is confounded by other variables and causal links are difficult to make.

Self-Regulated Dosing of Marijuana

Further research is needed to examine the potential effects and side effects of self-regulated dosing of marijuana, as is the practice in medical marijuana states in the United States (vs. doctor-controlled and doctor-prescribed dosing of THC). Due to lax medical marijuana law regulations, it is not a valid assumption to assume that benefits and levels of harm seen in controlled scientific studies will translate to benefits and levels of harm seen in an environment where patients control their own dosing and frequency of use of a substance that is habit-forming. Individuals left to use and dose on their own will often exceed the safety guidelines for medical marijuana and may miss therapeutic benefits seen at moderate doses that are potentially eclipsed at higher doses.

Difficulties in Placebo Control of Marijuana Studies

There are methodological challenges when medical marijuana studies use self-report measures. The first is that beyond the placebo effect of taking a medication that the user believes might help, there is an effect of intoxication on subjective reporting of all events. During a state of euphoria, neutral events are more likely to be rated positively, because of the neurobiologic alterations of the brain under the influence of THC. Activation of the ventral tegmental area and nucleus accumbens shell underlies the reinforcing properties of THC, and placebo effects have been shown to activate the nucleus accumbens as well. This means that subjective reports will be colored, typically toward the more positive during intoxication. Impairment of insight and awareness of errors has been shown with marijuana users (Hester, Nestor, & Garavan, 2009), and this may lead to underreporting of adverse effects of the drug on cognitive and behavioral performance. Pharmacologic studies of psychiatric medications rely on the blinded status of participants (not knowing which arm of the treatment study they have been allocated to), who are unaware of their medication states, to eliminate placebo effects. Participants in studies can sometimes accurately guess whether they have received active drug or placebo, and the use of cannabis and cannabinoids that take effect immediately raises a significant risk to double-blind studies, as users will often be able to tell that they are using a psychoactive cannabinoid (Lutge, Gray, & Siegfried, 2013).

It is very difficult to design a study in which an active marijuana user is unable to determine whether he or she had received marijuana or placebo—particularly when we are considering studies of smoked or vaporized cannabis that act rapidly on the central nervous system. For this reason, subjective reports of improvement are suspect if not corroborated by blinded raters' assessments of the individual's behaviors. Better potential exists for successful blinding with slow-release, oral forms of cannabis and cannabinoids that also probably have fewer central nervous system effects and greater therapeutic indices, meaning there is a larger margin for error between the dose that is medically effective and the dose that is dangerously toxic. Again, this highlights one of the major problems with medical marijuana. The question should not be whether inhaled whole-plant marijuana can positively affect any disease outcome; it is whether there is any value added to administering the smoked form of the drug to otherwise available oral forms.

DO MEDICAL MARIJUANA LAWS INCREASE USE?

Many studies seek to understand the relationship between approving norms of marijuana in a community and positive attitudes toward it and prevalence of its use, particularly among adolescents (Chilenski, Greenberg, & Feinberg, 2010; Hasin et al., 2015; Lipperman-Kreda, Grube, & Paschall, 2010; Stolzenberg, D'Alessio, & Dariano, 2016). While in many of the articles it has been stated as a conclusion that medical marijuana laws have not increased the use by adolescents, it is important to remember that this is very difficult to disprove, and failure to detect a difference does not prove a noneffect. The method of investigation has often been to determine whether the law enacted by the state changes adolescent use in that same state by controlling for pre-existing prevalence. While local laws would be expected to affect availability, changes in perception of harm are highly unlikely to stop at state borders. In assuming that they will do so, this approach ignores the realities of mass media culture, which brings the discussion of medical marijuana law changes in any state at a national level. Adolescents' perception of harm has gone down, and state-by-state data need to be analyzed to see how different forms of medicalization, commercialization, and legalization affect drug availability in that particular state. Not all medical marijuana laws are created equal, and those that increase cannabis supply by creating a commercial market might be expected to have a higher impact, as shown by Pacula, Powell, Heaton, and Sevigny (2015). Analysis of individual factors and features of each medical marijuana law is critical for determining the effects of the law on a population. For this reason, it has been suggested that we use a taxonomy of medical marijuana regimes to analyze their effects on the population more effectively (Chapman, Spetz, Lin, Chan, & Schmidt, 2016).

A common question people ask is whether marijuana use rates are sensitive to changes in policy? Theory suggests that passage of medical marijuana policies can increase demand for marijuana in at least three ways: (a) through changes in perceived harms, risks, or disapproval of the drug; (b) through changes in the ability to access marijuana; and (c) changes in the supply or production of marijuana that ultimately reduce its price (Pacula & Sevigny, 2013).

Challenges in Analyzing the Effects of Marijuana Laws

An added difficulty of measuring the effects of marijuana laws on perceived harms is that the message of less harm is often delivered most forcefully during the phase of campaigning for legislative change—that is, prior to the vote. Also, an electoral victory may change perceptions of social acceptance of a drug prior to the actual implementation of the law. Measuring local effects of marijuana laws is difficult because messages communicated in the marijuana debate often do not stay confined to locale where the law was being debated—due to much of the conversation being through national media. Likewise, there is difficulty measuring the effects of marijuana laws on supply and availability of marijuana because licitly produced drug in a looser medical marijuana laws state will often illicitly cross state lines, as has been reported by Rocky Mountain High Density Trafficking Area (2014) reports. Another potential bias is that legal changes to marijuana and medical marijuana laws may simply be a reflection of greater acceptance of the drug, and studies would need to account for the expected continued rate of change before and after a medical marijuana law was passed. Certainly, the issue is complicated and requires better studies.

Since there has been a generalized reduction in the rates of many different adolescent risk-taking behaviors (e.g., sexual behavior, smoking, drinking, other drug use), it is important to analyze any change in marijuana use in regards to the general trend for other drug use, teen pregnancy, and motor vehicle accidents. Also, the Internet and social media have greatly changed teen culture, and more people than ever are staying connected by Internet as opposed to real-life contacts. This new phenomenon might explain some of the changes in drug using patterns. The rewarding effects of social media may be a substitute for some youth to the effects of using drugs, a possibility that has even intrigued Nora Volkow, the director of the National Institute on Drug Abuse (Richtel, 2017). But we appreciate that mathematically modeling the contribution of online activities is very challenging.

EARLY EVIDENCE ON THE EFFECTS OF MEDICAL MARIJUANA LAWS

According to the 2014 National Survey on Drug Use and Health (NSDUH), the perceived risk of regularly (i.e., once or twice a week) using marijuana among Americans of all ages has been steadily declining, from approximately 51% in 2002 to 34% in 2014—a statistically significant difference in rates between the two years (Lipari, Kroutil, & Pemberton, 2015). Moreover, the 2014 Monitoring the Future survey data show that 23% of eighth graders associate risks and harm with marijuana use, compared to 29% in 2000 (Johnston, O'Malley, Miech, Bachman, & Schulenberg, 2014). Other studies have sought to examine the relationship between the availability of marijuana and prevalence of its use, yet the results remain mixed (Kim et al., 2016; Lucas & Walsh, 2017; Pardo, 2016).

Other correlations with medical marijuana laws have been found that are somewhat surprising, such as the effect on education based on medical marijuana law exposure (Plunk et al., 2016). It is important to analyze data such as these further, as was done by the authors of a study showing a correlation of medical marijuana laws and reduced fatality rates (Santaella-Tenorio et al., 2017). The authors noted that the heterogeneity of effects based on medical marijuana laws within states suggested that the reduction in traffic accidents was mediated by other factors. It is also important to analyze findings regarding traffic fatalities within the lens of decreasing rates of traffic fatalities over time

(NHTSA, 2016) for the entire nation and to examine effects of changes in ride-sharing availability and driving under the influence enforcement.

Harper et al. (2012) questioned the validity of Wall et al.'s (2011) conclusion that states that legalized medical marijuana had higher rates of adolescent marijuana use, declaring that it is "unable to validly isolate the causal effect of interest, which is the estimated difference in marijuana use that we would observe if we randomly assigned some states to pass a law" (p. 208). (An important note: Wall et al. use 2002–2008 NSDUH data while Harper et al. use 2002–2009 data, adding an additional year of data to their sample.) To account for this, Harper et al. used a difference-in-difference model to analyze the same data, estimating within-state changes in marijuana use, before and after medical marijuana legislation. They concluded that past-month marijuana use among adolescents actually decreased by 0.53 percentage points MML states with medical marijuana laws, though their findings was consistent with Wall et al. that the perception of marijuana's great risk decreased among youth in states with medical marijuana laws (Harper et al., 2012). Harper et al.'s analysis is problematic given that the estimated causal effect of marijuana was determined by changes observed in only 5 of the 16 states with medical marijuana laws. A further technical problem in the analysis is that difference-in-difference estimators are suited to a case-crossover design where all 50 states crossed over, rather than the analysis of 5 nonrandomly selected states among a group of 50. Furthermore, two of the five states used in their sample had abnormally high use rates in the year prior to legalization and removal of either of the states from the analysis would have yielded null results (Wall et al., 2012).

An analysis of combined state- and national-level Youth Risk Behavior Survey Surveillance between 1993 and 2011 found that medical marijuana legalization is associated with a decrease in the probability of past-month marijuana use among 12 to 17 year olds by 2.1 percentage points, though the study's sample does not include Washington State and Oregon—two states with medical marijuana laws during the study period (Anderson, Hansen, & Rees, 2012). Conversely, an all-50-states analysis, the National Epidemiologic Survey on Alcohol and Related Conditions found a higher rate of marijuana use and a higher rate of dependence in all 50 states (Cerda, Wall, Keys, Calea, & Hasin, 2012). The survey also failed to find a difference in cannabis use disorders using NSDUH dat, but still demonstrated higher rates of use in those states (Cerda et al., 2012).

Schuermeyer et al. (2014) showed a difference in perceived risk for all age groups, greater availability for those age 26 and older, and a trend toward increased rates of abuse and dependence after the onset of commercialization in Colorado. Over the past decade, while medical marijuana use has been widely discussed and debated, we have seen reductions of perceived risk from 2002 to 2012, with especially great reductions in risk from 2008 to 2012 (Pacek, Mauro, & Martins, 2015). While one cannot say for certain how much medicalization has led to this decreased risk, the decreased perception of harm has correlated with increased daily and nondaily use (Pacek et al., 2015). The conversation has taken place on the national stage, and common sense would assume to lead one to think that conversations in the national stage might affect an individual's perception of harm even outside of communities that have considered and enacted legislation.

A 2016 study published in the International Journal of Drug Policy (Stolzenberg et al., 2016) found that medical marijuana laws amplify youth marijuana use. The study, which utilized the largest national sample of drug users available, used five measurement periods calibrated in two-year intervals (2002–2003 to 2010–2011). The authors remarked,

> [Our] research design is advantageous in that it affords us the ability not only to assess the effect of the implementation of medical marijuana laws on juvenile drug use, but also to consider other state-specific factors that may explain variation in drug use that cannot be accounted for using a single time series. (p. 1)

Stolzenberg et al. also found that other salient predictors of juvenile marijuana use include perceived availability of marijuana, percent of juveniles skipping school, severity of perceived punishment for marijuana possession, alcohol consumption, percent of respondents with a father residing in household, and percent of families in the state receiving public assistance.

An analysis of the Monitoring the Future surveys, which contain annual representative data of 8th-, 10th-, and 12th-grade students in the United States between 1991 and 2014, finds that past-month marijuana use is more prevalent among all three grades in states with medical marijuana laws than states without such laws (Hasin et al., 2015). However, the researchers also reported that the risk of marijuana use in medical marijuana states before passing medical marijuana laws did not differ significantly from their risks after the law was passed. The study, published in *Lancet Psychiatry*, attracted considerable attention. However, key findings were omitted from the media reports. For example, the study found that 10th and 12th grade use in Colorado increased significantly after medical marijuana. This finding suggests that medical marijuana laws and their implementation vary drastically across the United States. Colorado has a large, well-established, commercialized medical marijuana program, often heralded as an example by legalization advocates. It is important to control for these vast differences and to look at what happened in states with more established laws and laws that allow for commercialization.

A similar study was conducted by Pacula et al. (2015) in which the authors evaluated the impact of differential medical marijuana provisions—such as allowing home cultivation, commercialization, or requiring users to register as cardholders—on youth and adult use rates. They postulated that medical marijuana laws that increase the availability of the drug reduce the costs associated with consuming it, such as search costs, legal risks, perceptions of associated health risks, and its price, and thus, as basic economic theory predicts, demand for the drug increases.

Wen, Hockenberry, and Cummings (2015) pooled nine years of cross-sectional data from a restricted-access version of the NSDUH data set, 2004 to 2012, and reported there were increases in (a) the probability of current marijuana use, regular marijuana use, and marijuana abuse/dependence among those ages 21 years and above and (b) in marijuana use initiation among those ages 12 to 20 years.

Using data from the Treatment Episode Data Set and the National Longitudinal Survey of Youth 1997, Pacula et al. (2015) reported that states that allow the existence of medical marijuana dispensaries are associated with a 15% increase in treatment admissions, though the associations between home cultivation and cardholder registration requirements do not yield significant results. Moreover, the authors found that legal protection of medical marijuana dispensaries is associated with a 2% increase in past-month marijuana use and that laws allowing home cultivation are associated with an increase in past-month use by 1.8% and raise the probability of heavy use (defined as using marijuana more than 20 times in the last 30 days) by 1%.

Location of Dispensaries

The location and density of marijuana dispensaries is also related to marijuana use prevalence. A study published in September 2015, analyzing panel data of marijuana-related hospitalizations in California between 2001 and 2012, finds that each additional dispensary per square mile is associated with a 6.8% increase in the number of marijuana-related hospitalizations (Mair, Freisthler, Ponicki, & Gaidus, 2015). With regards to the changing price of marijuana, evidence suggests that the availability and legality of medical marijuana are associated with a 9.8% decrease in the price of high-quality marijuana (Anderson, Hansen, & Rees, 2013). A 2015 study finds that exposure to medical marijuana advertising has effects on youth by increasing their intentions to use (D'Amico, Miles, & Tucker, 2015). Monte, Zane, and Heard (2015) reported that there were more medical marijuana dispensaries than McDonald's or Starbucks (Monte, Zane, & Heard, 2015).

Methodological Issues

Implementation of medical marijuana laws takes years, so what is needed is an analysis of the longer-term effects of these laws and their accompanying commercialization/regulation efforts. Colorado, for example, passed medical marijuana laws in 2000 but did not experience major changes until 2009, when commercialization began to flourish (Ghosh et al., 2015). Some studies only report a limited range of use frequency variables. For example, the *Lancet* study (Hasin et al., 2015) only reported past-year and past-30-day use and inexplicably did not include heavier (weekly or daily) use; such heavy use was the variables most associated with changes in marijuana laws in Pacula et al. (2015). Also, any

Monitoring the Future study that reports the 12th grade data is not going to reflect nationally representative of 18- and 19-year-olds given the relatively high rates of school dropout rates in many regions of the country.

EFFECT OF MEDICAL MARIJUANA LAWS ON OTHER SUBSTANCE USE

The reduction of opioid use in medical cannabis using individuals is frequently cited as a reason for allowing medical marijuana, and it is based on patients' self-reports of substitution of cannabis for opioids (Lucas & Walsh, 2017). An oft-cited statistic is that harmful opioid use went down in states with medical marijuana laws (Kim et al., 2016), but this was an effect inferred from a reduction only seen in 21- to 40-year-old males based on fatal overdose toxicity, when the data were aggregated across states, which does make it difficult to analyze whether concomitant changes in state-level opioid policy has mediated any of the decrease. There remain significant barriers to making causal assumption because there have been significant changes in state and federal policy regarding opioids recently, which have been found to reduce opioid use, particularly prescription monitoring programs (Pardo, 2016). There have not been any analyses that have examined the combined contribution of reduction in opioid use from prescription monitoring and medical marijuana and crackdowns on pill mills (clinics with very high rates of opioid prescribing) that would be expected to have a more direct effect on opioid use. Choi (2014) reported that alcohol abuse/dependence rates are sensitive to medical marijuana laws; these rates increased after marijuana legalization, suggesting the two drugs might be complements and not substitutes as is often assumed. Also, a similar increase in nicotine use has been observed after marijuana legalization (Choi, Dave, & Sabia, 2016).

CONCLUSION

The term *medical marijuana* implies that the whole marijuana plant is a safe and effective medicine established by scientific inquiry. It is easy to see how the term *medical opium* could have led to similar confusion in the past, and, today, it is important to clarify the debate to inform people that different constituent components of the cannabis plant, called cannabinoids, have different effects on different diseases, and many of the potential effects remain less well-established than others. The cannabinoid system is a potentially powerful system to modulate, and much investigation into this area is needed.

Medical marijuana's marketing to society, and the emphasis of potential positive benefits may have affected youth use. Moreover, the amplification of THC concentration since legalization and medical commercialization has led to a less-safe and less-standardized product because of protected indoor growing. Supply of marijuana is greater in these areas, and ill-effects of commercialization are not acted upon due to the powerful financial interests of recently legitimized medical marijuana growers allowing them to resist appropriate regulation. Recently, an attempt to collect signatures for a ballot initiative to require warning labels in Colorado was stifled by the industry paying the signature-collecting corporations not to collect signatures that were necessary for the referendum to head to a ballot ("Big Marijuana Trashes Democratic Process," 2016).

Some benefits of THC and CBD have been found in a handful of controlled clinical trials for a very limited number of health problems. Following on this success, dramatic claims for success and accusations of conspiratorial silencing of marijuana's benefits have led to an explosion in advertised benefits of medical marijuana, with frequently very little data backing up the claims, including claims seen in petri dishes that have been refuted in living organisms, as is the case of cancer. Effects of impure CBD preparations could lead many families to report effects of the preparation that are actually due to tranquilization secondary to THC intoxication. With a therapeutic dose range of 200 to 600 mg for CBD, even a residual 20:1 CBD:THC ratio could intoxicate a young person at a dose of 10 to 30 mg of THC.

When we look at the unintended effects of medical marijuana laws on health outcomes, an important caveat is that we must not assume that the effects of legalization and medicalization do not cross state lines. Youth and adults are well aware of the messages being transmitted in Colorado, California, and other states through the national media. We have seen marijuana being trafficked out of Colorado and California, and provisions allowing retail dispensaries have been associated with a subsequent increase in marijuana potency (Sevigny, Pacula, & Heaton, 2014). Due to illegal trafficking of legally produced marijuana in Colorado and California, it remains to be seen whether this will also increase the supply of high-potency THC across the country. Finally, another policy dimension that becomes incredibly complicated to study is the effect of domestic marijuana production on the rates of importation of cocaine, methamphetamine, and heroin. There is evidence for crop substitution in Mexico, with illegal traffickers switching from cannabis to opioids (Miroff, 2015).

The effects of medicalization have not been studied in depth, despite legalization and medicalization proponents claims that such policy changes would aid research. For example, money earmarked for research in California was not spent studying the effects of the legalized medical marijuana in humans. Unartful legislative drafting has not specified a practical monitoring mechanism for the drug, and the effects of legalization on testing have not been shown. The fast-tracking of research and collecting of data are highly important. None of the states that allow marijuana and extracts to be used as medicine have implemented adequate data collection tools. Part of this deficiency may be due to state governments not possessing the regulatory apparatus and expertise of the federal government, which are needed to ensure that measures are put in place to determine the efficacy and safety of pharmaceutical products. It has only been recently, and only with marijuana, that states have taken on the regulatory role of determining safety and efficacy of a pharmaceutical product. Furthermore, authors of the bills for regulation have not included experts in all of the relevant fields to legalization. The effects of medicalization that remain unexplored are those involving the substitution of medical marijuana for other treatments, the effect of regular marijuana use on compliance with other prescribed medical regimens, the adherence of medical marijuana patients to their prescribed regimens of marijuana, and the potential confounds of unblinding caused by the noticeable physical effects of marijuana.

REFERENCES

Abrams, D. I., Jay, C. A., Shade, S. B., Vizoso, H., Reda, H., Press, S., . . . Petersen, K. L. (2007). Cannabis in painful HIV-associated sensory neuropathy. *Neurology*, *68*, 515–521. http://dx.doi.org/10.1212/01.wnl.0000253187.66183.9c

Anderson, D. M., Hansen, B., & Rees, D. I. (2012). *Medical marijuana laws and teen marijuana use*. IZA Discussion Papers No. 6592.

Anderson, D. M., Hansen, B., & Rees, D. I. (2013). Medical marijuana laws, traffic fatalities, and alcohol consumption. *Journal of Law and Economics*, *56*, 333–369. http://dx.doi.org/10.1086/668812

Andreae, M. H., Carter, G. M., Shaparin, N., Suslov, K., Ellis, R. J., Ware, M. A., . . . Saks, H. S. (2015). Inhaled cannabis for chronic neuropathic pain: A meta-analysis of individual patient data. *Journal of Pain*, *16*, 1221–1232. http://dx.doi.org/10.1016/j.jpain.2015.07.009

Aragona, M., Onesti, E., Tomassini, V., Conte, A., Gupta, S., Gilio, F., . . . Inghilleri, M. (2009). Psychopathological and cognitive effects of therapeutic cannabinoids in multiple sclerosis: A double-blind, placebo controlled, crossover study. *Clinical Neuropharmacology*, *32*, 41–47. http//dx.doi.org/10.1097/WNF.0B013E3181633497

Bestrashniy, J., & Winters, K. C. (2015). Variability in medical marijuana laws in the United States. *Psychology of Addictive Behaviors*, *29*, 639–642. http://dx.doi.org/10.1037/adb0000111

Big marijuana trashes democratic process. (2016, July 8). *The Gazette* [Editorial]. Retrieved from http://gazette.com/editorial-big-marijuana-trashes-democratic-process/article/1579890

Boehnke, K. F., Litinas, E., & Clauw, D. J. (2016). Medical cannabis use is associated with decreased opiate medication use in a retrospective cross-sectional survey of patients with chronic pain. *Journal of Pain*, *17*, 739–744. http://dx.doi.org/10.1016/j.jpain.2016.03.002

Bradford, A. C., & Bradford, W. D. (2016). Medical marijuana laws reduce prescription medication use in Medicare Part D. *Health Affairs*, *35*, 1230–1236. http://dx.doi.org/10.1377/hlthaff.2015.1661

Budney, A. J., Hughs, J. R., Moore, B. A., & Vandrey, R. (2004). Review of the validity and significance of cannabis withdrawal syndrome. *American Journal of Psychiatry*, *161*, 1967–1977. http://dx.doi.org/10.1176/appi.ajp.161.11.1967

Cerda, M., Wall, M., Keys, K. M., Calea, S., & Hasin, D. (2012). Medical marijuana laws in 50 states: Investigating the relationship between state legalization of medical marijuana and marijuana use, abuse and dependence. *Drug and Alcohol Dependence*, *120*, 22–27. http://dx.doi.org/10.1016/j.drugalcdep.2011.06.011

Chapman, S. A., Spetz, J., Lin, J., Chan, K., & Schmidt, L. A. (2016). Capturing heterogeneity in medical marijuana policies: A taxonomy of regulatory regimes across the United States. *Subtance Use & Misuse, 51*, 1174–1184. http://dx.doi.org/10.3109/10826084.2016.1160932

Cherif, H., Argaw, A., Cécyre, B., Bouchard, A., Gagnon, J., Javadi, P., . . . Bouchard, J.-F. (2015). Role of GPR55 during axon growth and target innervation. *eNeuro, 2*(5). http://dx.doi.og/10.1523/ENEURO.0011-15.2015

Chilenski, S. M., Greenberg, M. T., & Feinberg, M. E. (2010). The community substance use environment: The development and predictive ability of a multi-method and multiple-reporter measure. *Journal of Community & Applied Social Psychology, 20*, 57–71. http://dx.doi.org/10.1002/casp.1014

Choi, A. (2014). *The impact of medical marijuana laws on marijuana use and other risky health behaviors.* Paper presented at the ASHEcon 2015, Los Angeles.

Choi, A., Dave, D., & Sabia, J. J. (2016). *Smoke gets in your eyes: Medical marijuana laws and tobacco use.* NBER Working Paper No. w22554.

Colorado Department of Public Health and Environment. (2015). *Medical Marijuana Registry Program Statistics: June 30, 2015.* Retrieved from https://www.colorado.gov/pacific/sites/default/files/06_2015_MMR_report.pdf

Compassionate Use Act of 1996. Proposition 215. California Health & Safety Code 11362.5.

Corey-Bloom, J., Wolfson, T., Gamst, A., Jin, S., Marcotte, T. D., Bentley, H., & Gouaux, B. (2012). Smoked cannabis for spasticity in multiple sclerosis: A randomized, placebo-controlled trial. *Canadian Medical Association Journal, 184*, 1143–1150. http://dx.doi.org/10.1503/cmaj.110837

Cutando, L., Busquets-Garcia, A., Puighermanal, E., Gomis-González, M., Delgado-García, J. M., Gruart, A., . . . Ozaital, A. (2013). Microglial activation underlies cerebellar deficits produced by repeated cannabis exposure. *Journal of Clinical Investigation, 123*, 2816–2831. http://dx.doi.org/10.1172/jci67569

D'Amico, E. J., Miles, J. N., & Tucker, J. S. (2015). Gateway to curiosity: Medical marijuana ads and intention and use during middle school. *Psychology of Addictive Behaviors, 29*, 613–619. http://dx.doi.org/10.1037/adb0000094

Devinsky, O., Cilio, M. R., Cross, H., Fernandez-Ruiz, J., French, J., Hill, C., . . . Friedman, D. (2014). Cannabidiol: Pharmacology and potential therapeutic role in epilepsy and other neuropsychiatric disorders. *Epilepsia, 55*, 791–802. http://dx.doi.org/10.1111/epi.12631

Devinsky, O., Marsh, E., Friedman, D., Thiele, E., Laux, L., Sullivan, J., . . . Cilio, M. R. (2016). Cannabidiol in patients with treatment-resistant epilepsy: an open-label interventional trial. *The Lancet, 15*, 270–278. http://dx.doi.org/10.1016/S1474-4422(15)00379-8

Felder, C. C., & Glass, M. (1998). Cannabinoid receptors and their endogenous agonists. *Annual Review of Pharmacology and Toxicology, 38*, 179–200. http://dx.doi.org/10.1146/annurev.pharmtox.38.1.179

Forti, M. D., Marconi, A., Carra, E., Fraietta, S., Trotta, A., Bonomo, M., . . . Murray, R. M. (2015). Proportion of patients in south London with first-episode psychosis attributable to use of high potency cannabis: a case-control study. *The Lancet, 2*, 233–238. http://dx.doi.org/10.1016/S2215-0366(14)00117-5

Fraser, G. A. (2009). The use of a synthetic cannabinoid in the management of treatment-resistant nightmares in posttraumatic stress disorder (PTSD). *CNS Neuroscience & Therapeutics, 15*, 84–88. http://dx.doi.org/10.1111/j.1755-5949.2008.00071.x

Ghosh, T. S., Dyke, M. V., Maffey, M., Whitley, E., Erpelding, D., & Wolk, L. (2015). Medical marijuana's public health lessons: Implications for retail marijuana in Colorado. *New England Journal of Medicine, 372,* 991–993. http://dx.doi.org/10.1056/NEJMp1500043

Gupta, S. (writer). (2013). *CNN weed 1: A special report by Dr. Sanjay Gupta* [television episode] Atlanta: CNN.

Harper, S., Stumpf, E. C., & Kaufman, J. S. (2012). Do medical marijuana laws increase marijuana use? Replication study and extension. *Annals of Epidemiology, 22,* 207–212. http://dx.doi.org/10.1016/j.annepidem.2011.12.002

Hasin, D., Wall, M., Keys, K. M., Cerda, M., Schulenberg, H., O'Malley, P. M., . . . Feng, T. (2015). Medical marijuana laws and adolescent marijuana use in the USA from 1991 to 2014: Results from annual, repeated cross-sectional surveys. *The Lancet, 2,* 601–608. http://dx.doi.org/10.1016/S2215-0366(15)00217-5

Hester, R., Nestor, L., & Garavan, H. (2009). Impaired error awareness and anterior cingulate cortex hypoactivity in chronic cannabis users. *Neuropsychopharmacology, 34,* 2450–2458. http://dx.doi.org/10.1038/npp.2009.67

Hill, A. J., Mercier, M. S., Hill, T. D., Glyn, S. E., Jones, N. A., Yamasaki, Y., . . . Whalley, B. J. (2012). Cannabidivarin is anticonvulsant in mouse and rat. *British Journal of Pharmacology, 167,* 1629–1642. http://dx.doi.org/10.1111/j.1476-5381.2012.02207.x

Hill, T. D., Cascio, M.-G., Romano, B., Duncan, M., Pertwee, R. G., Williams, C. M., . . . Hill, A. J. (2013). Cannabidivarin-rich cannabis extracts are anticonvulsant in mouse and rat via a CB1 receptor-independent mechanism. *British Journal of Pharmacology, 170,* 679–692. http://dx.doi.org/10.1111/bph.12321

Hindocha, C., Freeman, T. P., Schafer, G., Gardener, C., Das, R. K., Morgan, C. J., & Curran, H. V. (2014). Acute effects of delta-9-tetrahydrocannabinol, cannabidiol and their combination on facial emotion recognition: A randomised, double-blind, placebo-controlled study in cannabis users. *European Neuropsychopharmacology, 25*(3), 325–334. http://dx.doi.org/10.1016/j.euroneuro.2014.11.014

Hoffman, D., Brunneman, K. D., Gori, G. B., & Wynder, E. L. (1975). On the carcinogenicity of marijuana smoke. In V. C. Runeckles (Ed.), *Recent advances in phytochemistry* (Vol. 9, pp. 63–81). New York: Plenum.

Honarmand, K., Tierney, M. C., O'Connor, P., & Feinstein, A. (2011). Effects of cannabis on cognitive function in patients with multiple sclerosis. *Neurology, 76,* 1153–1160. http://dx.doi.org/10.1212/WNL.0b013e318212ab0c

Hunault, C. C., Mensinga, T. T., Vries, I. d., Kelholt-Dijkman, H. H., Hoek, J., Kruidenier, M., . . . Meulenbelt, J. (2008). Delta-9-tetrahydrocannabinol (THC) serum concentrations and pharmacological effects in males after smoking a combination of tobacco and cannabis containing up to 69 mg THC. *Psychopharmacology, 201,* 171–181. http://dx.doi.org/10.1007/s00213-008-1260-2

Iversen, L. L. (2007). *The science of marijuana.* Oxford: Oxford University Press.

Jetley, R., Heber, A., Fraser, G., & Boisvert, D. (2015). The efficacy of nabilone, a synthetic cannabinoid, in the treatment of PTSD-associated nightmares: A preliminary randomized, double-blind, placebo-controlled cross-over design study. *Psychoneuroendocrinology, 51,* 585–588. http://dx.doi.org/10.1016/j.psyneuen.2014.11.002

Johnson, J. R., Burnell-Nugent, M., Lossignol, D., Ganae-Motan, E. D., Potts, R., & Fallon, M. T. (2010). Multicenter, double-blind, randomized, placebo-controlled, parallel-group study of the efficacy, safety, and tolerability of THC: CBD extract and THC extract in patients with intractable cancer-related pain. *Journal of Pain and Symptom Management*, 39, 167–179. http://dx.doi.org/10.1016/j.jpainsymman.2009.06.008

Johnston, L. D., O'Malley, P. M., Miech, R. A., Bachman, J. G., & Schulenberg, J. E. (2014). *Monitoring the Future national survey results on drug use: 1975–2013: Overview, key findings on adolescent drug use.* Ann Arbor: Institute for Social Research, University of Michigan.

Joy, J. E., Jr., Watson, S. J., & Benson, J. A., Jr. (1999). *Marijuana and medicine: Assessing the evidence base.* Washington: National Academies Press.

Karschner, E. L., Darwin, W. D., McMahon, R. P., Liu, R., Wright, S., Goodwin, R. S., & Huestis, M. A. (2011). Subjective and physiological effects after controlled Sativex and oral THC administration. *Clinical Pharmacology and Therapeutics*, 89, 400–407. http://dx.doi.org/10.1038/clpt.2010.318

Kim, H. S., Anderson, J. D., Saghafi, O., Heard, K. J., & Monte, A. A. (2015). Cyclic vomiting presentations following marijuana liberalization in Colorado. *Academic Emergency Medicine*, 22, 694–699. http://dx.doi.org/10.1111/acem.12655

Kim, J. H., Santaella-Tenorio, J., Mauro, C., Wrobel, J., Cerda, M., Keys, K. M., . . . Li, G. (2016). State medical marijuana laws and the prevalence of opioids detected among fatally injured drivers. *American Journal of Public Health*, 106, 2032–2037. http://dx.doi.org/10.2105/ajph.2016.303426

Kraft, B., Frcikey, N. A., Kaufmann, R. M., Reif, M., Frey, R., Gustorff, B., & Kress, H. G. (2008). Lack of analgesia by oral standardized cannabis extract on acute inflammatory pain and hyperalgesia in volunteers. *Anesthesiology*, 109, 101–110. http://dx.doi.org/10.1097/ALN.0b013e31817881e1

Langford, R. M., Mares, J., Novotna, A., Vachova, M., Novakova, I., Notcutt, W., & Ratcliffe, S. (2013). A double-blind, randomized, placebo-controlled, parallel-group study of THC/CBD oromucosal spray in combination with the existing treatment regimen, in the relief of central neuropathic pain in patients with multiple sclerosis. *Journal of Neurology*, 260, 984–997. http://dx.doi.org/10.1007/s00415-012-6739-4

Lankenau, S. E., Fedorova, E. V., Reed, M., Schrager, S. M., Iverson, E., & Wang, C. F. (2017). Marijuana practices and patterns of use among young adult medical marijuana patients and non-patient marijuana users. *Drug and Alcohol Dependence*, 170, 181–188. http://dx.doi.org/10.1016/j.drugalcdep.2016.10.025

Laprairie, R. B., Bagher, A. M., Kelly, M. E., & Denovan-Wright, E. M. (2015). Cannabidiol is a negative allosteric modulator of the cannabinoid CB1 receptor. *British Journal of Pharmacology*, 172, 4790–7805. http://dx.doi.org/10.1111/bph.13250

Lipari, R., Kroutil, L. A., & Pemberton, M. R. (2015). Risk and protective factors and initiation of substance use: Results from the 2014 National Survey on Drug Use and Health. Retrieved from https://www.samhsa.gov/data/sites/default/files/NSDUH-DR-FRR4-2014rev/NSDUH-DR-FRR4-2014.pdf.

Lipperman-Kreda, S., Grube, J. W., & Paschall, M. J. (2010). Community norms, enforcement of minimum legal drinking age laws, personal beliefs and underage drinking: An explanatory model. *Journal of Community Health*, 35, 249–257. http://dx.doi.org/10.1007/s10900-010-9229-6

Lucas, P., & Walsh, Z. (2017). Medical cannabis access, use, and substitution for prescription opioids and other substances: A survey of authorized medical cannabis patients. *International Journal of Drug Policy, 42*, 30–35. htpp://dx.doi.org/10.1016/j.drugpo.2017.01.011

Lutge, E. E., Gray, A., & Siegfried, N. (2013). The medical use of cannabis for reducing morbidity and mortality in patients with HIV/AIDS. *Cochrane Database of Systematic Reviews, 4*, CD005175. http://dx.doi.org/10.1002/14651858.CD005175.pub3

Mair, C., Freisthler, B., Ponicki, W. R., & Gaidus, A. (2015). The impacts of marijuana dispensary density and neighborhood ecology on marijuana abuse and dependence. *Drug and Alcohol Dependence, 154*, 111–116. http://dx.doi.org/10.1016/j.drugalcdep.2015.06.019

Mathern, G. W., Beninsig, L., & Nehlig, A. (2014). From the editors: Epilepsia's 2014 Operational Definition of Epilepsy Survey. *Epilepsia, 55*, 1683–1687. http://dx.doi.org/10.1111/epi.12812

Miroff, N. (2015, January 11). Losing marijuana business, Mexican cartels push heroin and meth. *The Washington Post*. Retrieved from https://www.washingtonpost.com/world/the_americas/losing-marijuana-business-mexican-cartels-push-heroin-and-meth/2015/01/11/91fe44ce-8532-11e4-abcf-5a3d7b3b20b8_story.html?utm_term=.5f517112ed0a&wprss=rss_homepage

Monte, A. A., Zane, R. D., & Heard, K. J. (2015). The implications of marijuana legalization in Colorado. *Journal of the American Medical Association, 313*, 241–242. http://dx.doi.org/10.1001/jama.2014.17057

Moore, B. A., Augustson, E. M., Moser, R. P., & Budney, A. J. (2005). Respiratory effects of marijuana and tobacco use in a U.S. sample. *Journal of General Internal Medicine, 20*, 33–37. http://dx.doi.org/10.1111/j.1525-1497.2004.40081.x

Morgan, C. J. A., Freeman, T. P., Schafer, G. L., & Curran, H. V. (2010). Cannabidiol Attenuates the appetitive effects of Δ9-Tetrahydrocannabinol in humans smoking their chosen cannabis. *Neuropsychopharmacology, 35*, 1879–1885. http://dx.doi.org/10.1038/npp.2010.58

Munro, S., Thomas, K. L., & Abu-Shaar, M. (1993). Molecular characterization of a peripheral receptor for cannabinoids. *Nature, 365*, 61–65. http://dx.doi.org/10.1038/365061a0

Murthy, N. V., Vassell, M., Melville, G. N., Wray, S. R., Shah, D., Wynter, H. H., & West, M. (1985). Long-term effects of marihuana smoke on uterine contractility and tumour development in rats. *West Indian Medical Journal, 34*, 244–247.

National Academies of Sciences, E., and Medicine. (2017). *The health effects of cannabis and cannabinoids: The current state of evidence and recommendations for research.* Washington, DC: National Academies Press.

National Council of State Legislatures. (2017). *State medical marijuana laws.* Retrieved from http://www.ncsl.org/research/health/state-medical-marijuana-laws.aspx

National Highway Traffic Safety Administration. (n.d.). *Fatality analysis reporting system (FARS) encyclopedia: National statistics.* Retrieved from https://www-fars.nhtsa.dot.gov/Main/index.aspx

Nelson, S. (2016, June 6). Debate over? 89 percent support medical pot in new poll. *U.S. News and World Report.* Retrieved from https://www.usnews.com/news/articles/2016-06-06/debate-over-89-percent-support-medical-pot-in-new-poll

Nguyen, T., Li, J.-X., Thomas, B. F., Wiley, J. L., & Kenakin, T. P. (2016). Allosteric modulation: An alternate approach targeting the cannabinoid CB1 receptor. *Medicinal Research Reviews, 37*, 441–474. http://dx.doi.org/10.1002/med.21418

NHTSA. (2016). https://www.nhtsa.gov/press-releases/traffic-fatalities-sharply-2015

Novotna, A., Mares, J., Ratcliffe, S., Novakova, I., Vachova, M., Zapletalova, O., . . . Sativex Spasticity Study Group. (2011). A randomized, double-blind, placebo-controlled, parallel-group, enriched-design study of nabiximols (Sativex®), as add-on therapy, in subjects with refractory spasticity caused by multiple sclerosis. *European Journal of Neurology, 18,* 1122–1131. http://dx.doi.org/10.1111/j.1468-1331.2010.03328.x

Nunberg, H., Kilmer, B., Pacula, R. L., & Burgdorf, J. R. (2011). An analysis of applicants presenting to a medical marijuana specialty practice in California. *Journal of Drug Policy Analysis, 4.* http://dx.doi.org/10.2202/1941-2851.1017

Nussbaum, A. M., Thurstone, C., McGarry, L., Walker, B., & Sabel, A. L. (2015). Use and diversion of medical marijuana among adults admitted to inpatient psychiatry. *American Journal of Drug and Alcohol Abuse, 41,* 166–172. http://dx.doi.org/10.3109/00952990.2014.949727

O'Connell, T. J., & Bou-Matar, C. B. (2007). Long term marijuana users seeking medical cannabis in California (2001–2007): Demographics, social characteristics, patterns of cannabis and other drug use of 4117 applicants. *Harm Reduction Journal, 4.* http://dx.doi.org/10.1186/1477-7517-4-16

Oleson, E. B., & Cheer, J. F. (2012). A brain on cannabinoids: The role of dopamine release in reward weeking. *Cold Spring Harbor Perspectives in Medicine, 2,* a012229. http://dx.doi.org/10.1101/cshperspect.a012229

Oregon Health Authority. (2015). *Oregon medical marijuana program: Statistical snapshot July, 2015.* Retrieved from https://public.health.oregon.gov/DiseasesConditions/ChronicDisease/MedicalMarijuanaProgram/Documents/ed-materials/ommp_stats_snapshot.pdf

Pacek, L. R., Mauro, P. M., & Martins, S. S. (2015). Perceived risk of regular cannabis use in the United States from 2002 to 2012: Differences by sex, age, and race/ethnicity. *Drug and Alcohol Dependence, 149,* 232–244. http://dx.doi.org/10.1016/j.drugalcdep.2015.02.009

Pacula, R., Powell, D., Heaton, P., & Sevigny, E. (2015). Assessing the effects of medical marijuana laws on marijuana use: The devil is in the details. *Journal of Policy Analysis and Management, 34,* 7–31. http://dx.doi.org/10.1002/pam.21804

Pacula, R., & Sevigny, E. (2013). Marijuana liberalization policies: Why we can't learn much from policy still in motion. *Journal of Policy Analysis and Management, 33,* 212–221. http://dx.doi.org/10.1002/pam.21726

Pardo, B. (2017). Do more robust prescription drug monitoring programs reduce prescription opioid overdose? *Addiction, 112,* 1773–1783. http://dx.doi.org/10.1111/add.13741

Pertwee, R. G. (1999). Evidence for the presence of CB1 cannabinoid receptors on peripheral neurones and for the existence of neuronal non-CB1 cannabinoid receptors. *Life Sciences, 65,* 597–605. http://dx.doi.org/10.1016/S0024-3205(99)00282-9

Pertwee, R. G. (2006). The pharmacology of cannabinoid receptors and their ligands: An overview. *International Journal of Obesity, 30,* S13–S18. http://dx.doi.org/10.1038/sj.ijo.0803272

Pertwee, R. G. (2008). The diverse CB1 and CB2 receptor pharmacology of three plant cannabinoids: delta9-tetrahydrocannabinol, cannabidiol and delta9-tetrahydrocannabivarin. *British Journal of Pharmacology, 153,* 199–215. http://dx.doi.org/10.1038/sj.bjp.0707442

Pertwee, R. G., Thomas, A., Stevenson, L. A., Ross, R. A., Varvel, S. A., Lichtman, A. H., . . . Razdan, R. K. (20007). The psychoactive plant cannabinoid, Δ9-tetrahydrocannabinol, is antagonized by Δ8- and Δ9-tetrahydrocannabivarin in mice in vivo. *British Journal of Pharmacology, 15*, 586–594. http://dx.doi.org/586-594. doi: 10.1038/sj.bjp.0707124

Petrocellis, L. D., Orlando, O., Moriello, A. S., Aviello, G., Stott, C., Izzo, A. A., & Marzo, V. D. (2012). Cannabinoid actions at TRPV channels: effects on TRPV3 and TRPV4 and their potential relevance to gastrointestinal inflammation. *Acta Physiologica, 204*, 255–266. http://dx.doi.org/10.1111/j.1748-1716.2011.02338.x

Picone, R. P., & Kendall, D. A. (2015). Minireview: From the bench, toward the clinic: Therapeutic opportunities for cannabinoid receptor modulation. *Molecular Endocrinology, 29*, 801–813. http://dx.doi.org/10.1210/me.2015-1062

Platt, B., Kamboj, S., Morgan, C. J., & Curran, H. V. (2010). Processing dynamic facial affect in frequent cannabis-users: Evidence of deficits in the speed of identifying emotional expressions. *Drug and Alcohol Dependence, 112*, 27–32. http://dx.doi.org/10.1016/j.drugalcdep.2010.05.004

Plunk, A. D., Agrawal, A., Harrell, P. T., Tate, W. F., Will, K. E., Mellor, J. M., & Grucza, R. A. (2016). The impact of adolescent exposure to medical marijuana laws on high school completion, college enrollment and college degree completion. *Drug and Alcohol Dependence, 168*, 320–327. http://dx.doi.org/10.1016/j.drugalcdep.2016.09.002

Porter, B. E., & Jacobson, C. (2015). Report of a parent survey of cannabidiol-enriched cannabis use in pediatric treatment-resistant epilepsy. *Epilepsy & Behavior, 29*, 574–577. http://dx.doi.org/10.1016/j.yebeh.2013.08.037

Press, C. A., Knupp, K. G., & Chapman, K. E. (2015). Parental reporting of response to oral cannabis extracts for treatment of refractory epilepsy. *Epilepsy & Behavior, 45*, 49–52. http://dx.doi.org/10.1016/j.yebeh.2015.02.043

Reinarman, C., Nunberg, H., Lanthier, F., & Heddleston, T. (2011). Who are medical marijuana patients? Population characteristics from nine California assessment clinics. *Journal of Psychoactive Drugs, 43*, 128–135. http://dx.doi.org/10.1080/02791072.2011.587700

Richtel, M. (2013, March 13). Are teenagers replacing drugs with smartphones? *New York Times*. Retrieved from https://www.nytimes.com/2017/03/13/health/teenagers-drugs-smartphones.html?_r=0

Rocky Mountain High Density Trafficking Area. (2014). *Legalization of marijuana in Colorado: The Impact*. Retrieved from http://www.rmhidta.org/html/august%20 2014%20legalization%20of%20mj%20in%20colorado%20the%20impact.pdf

Sabet, K. A., & Grossman, E. (2014). Why do people use medical marijuana? The medical conditions of users in seven U.S. states. *Journal of Global Drug Policy and Practice, 8*(2).

Sallan, S. E., Cronin, C., Zelen, M., & Zinberg, N. E. (1980). Antiemetics in patients receiving chemotherapy for cancer: A randomized comparison of delta-9-tetrahydrocannabinol and prochlorperazine. *New England Journal of Medicine, 302*, 135–138. http://dx.doi.org/10.1056/nejm198001173020302

Santaella-Tenorio, J., Mauro, C., Wall, M., Kim, J. H., Cerda, M., Keys, K. M., . . . Martins, S. S. (2017). US traffic fatalities, 1985–2014, and their relationship to medical marijuana laws. *American Journal of Public Health, 107*, 336–342. http://dx.doi.org/10.2105/ajph.2016.303577

Schuermeyer, J., Salomonsen-Sautel, S., Price, R. K., Balan, S., Thurstone, C., Min, S. J., & Sakai, J. T. (2014). Temporal trends in marijuana attitudes, availability and use in Colorado compared to non-medical marijuana states: 2003–11. *Drug and Alcohol Dependence, 140,* 145–155. http://dx.doi.org/10.1016/j.drugalcdep.2014.04.016

Schwartz, R. H., & Beveridge, R. A. (1994). Marijuana as an antiemetic drug: How useful is it today? Opinions from clinical oncologists. *Journal of Addictive Diseases, 13,* 53–65. http://dx.doi.org/10.1300/J069v13n01_05

Selvarajah, D., Gandhi, R., Emery, C. J., & Tesfaye, S. (2010). Randomized placebo-controlled double-blind clinical trial of cannabis-based medicinal product (Sativex) in painful diabetic neuropathy: Depression is a major confounding factor. *Diabetes Care, 33,* 128–130. http://dx.doi.org/10.2337/dc09-1029

Serpell, M. G., Notcutt, W., & Collin, C. (2013). Sativex long-term use: An open-label trial in patients with spasticity due to multiple sclerosis. *Journal of Neurology, 260,* 285–295. http://dx.doi.org/10.1007/s00415-012-6634-z

Sevigny, E., Pacula, R., & Heaton, P. (2014). The effects of medical marijuana laws on potency. *International Journal of Drug Policy, 25,* 308–319. http://dx.doi.org/10.1016/j.drugpo.2014.01.003

St. Pierre, A. (2009) *CNN Newsroom* [Interview by Don Lemon]. Atlanta: CNN.

Stolzenberg, L., D'Alessio, S. J., & Dariano, D. (2016). The effect of medical cannabis laws on juvenile cannabis use. *International Journal of Drug Policy, 27,* 82–88. http://dx.doi.org/10.1016/j.drugpo.2015.05.018

Strasser, F., Luftner, D., Possinger, K., Ernst, G., Ruhstaller, T., Meissner, W., . . . Cerny, T. (2006). Comparison of orally administered cannabis extract and delta-9-tetrahydrocannabinol in treating patients with cancer-related anorexia-cachexia syndrome: A multicenter, phase III, randomized, double-blind, placebo-controlled clinical trial from the Cannabis-in-Cachexia-Study-Group. *Journal of Clinical Oncology, 24,* 3394–3400. http://dx.doi.org/10.1200/JCO.2005.05.1847

NORML chairman Keith Stroup talks on pot issues. (1979, February 6). *Emory Wheel,* pp. 18–19

Thomas, A., Stevenson, L. A., Wease, K. N., Price, M. R., Baillie, G., Ross, R. A., & Pertwee, R. G. (2005). Evidence that the plant cannabinoid Delta9-tetrahydrocannabivarin is a cannabinoid CB1 and CB2 receptor antagonist. *British Journal of Pharmacology, 146,* 917–926. http://dx.doi.org/10.1038/sj.bjp.0706414

Tomida, I., Azuara-Blanco, A., House, H., Flint, M., Pertwee, R. G., & Robson, P. J. (2006). Effect of sublingual application of cannabinoids on intraocular pressure: A pilot study. *Journal of Glaucoma, 15,* 349–353. http://dx.doi.org/10.1097/01.ijg.0000212260.04488.60

Trojano, M., & Vila, C. (2015). Effectiveness and tolerability of THC/CBD oromucosal spray for multiple sclerosis spasticity in Italy: First data from a large observational study. *European Journal of Neurology, 74,* 178–185. http://dx.doi.org/10.1159/000441619

Tuo, W., Leleu-Chavain, N., Spencer, J., Sansook, S., Millet, R., & Chavatte, P. (2017). Therapeutic potential of fatty acid amide hydrolase, monoacylglycerol lipase, and N-acylethanolamine acid amidase inhibitors. *Journal of Medicinal Chemistry, 60,* 4–46. http://dx.doi.org/10.1021/acs.jmedchem.6b00538

US Food and Drug Administration. (n.d.). *2016 warning letters and test results for cannabidiol-related products.* Retrieved from https://www.fda.gov/NewsEvents/PublicHealthFocus/ucm484109.htm

Volkow, N. (February 28, 2017). NASEM Report Recommends Removing Barriers to Cannabis Research https://www.drugabuse.gov/about-nida/noras-blog/2017/02/nasem-report-recommends-removing-barriers-to-cannabis-research

Wade, D. T., Collin, C., Stott, C., & Duncombe, P. (2010). Meta-analysis of the efficacy and safety of Sativex (nabiximols), on spasticity in people with multiple sclerosis. *Multiple Sclerosis*, *16*, 707–714. http://dx.doi.org/10.1177/1352458510367462

Wall, M., Poh, E., Cerda, M., Keys, K. M., Galea, S., & Hasin, D. (2011). Adolescent marijuana use from 2002 to 2008: Higher in states with medical marijuana laws, cause still unclear. *Annals of Epidemiology*, *21*, 714–716. http://dx.doi.org/10.1016/j.annepidem.2011.06.001

Wall, M., Poh, E., Cerda, M., Keys, K. M., Galea, S., & Hasin, D. (2012). Do medical marijuana laws increase marijuana use? Replication study and extension. *Annals of Epidemiology*, *22*, 536–537. http://dx.doi.org/10.1016/j.annepidem.2012.03.003

Wallace, M., Schulteis, G., Atkinson, J. H., Wolfson, T., Lazzaretto, D., Bentley, H., . . . Abramson, I. (2007). Dose-dependent effects of smoked cannabis on capsaicin-induced pain and hyperalgesia in healthy volunteers. *Anesthesiology*, *107*, 785–796. http://dx.doi.org/10.1097/01.anes.0000286986.92475.b7

Wallace, M. S., Marcotte, T. D., Umlauf, A., Gouaux, B., & Atkinson, J. A. (2015). Efficacy of inhaled cannabis on painful diabetic neuropathy. *Journal of Pain*, *16*, 616–627. http://dx.doi.org/10.1016/j.jpain.2015.03.008

Walton, R. P. (1938). Description of the hashish experience. *Marihuana: Americas new drug problem*. Philadelphia: Lippincott.

Ward, A., & Holmes, B. (1985). Nabilone: A preliminary review of its pharmacological properties and therapeutic use. *Drugs*, *30*, 127–144.

Wehner, F. C., Renseburg, S. J. v., & Thiel, P. G. (1980). Mutagenicity of marijuana and Transkei tobacco smoke condensates in the Salmonella/microsome assay. *Mutation Research*, *77*, 135–142.

Wen, H., Hockenberry, J. M., & Cummings, J. R. (2015). The effect of medical marijuana laws on adolescent and adult use of marijuana, alcohol, and other substances. *Journal of Health Economics*, *42*, 64–80. http://dx.doi.org/10.1016/j.jhealeco.2015.03.007

Whiting, P. F., Wolff, R. F., Deshpande, S., Duffy, M., Hernandez, A. V., Keurentjes, J. C., . . . Keijnen, J. (2015). Cannabinoids for medical use: A systematic review and meta-analysis. *Journal of the American Medical Association*, *313*, 2456–2473. http://dx.doi.org/10.1001/jama.2015.6358

Wilsey, B., Marcotte, T. D., Deutsch, R., Zhao, H., Prasad, H., & Phan, A. (2016). An exploratory human laboratory experiment evaluating vaporized cannabis in the treatment of neuropathic pain from spinal cord injury and disease. *Journal of Pain*, *17*, 982–1000. http://dx.doi.org/10.1016/j.jpain.2016.05.010

Yi, P., & Pryzbylkowski, P. (2015). Opioid induced hyperalgesia. *Pain Medicine*, *16*(Suppl 1), S32–S36. http://dx.doi.org/10.1111/pme.12914

Zajicek, J. P., Sanders, H. P., Wright, D. E., Vickery, P. J., Ingram, W. M., Reilly, S. M., . . . Thompson, A. J. (2005). Cannabinoids in multiple sclerosis (CAMS) study: Safety and efficacy data for 12 months follow up. *BMJ Journal of Neurology, Neurosurgery & Psychiatry*, *76*, 1664–1669. http://dx.doi.org/10.1136/jnnp.2005.070136

11

Policy Implications

KEVIN A. SABET AND KEN C. WINTERS

INTRODUCTION

The landscape in terms of what we know about marijuana, as well has attitudes and perceptions about the drug, have changed significantly compared to the 1960s and 1970s. Our scientific understanding of marijuana has also changed dramatically in the last 50 years. We are in an era where a significant debate about marijuana is underway, and this is manifested by variability among US states and other countries pertaining to laws about medical and recreational use. Interestingly, it has been the United States—not Europe, home of the famous Dutch marijuana policy experiment—that has experienced rapid, drastic marijuana policy changes in a short period of time. Following the 2016 November election, 29 states have legalized the use of medical marijuana, 8 states permit the retail consumption of marijuana for adults age 21 and older, and a number of states have also decriminalized the possession of small amounts of marijuana. The District of Columbia has legalized marijuana for medical and recreational purposes. Some states have shown a promarijuana stance but had such efforts halted by the influence of grassroots groups (e.g., Vermont). Among states that allow medical marijuana use, there is great variability. At one end are the relatively constrained regulations in Minnesota (limited number of qualifying medical conditions, rigorous review process to determine patient eligibility, prescribed by a state licensed practitioner registered in the state medical marijuana program, and available only in nonsmokeable forms [pill, liquid, or oil for vaporizer]), whereas at the other end are more permissive regulations in California (e.g., broad allowances for cultivation and dispensing; physicians can recommend marijuana for hundreds of indications, including such common complaints as insomnia, premenstrual syndrome, posttraumatic stress, depression, and substance abuse; California NORML, 2017). There is even wide variation as to what most people desire as their preferred "new" policy. In one poll conducted by Emerson College, 60% of respondents expressed approval for legalization; one week later the poll was updated by Emerson to include more than just a binary "legalization v prohibition" question. When likely voters were given policy choice, support for legalization fell 20 points; most people preferred decriminalizing small amounts of marijuana for personal use or medical use (cite Humphreys, K, https://www.washingtonpost.com/news/wonk/wp/2017/12/12/what-voters-really-mean-when-they-say-they-support-marijuana-legalization/?utm_term=.fc3927015ed9 *Washington Post* Dec 12 2017).

The United States is in the very early stages of a real-world experiment. For those states with at least a few years of legal recreational use, what do they make of the evidence associated with these real-life public health tests? Moreover, to what extent will other states who may consider prolegalization legislation take into account the extant public health data, and how will they balance these issues with perceptions of economic benefits from a marijuana market? And, perhaps most important, if we are to call these *experiments*, then to what extent are states actually designing data systems to track possible consequences?

Four of our chapters specifically addressed marijuana use and these possible impacts on the health of the user: development of a substance use disorder, structure and function in a developing brain, mental health, lung functioning, functioning while driving, and rates of dependence. In all of these chapters, the authors conclude, albeit with caution, that there is mounting evidence that marijuana use contributes to deleterious health effects. Moreover, as noted in the chapter by Compton et al., there is considerable evidence also linking marijuana use to several adverse life-functioning variables, including lower educational attainment, lower income, criminal behavior, and lower life satisfaction. The book's general conclusion that marijuana use is harmful across multiple health outcomes is consistent with the recent report by the National Academies of Sciences, Engineering, and Medicine (2017).

Admittedly, science-based research on how marijuana impacts health is still evolving, and we still do not know the extent to which and nature of the associations of marijuana use and negative impacts are causal. But the current expansion of promarijuana laws in the United States certainly exceeds what we know about the drug. As legalization expands and the social stigma of marijuana use is reduced, history tells us that proportionally more individuals will perceive that the drug is not harmful and that using the drug is relatively normative. As detailed in the chapter by Cottler et al., there are indications that the prevalence of marijuana use increases in some states (but not all) that have legalized marijuana for recreational purposes. (For a detailed analysis of trend changes in Colorado and Washington, two states who have recently legalized recreational use of marijuana, see Smart Approaches to Marijuana, 2016.) These influences and changes in societal attitudes are a recipe for a trend of more use of marijuana by more individuals and may diminish the influence of science-based information.

HOW DID WE GET HERE?

Several factors likely have contributed to the fact that there is wide policy experimentation and changing cultural attitudes toward marijuana, especially in the United States. We highlight three.

Marijuana as Medicine

Laws emphasizing enforcement and punitiveness seemed like overkill to many Americans who perceived marijuana to be the soft drug of Woodstock and the college experience during the 1960s and 1970s. Capitalizing on this sentiment, well-funded campaigns began in the 1990s touting marijuana on compassionate grounds for sick and dying and as a legitimate alternative to various chronic illnesses, such as intractable epilepsy and multiple sclerosis. Once marijuana was seen as medicine, stigma against the drug declined.

Enforcement Polices of the Federal Government

From a policy perspective, despite the fact that the vast majority of medical marijuana cases did not involve the terminally ill, the concept picked up steam, and the de-escalation of marijuana enforcement began in earnest in 2009, with a formal memo issued by the Deputy Attorney General, David Ogden. The so-called Ogden memo of 2009 explained that federal prosecutions would not target individual users of marijuana or their caregivers. Although individual marijuana enforcement (especially among sick people) was never part of federal enforcement, legalization groups cheered, since it signaled the formal change of posture they had been after for decades. The number of marijuana stores selling the drug as medicine skyrocketed in several states, including Colorado, California, and Montana. For example, Colorado had roughly 2,000 medical marijuana users in January of 2008. That jumped to 55,469 by the end of January 2010, making the adult medical marijuana users about 1.4% of the total adult population.

Even with the Ogden memo in place, US attorneys under President Barack Obama, in several jurisdictions began to ramp up enforcement against large medical marijuana production and retail operations. In one jurisdiction, US attorneys even implied that state employees could be subject to prosecution (see http://www.thestranger.com/images/blogimages/2011/04/14/1302831694-usa_letter_4-14-2011.pdf). After several federal lawsuits and threats of enforcement action, the administration released in 2011 a follow-up memo by the now new Deputy Attorney General, James Cole. In the Cole memo, the department of Justice discussed how the Ogden memo had been misinterpreted as a green light for marijuana selling and that the United States would continue to pursue larger marijuana trafficking cases, even in instances where medical marijuana was claimed.

Though several laws had been passed governing the decriminalization of marijuana on the state level, no laws had ever been passed on the state level authorizing the retail sales and production of the drug until 2012. After five decades of attempts to legalize marijuana, including losses in Nevada in 2006 and California in 2010, legalization advocates claimed victory in Washington and Colorado (and a loss in Oregon). By margins of 55% in both states, voters agreed with the multimillion-dollar campaigns that the sales of marijuana should be legal.

After almost a year of virtually no response from the federal government, on August 29, 2013, James Cole released a new memo indicating that the Justice

Department would not prosecute states "right now" for breaching the Controlled Substances Act. This was met with adulation from legalization advocates and ire from opponents. In the new memo, Cole listed eight enforcement priorities the Department of Justice (DOJ) would focus on when determining future courses of action with respect to marijuana laws (see https://www.justice.gov/iso/opa/resources/3052013829132756857467.pdf).

As of this writing—five years after the Cole memo was released—the DOJ has yet to follow up on anything mentioned in the memo. The independent, non-partisan US Government Accountability Office (2015; GAO) released a report recommending the DOJ implement a specific plan for documenting the effects of state marijuana legalization, since they have yet to do so.

The GAO (2015) report, which a bipartisan group of US senators requested, states that DOJ has not "documented their monitoring process or provided specificity about key aspects of it" (p. 31). This lack of specificity includes missing information about "potential limitations of the data [DOJ officials] report using and how they will use the data to identify states that are not effectively protecting federal enforcement priorities" (p. 38).

When asked about how DOJ is doing at tracking its priorities, the lead GAO author responded, "It's hard to tell, because DOJ has not documented its plan for monitoring the effects of the state marijuana legalization."

The GAO (2015) report also highlights unusual attitudes and behavior by DOJ officials concerning monitoring of the agency's own priorities concerning marijuana, including:

- "Officials reported that they did not see a benefit in DOJ documenting how it would monitor the effects of state marijuana legalization relative to the August 2013 [Office of the Deputy Attorney General] guidance" (p. 31).
- DOJ field offices "do not consistently enter information" in a "key source of information for monitoring," thus ensuring that the database "would not provide reliable information regarding the extent of marijuana-related cases" (p. 30).
- Drug Enforcement Administration and DOJ officials from California, Colorado, Oregon, and Washington reported that they had not sent warning letters to owners and lien holders of medical marijuana dispensaries since DOJ issued the August 2013 guidance on marijuana (p. 37).

The Business of Marijuana

Another factor is the vigorous efforts by the marijuana industry to advance a narrative on the public that legalization of marijuana will deliver many economic, social, and health benefits and few, if any, negative outcomes. Legalization for recreational purposes may appeal to some with a libertarian viewpoint, but it is hard to argue against the view that the legalization movement is primarily driven by monetary benefits for a few (mainly the financiers and owners of marijuana-related businesses). A host of business interests have been involved with the legal marijuana trade in states that have already approved legalization, and they are working in states that are considering law changes. These promarijuana business interests establish private equity firms and fundraising organizations in order to attract investors, they advance the rhetoric that marijuana is not harmful and has indisputable medical value and that it will be available in many forms to satisfy a diverse marketplace (food items, oils, and other products). Will the marijuana industry follow the tobacco industry and target the poor and disenfranchised? We are not being cynical in predicting a "yes" if it can be expected that doing so will increase profits. The irony in all of this is that as tobacco users are increasingly shunned—and its lobby reduced to a national anathema—an aggressive Big Pot industry is gaining steam. We note with anxiety the growing practice of state marijuana regulatory officials fleeing public service for work in the marijuana industry (Fallon, 2017).

IMPLICATIONS FOR DRUG POLICY REFORM

Policymakers must deal with several social, economic, and health issues unique to marijuana. These issues frequently pit science versus promarijuana claims; several prominent ones are discussed in Table 11.1.

KEEPING MARIJUANA POLICY ACCOUNTABLE

Currently, the US government has no plans for a robust system to track marijuana policy outcomes. This should change. There is much we still do not know about these policy changes. The Institute of Behavior and Health, founded by the first director of the National Institute on Drug Abuse and former White House drug chief, Bob DuPont, provides the following guide and rationale.

- Congress should take the necessary steps to request the National Academies of Sciences, Engineering, and Medicine to establish a Scientific Committee to Monitor the Effects of Marijuana Policy Changes.
- The National Academies of Sciences, Engineering, and Medicine would be solely responsible for selecting the members of the Scientific Committee, who would be drawn from the full range of scientific disciplines, including but not limited to policy, epidemiology, statistics, economics, psychology, law, and medicine.
- The charge of the Scientific Committee would include:

Table 11.1 BIG MARIJUANA CLAIMS VERSUS SCIENTIFIC FACTS

Big Marijuana Claims	Scientific Facts
Marijuana can't kill or hurt you.	Marijuana may not produce direct overdoses, but tobacco rarely, if ever, does either. But we would not say tobacco can't kill or hurt you, and we would not say marijuana cannot do these things either. Emergency room admissions for marijuana use now exceed those for heroin and are continuing to rise (Center for Behavioral Health Statistics and Quality, 2011). The link between suicide and marijuana is strong, as are car accidents—too many of which result in death.
Marijuana does not affect the workplace.	Marijuana use impairs the ability to function effectively and safely on the job and increases work-related absences, tardiness, accidents, compensation claims, and job turnover (National Institute on Drug Abuse, 2012).
Marijuana users are clogging our prisons.	There are very few people in state or federal prison for marijuana-related crimes. It is useful to look at all drug offenses for context. In 2004, the percentage of drug offenders in State prisons serving time for drug law violations involving marijuana was 12%; this compares to 19% for stimulants and 62% for cocaine (Mumola & Karberg, 2006). Among sentenced prisoners under state jurisdiction in 2008, 18% were sentenced for drug offenses (West, Sabol, & Greenman, 2010). Other independent research has shown that the risk of arrest for each "joint," or marijuana cigarette, smoked is about 1 arrest every 12,000 joints (Kilmer, Caulkins, Pacula, MacCoun, & Reuter, 2010).
Marijuana is medicine.	Marijuana may contain medical components, like opium does. But we don't smoke opium to get the effects of morphine. Similarly we don't need to smoke marijuana to get its potential medical benefit (Watson, Benson, & Joy, 2000). We need more research.
The sick and dying need medical marijuana programs to stay alive.	Research shows that very few of those seeking a recommendation for medical marijuana have cancer, HIV/AIDS, glaucoma, or multiple sclerosis (Nunberg, Kilmer, Pacula, & Burgdorf, 2011); and in most states that permits the use of medical marijuana, less than 2% to 3% of users report having cancer, HIV/AIDS, glaucoma, multiple sclerosis, or other life-threatening diseases (Colorado Department of Public Health, 2012).

Table 11.1 Continued

Big Marijuana Claims	Scientific Facts
Marijuana should be rescheduled to facilitate its medical and legitimate use.	Rescheduling is a source of major confusion. Marijuana meets the technical definition of Schedule I because it is not an individual product with a defined dose. You can't dose anything that is smoked or used in a crude form. However, components of marijuana can be scheduled for medical use, and that research is fully legitimate. That is very different than saying a joint is medicine and should be rescheduled (see Sabet, 2013). It is important to note, too, that rescheduling does not generally correspond with criminalization or penalization. So if your target is to reduce penalties for use, focusing on rescheduling is the wrong target.
Alcohol is legal, why shouldn't marijuana also be legal?	Our currently legal drugs—alcohol and tobacco— provide a good example, since both youth and adults use them far more frequently than illegal drugs. According to recent surveys, alcohol use is used by 52% of Americans and tobacco is used by 27% of Americans, but marijuana is used by only 8% (see Smart Approaches to Marijuana, 2014).
We can get tax revenue if we legalize marijuana.	Because marijuana legalization would increase use, any tax revenue gained from legal marijuana would be quickly offset by the social costs. One example with a legal drug—alcohol—provides some clarity. Federal excise taxes collected on alcohol in 2007 totaled around $9 billion; states collected around $5.5 billion. Combined, these amounts are less than 10% of the estimated $185 billion in alcohol-related costs to health care, criminal justice, and the workplace in lost productivity (Tax Policy Center, 2017). And so far in Colorado, tax revenue has fallen short of expectations.
Legalization would remove the black market and stop enriching gangs.	Criminal enterprises do not receive the majority of their funding from marijuana. Furthermore, with legal marijuana taxed and only available to adults, a black market will continue to thrive. The black market and illegal drug dealers will continue to function—and even flourish (Baca, 2014; Gurman, 2014; Jones, 2014)—under legalization, as people seek cheaper, untaxed marijuana.

1. To assemble, synthesize and interpret available federal and state data and research pertaining to the effects of marijuana use and the effects of changes in marijuana policy in the United States;
2. To recommend improvements in data collection by public and private agencies and organizations;

3. To recommend priorities in research on the effects of marijuana use and the effects of changes in marijuana policy, directed to federal and states agencies, foundations and other entities that fund research; and

4. To issue annual reports setting forth findings regarding the effects of marijuana use and the effects of changes in marijuana policy. (Institute for Behavior and Health, 2016, p. 2)

ISSUES FOR STATES WITH LEGALIZATION

Our instincts are to urge states to abide by both federal and international law and not legalize marijuana. But for the several states that already have, great care should be taken as to how legalization is implemented. Here are some guidelines that should be broadly followed:

- **Public health and safety advocates should hold the majority of seats on the advisory committees related to the proposition.** It is imperative that these advisory committees not go the way of their cousins in Colorado, which were dominated by industry voices. As a result, Colorado regulation of potency, edibles, and other important public health issues was—and remains—extremely weak. Ensure that strong voices for the public interest hold a majority of the seats on these bodiesand, if not, establish independent oversight panels.
- **Demand a strong standard for driving while high.** Following in the footsteps of Colorado and Washington, other legal states should expect a surge in fatalities related to driving while high. A strong standard for driving while high is critical to preventing at least some of these needless deaths. This standard can include a behavioral test combined with oral testing that can detect recent use. A major anti-stoned driving campaign should also be implemented.
- **Establish an independent oversight office, staffed solely by public health experts, to track data related to marijuana use.** Following the adage of "you can't manage what you can't measure," an independent office staffed solely by public health professionals needs to gather and track data related to the health impacts of marijuana use. The advisory committees previously referenced are not enough—their objective is to make recommendations, not to collect data, and they will also be subject to tremendous political pressure by a powerful pot lobby. An independent body is needed, staffed with experts with deep expertise in addictive substances like that of the University of California–San Francisco's Stanton Glantz. Otherwise, the marijuana industry can override and influence political appointees, and there will be no robust data collection to track the industry's impact.
- **Set up a statewide law enforcement office to measure black market and cartel activity and coordinate with neighboring states.** Colorado

has seen an unprecedented rise in black market activity since legalization. The state had one organized crime filing in 2007 and 40 in 2015. Recently, reports of Mexican cartel activity even began to filter in, indicating that they are taking advantage of these lax laws to hide in plain sight. Gathering data on their activity will be critical, and the industry will not shoulder that burden.

- **Pass strong product liability and dram shop laws for marijuana.** Although the marijuana industry claims to want to be regulated like other intoxicants, they have so far been curiously exempt from accountability in the form of product liability lawsuits and dram shop laws. Shops that sell marijuana to individuals who are clearly impaired should be strictly liable to anyone injured by that person. Also, manufacturers, distributors, and retailers should be liable to those who have adverse reactions from using their product. Municipalities planning on restricting marijuana sales should lawyer up now.

- **Restrict edibles and concentrates as much as possible.** The most serious danger to public health with respect to legal marijuana products are edibles and concentrate products. Their high potency, resemblance to nonlaced consumer products (candy, topical lotions, etc.) and ease of use create particular problems. They should be heavily regulated, or banned outright until we know more about their effects, to discourage their advertising, sales, and use.

- **Advertising restrictions.** Like alcohol and tobacco, underage users are a very profitable market for the marijuana industry, even if sales to them are illegal. Early-onset users are more likely to become highly profitable heavy users, and brand loyalty is generally developed and solidified when users are younger. Advertising is therefore an important component to targeting and capturing these users, as this country's experience with tobacco has demonstrated. To the extent possible, therefore, advertising should be heavily regulated and restricted. Moreover, simple prohibitions on ads targeting minors has an empirically poor track record—there is too much legal room to debate on what targets minors and what does not. Good restrictions must go farther than that and be general in nature. Also, keep in mind that any such restrictions must also be compatible with First Amendment protections on commercial speech, but it is unclear whether that protection would apply to activities that are illegal under federal law. Additionally, litigation over advertising restrictions is likely to cast the marijuana industry in a bad light as it claims a right to advertise an addictive substance.

- **Heavy penalties for advertising or selling to minors.** Given the importance of keeping marijuana out of the hands of minors, this is a critical, if not obvious, component of a strong regulatory policy.

- **Targeting investors with enforcement actions.** Strong enforcement should address those financing noncompliant marijuana operations as well as the operators.

REFERENCES

Baca, R. (2014, 26 February). Drug dealer says legal pot helps his business (Video). *The Cannabist*. Retrieved from http://www.thecannabist.co/2014/02/26/drug-dealer-anything-legalization-helped-business-video/5581/

California NORML. (2017). *Patients' guide to medical marijuana law in California*. Retrieved from http://www.canorml.org/medical-marijuana/patients-guide-to-california-law

Center for Behavioral Health Statistics and Quality. (2011). *Drug abuse warning network, 2008: National estimates of drug-related emergency department visits* (HHS Publication No. SMA 11-4618). Rockville, MD: Substance Abuse and Mental Health Services Administration.

Colorado Department of Public Health. (2012). *Medical marijuana registry program update (as of September 30, 2012)*. Retrieved January 2013 from http://www.cdphe.state.co.us/hs/medicalcannabis/statistics.html

Fallon, J. (2017, January 17). *Regulators get cozy with cannabis: How can they police the very industry that will line their pockets?* Retrieved from https://www.lifezette.com/healthzette/regulators-get-cozy-with-cannabis/

Gurman, S. (2014, April 4). *Legal pot in Colorado hasn't stopped black market*. Retrieved from http://bigstory.ap.org/article/legal-pot-colorado-hasnt-stopped-black-market.

Institute for Behavior and Health. (2016). *A strategy to assess the consequences of marijuana legalization*. Retrieved from https://static1.squarespace.com/static/575830e0b09f958d96b6e4df/t/5851956b37c5818ff6361247/1481741676936/IBH_Marijuana_Strategy_Revision_December_2016.pdf

Jones, O. (2014). Pot is legal in Colorado, so why is the black market for it thriving? Retrieved from http://bigthink.com/ideafeed/pot-is-legal-in-colorado-so-why-is-the-black-market-for-it-thriving

Kilmer, B., Caulkins, J. P., Pacula, R. L., MacCoun, R. J., & Reuter, P. (2010). *Altered state? Assessing how marijuana legalization in California could influence marijuana consumption and public budgets*. Santa Monica, CA: RAND.

Mumola, C. J., & Karberg, J. C. (2006). *Drug use and dependence: State and federal prisoners, 2004*. Washington, DC: US Department of Justice, Office of Justice Programs, Bureau of Justice Statistics.

National Academies of Sciences, Engineering, and Medicine. (2017). *The health effects of cannabis and cannabinoids: The current state of evidence and recommendations for research*. Washington, DC: Author.

National Institute on Drug Abuse. (2012). *Marijuana abuse* (NIH Publication No. 12-3859). Washington, DC: Author.

Nunberg, H., Kilmer, B., Pacula, R. L., & Burgdorf, J. R. (2011). An analysis of applicants presenting to a medical marijuana specialty practice in California. *Journal of Drug Policy Analysis, 4*, 1–16. http://dx.doi.org/10.2202/1941-2851.1017

Sabet, K. (2013, October 12). Should marijuana be rescheduled? *Huffington Post*. Retrieved from https://www.huffingtonpost.com/kevin-a-sabet-phd/should-marijuana-be-resch_b_3745354.html

Smart Approaches to Marijuana (2014). *4/20 report card: Colorado*. Retrieved from https://learnaboutsam.org/wp-content/uploads/2014/04/CO-420-doc-final2.pdf

Smart Approaches to Marijuana (2016). *Lessons learned after 4 years of marijuana legalization*. Retrieved from https://learnaboutsam.org/wp-content/uploads/2016/11/SAM-report-on-CO-and-WA-issued-31-Oct-2016.pdf

Tax Policy Center. (2017, October 16). *Alcohol tax revenue: 1977 to 2015.* Retrieved from http://www.taxpolicycenter.org/statistics/alcohol-tax-revenue

US Government Accountability Office. (2016). *State marijuana laws* [transcript of interview with J. Glover]. Retrieved from http://www.gao.gov/assets/680/674577.txt

US Government Accountability Office. (2015). *State marijuana legalization: DOJ should document its approach to monitoring the effects of legalization.* Retrieved from http://www.gao.gov/products/GAO-16-1

Watson, S. J., Benson, J. A., & Joy, J. E. (2000). Marijuana and medicine: assessing the science base: a summary of the 1999 Institute of Medicine report. *Archives of General Psychiatry, 57,* 547–552.

West, H. C., Sabol, W. J., & Greenman, S. J. (December, 2010). *Prisoners in 2009: Bureau of Justice Statistics Bulletin.* Washington, DC: US Department of Justice, Office of Justice Programs, Bureau of Justice Statistics.

INDEX

Note: Page numbers followed by the italicized letters *b, f,* or *t,* indicate material found in boxes, figures or tables.

abstinence
  cognitive function and, 4–5
  memory functioning and, 99
  withdrawal symptoms and, 76
  working memory and, 100–101
abuse, of marijuana. *See also* cannabis use disorder (CUD)
  after commercialization, 281
  bipolar disorder and, 141
  data collection on, 208
  drugged driving and, 210
  in DSM criteria, 76–78, 82
  gender differences in, 80
  genetic influences and, 226
  interventions for, 243–244
  panic episodes and, 142
  prevalence of marijuana use, 24, 31–32, 32*f,* 35
  risk/protective factors for, 227–228
  schizophrenia spectrum disorders and, 127–128, 136
  state laws and, 198–199
  suicide attempts and, 145, 148
access
  to CBD preparations, 272, 274
  to effective interventions, 249–250
  to health services, 43
  to marijuana, vii, 227, 237, 279
  of states to testing kits, 207
  to treatment services, 242, 244*b,* 247*b*

addiction/addictive properties. *See also* cannabis use disorder (CUD)
  changing laws and, 237
  core features of, 75–77
  data collection on, 302
  of marijuana, 3
  THC levels and, 176
  transition to, 74
Addiction Severity Index, 239
administrative license removal (ALR), 207–208
adolescence, neurocognitive profile during. *See also* global intellectual neurocognitive functioning
  aberrant brain structure and, 107
  age inclusion, variability in, 103–104
  cannabis exposure thresholds, 104–105
  causation inference and, 107–108
  control group comparisons, 106
  domains of neurocognition and, 107
  examination of residual effects, 105–106
  functioning abnormalities, 96–97
  future research recommendations, 108–109
  high-risk populations, 105
  potency of cannabis and, 106
  structural abnormalities, 94–96

adolescent marijuana use, risk factors for
  community, 221–222
  conceptual issues in, 220–221
  family, 223–224
  individual, 224
  longitudinal studies on, 219–220
  peers, 224
  research directions for, 226–229
  school, 222–223
  society, 221
adolescents
  cannabis use among, 91–92
  central nervous system development
    of, 92–93
  cognitive deficits and, 5
  DSM-based cannabis symptoms in, 78
  heavy marijuana use by, 31f
  lifetime prevalence rates, 18
  past 12-month prevalence by, 20
  past 30-day prevalence by, 22
  psychosocial treatment literature
    on, 242b
adults
  CUD in, 78
  DSM-based cannabis symptoms in, 78
  lifetime prevalence rates, 18–19
  past 12-month prevalence by, 20–21
  past 30-day prevalence by, 22
  psychosocial treatment literature on,
    238–239, 240b
Advanced Roadside Impaired Driving
  Enforcement, 206
adverse effects, of marijuana, 105, 109,
  256, 268–269, 274–276, 278
advertising restrictions, 303
advisory committees, guidelines for, 302
AIDS/AIDS patients, 15, 175, 256,
  265–266, 271, 275, 300t
Alaska, medical marijuana laws in, 260t
alcohol/alcohol use
  BAC threshold for, 201
  brain activity with, 101–102
  data collection on, 204–205, 208
  dead/injured drivers and, 188, 190, 192f
  dependence on, 75, 92
  by drivers, 183–184
  DUI arrests and, 207

  early studies on, 47
  gender and, 60, 62f
  intervention/treatment for, 209,
    243, 245
  laws/regulations on, 197, 198, 237
  marijuana/alcohol comparison, 149,
    185, 301t
  with marijuana use, 80, 99, 187,
    191–193, 225, 282
  medical marijuana laws and, 284
  neurocognitive function with, 98
  by parents, 223, 228
  public education on, 194–196
  schizophrenia onset and, 127–129
  Standardized Field Sobriety Test
    (SFST) for, 206
  suicidal ideation/attempts and, 146–148
  24/7 Sobriety Program for, 210
American Academy of Neurology, 273
American Association of Motor Vehicle
  Administrators, 194
American Automobile Association, 194
American Glaucoma Society, 6
anandamide, 2
anxiety
  from different cannabinoid drugs,
    275–276
  gender differences in, 224
  marijuana use and, 142–143
  as mood reaction, 268
  research needs and, 148
  as THC side effect, 271
  during withdrawal, 76–77, 144–145
Argentina, epidemiological field survey
  estimates for, 53, 54f
Arizona, medical marijuana laws in, 260t
Arkansas, medical marijuana laws in, 260t
attention/attentional compromise, 99–100
attitudes, toward marijuana use, 34–35
Australia
  computer-delivered MET/CBT
    programs in, 245
  CUD prevalence in, 77, 78
  effects of legalization in, 221
  epidemiological field survey estimates
    for, 59–60, 61f
  medical marijuana laws in, 265

onset/progression of use in, 74
TMCU use in, 244
Australian Adolescent Cannabis
  Check-Up, 244

Big Marijuana claims, vs. scientific facts,
  300–301*t*
bipolar disorder, 5, 140–142. *See also*
  mental health/mental health
  disorders
Birchfield v. North Dakota, 204
black market/cartel activity, 302–303
bronchitis symptoms, marijuana use and,
  167, 167*t*, 171, 176, 277
Bulgaria, epidemiological field survey
  estimates for, 58–59, 60*f*

California
  Callaghan's study in, 128
  Compassionate Use Act, 259, 265
  data collection in, 302
  eligibility for medical marijuana, 265
  enforcement policies and, 297–298
  legalization of medical marijuana use,
    1, 33, 265
  location of dispensaries in, 283
  medical marijuana laws in, 260*t*
  Monitoring the Future (MTF)
    survey in, 34
  regulations in, 295
  respiratory cancer studies in, 174
  state laws in, 260*t*
  trafficking of marijuana from, 285
California Behavioral Risk Factor
  Surveillance System, 33
Canada
  epidemiological field survey estimates
    for, 49, 49*f*
  medical marijuana laws in, 265
cancer, respiratory, 165, 172–174, 176
cannabidiol. *See* CBD (cannabidiol)
cannabidivarin, 275
cannabinoid-containing products, 2
cannabinoid receptors, 2, 14, 93, 269–270
cannabinoids. *See also* CB1/CB2
  receptors; medical marijuana;
  randomized control trials

antitumoral effect of, 173
cannabis distinction, 7
efficacy of, 270, 272
endogenous/nonendogenous, 6, 147
exogenous, 2, 94
inhalation of, 65
in medical products, 258–259
in neuropathic pain, 277
oral solutions, 7, 276
placebo control and, 278
political controversy over, 259
in prefrontal cortex, 3
in presence of fatal crashes, 190, 192
saliva tests for, 56
term use/meaning, 14, 40
therapeutic applications for, 6–8
cannabis use disorder (CUD). *See also*
  cannabis withdrawal
  in adolescents/adults, 78
  clinical characteristics of, 72–73
  core features of, 75–77
  course of, 81–82
  cross-national comparisons in, 80
  definition of, 77
  DSM-based cannabis symptoms,
    78–81, 79*t*
  gender differences in, 80
  heterogeneity in course of, 75
  increase in, 237
  legalization differences in, 73–74
  onset/progression of use in, 74–75
  prevalence of DSM-IV CUD, 77–78
  relapse risk, 82
  remission/recovery from, 82–83
  research/treatment gaps in, 83
  subgroup differences in, 73
cannabis use disorder (CUD), treatment of
  clinical epidemiology, 236
  future research recommendations,
    249–250
  non-clinical interventions, 242–244
  number of people seeking
    treatment, 237
  pharmacotherapy for, 246–249
  research literature on, 237–238
  technology-delivered interventions in,
    245–246

cannabis withdrawal, 72, 76–77, 80–83, 238. *See also* withdrawal symptoms

Cannabis Youth Treatment (CYT) study, 241

cartel/black market activity, 302–303

CB1/CB2 receptors, 14–15, 93–94, 166, 247, 248, 249*b*, 250, 269–270, 274–275

CBD (cannabidiol)
    adverse effects of, 269
    combining other components with, 270
    contents/properties of, 2
    dosage issues, 274–276, 285
    impact on cognitive function/mental health, 4–5
    medicinal properties/value of, 143, 272–274

Centers for Disease Control and Prevention, 16

central nervous system development, among adolescents, 92–93

Cesamet (Nabilone), 272

Chile, epidemiological field survey estimates for, 52–53, 54*f*

chronic obstructive pulmonary disease (COPD), 165–167, 169–170, 171, 176. *See also* lung function

chronic pain, treatment of, 266–268

cigarettes. *See* lung function

CNN (news network), 273

cognitive-behavioral therapy (CBT), 237–239, 240*b*, 241–242, 242*b*, 245–246

cognitive function. *See also* neurocognitive profile, during adolescence
    executive functioning, 100–103
    marijuana's impact on, 4–6

Colombia
    CUD cross-national comparisons, 80
    epidemiological field survey estimates for, 51, 52*f*

Colorado
    first-time marijuana use in, 3
    legalization in, 4, 282
    marijuana-related traffic deaths in, 189*t*

medical marijuana laws in, 260–261*t*, 266

postlegalization traffic safety data, 188–189, 190*f*

recreational laws in, 34

Community Anti-Drug Coalitions of America, 195

community domain, in substance use, 221–222. *See also* risk and protective factors

Compassionate Use Act (California), 259, 265

compensatory neural effort, 107

Connecticut, medical marijuana laws in, 261*t*

Consumer Product Safety Commissions, 65

contingency management (CM), 237–242, 240*b*, 242*b*, 245

Controlled Substances Act, 198, 298

"Core Data for Epidemiological Studies of Nonmedical Drug Use" (Hughes), 47

Costa Rica, epidemiological field survey estimates for, 51, 52*f*

cumulative incidence proportion (CIP), 44–46, 49–53, 55–56, 58–65

daily marijuana use, 4, 30, 31*f*, 32*f*, 33*f*, 187, 269

data collection, 208–209

data sources, for epidemiological trends. *See also* Monitoring the Future (MTF); National Survey on Drug Use and Health (NSDUH)
    National Monitoring of Adolescent Prescription Stimulants (N-MAPSS), 15, 17–18, 25, 29, 35
    Youth Risk Behavior Surveillance System (YRBSS), 15, 16, 24–25, 25*t*, 281

decision-making, in adolescents, 102–103

Delaware, medical marijuana laws in, 261*t*

delta-9-tetrahydrocannabinol. *See* THC (delta-9-tetrahydrocannabinol)

demographic characteristics
    in CUD prevalence, 77–78
    lifetime prevalence rates by, 19*t*

past 12-month prevalence by, 21*t*
past 30-day prevalence by, 23*t*
Denmark, epidemiological field survey
    estimates for, 56, 58, 58*f*
Department of Justice (DOJ), 298
dependence, on marijuana. *See also*
    cannabis use disorder (CUD)
    as adverse effect, 268
    among adolescents, 35
    decision-making capacity and, 103
    depressive disorders and, 144
    DSM-based symptoms, 77–78
    gender and, 80
    genetic factors and, 226
    legalization and, 281, 283, 284
    lifetime risk of, 92
    onset of, 81
    panic disorders and, 142
    prevalence of, 31–32, 32*f*
    psychosocial treatments and, 239–240
    sustained abstinence and, 98
    thresholds of exposure and, 104
    transition to, 74–75
dependence syndrome, 75–77
depression. *See also* anxiety; mental
    health/mental health disorders
    incidence of, 143–144
    withdrawal and, 144–145
Diagnostic and Statistical Manual of
    Mental Disorders (DSM-IV), on
    marijuana abuse, 31
dispensaries
    DOJ guidance on, 298
    FDA warnings and, 273
    location of, 283
    marijuana use increases and, 283
    state laws' allowance of, 260–264*t*,
    265, 285
District of Colombia, 260, 261*t*, 295
driving. *See* marijuana-impaired driving
driving standards, guidelines for, 302
driving under the influence (DUI), 184,
    188–189, 191, 193, 197, 202, 204–206
driving while intoxicated (DWI) courts,
    209, 211
Dronabinol (Marinol and Syndros), 8,
    247–248, 271

Drug Enforcement Administration, 40
Drug Evaluation and Classification
    Program, 206
drugged driving. *See* marijuana-
    impaired driving
Drug-Impaired Driving—A Guide For
    What States Can Do (GHSA), 196
Drug Recognition Expert (DRE)
    training, 203, 206
drug tests/drug testing, 184, 186, 191,
    193, 201, 204–206, 208

edibles/concentrates, 1, 4, 14, 185, 260*t*,
    302, 303
educational level
    lifetime prevalence rates by, 19*t*
    past 12-month prevalence by, 21*t*
    past 30-day prevalence by, 23*t*
Egelhoff, Montana v., 202
Emerson College, 295
employment (current)
    lifetime prevalence rates by, 19*t*
    past 12-month prevalence by, 21*t*
    past 30-day prevalence by, 23*t*
endocannabinoids, therapeutic
    applications for, 6–7
endocannabinoid system, 2, 6, 93–95,
    247, 270, 275
endogenous cannabinoid ligands, 2
epidemiological field survey estimates
    for Argentina, 53, 54*f*
    for Australia, 59–60
    for Bulgaria, 58–59, 60*f*
    for Canada, 49, 49*f*
    for Chile, 52–53, 54*f*
    for Columbia, 51, 52*f*
    for Costa Rica, 51, 52*f*
    for Denmark, 56, 58, 58*f*
    for France, 58, 59*f*, 62
    for Germany, 58, 58*f*
    for Ireland, 56, 57*f*
    MAS estimate use, 48
    for Mexico, 50–51, 50*f*
    for Northern Ireland, 56
    for Peru, 51–52, 53*f*
    for Scotland, 56, 56*f*
    for United Kingdom, 56, 57*f*

epidemiological field survey
   estimates (*cont.*)
   for United States, 49–50, 50*f*
   vs. UN official statistics, 48
   for Uruguay, 53, 54*f*, 55
epidemiological studies/trends
   data sources on, 15–18
   on initiation of marijuana use, 26–35
   on prevalence of marijuana use, 18–26
   on psychotic disorders, 5
Epidiolex (oral solution cannabidiol), 8,
   272–273
Epilepsia, 273
epilepsy, 272–274, 297
Episode Data Set and the National
   Longitudinal Survey of Youth, 283
European School Survey Project on
   Alcohol and Other Drugs (ESPAD),
   39, 61, 64
exogenous cannabinoids, 2, 94

family domain, in substance use. *See* risk
   and protective factors
family risk/protective factors, 223–224
Fatality Analysis Reporting System
   (FARS), 188, 208
federal law
   enforcement policies under, 297–298
   FARS testing/reporting under, 208
   marijuana under, 1–2, 197–199, 202, 303
Finland, 62, 131
first-time marijuana use. *See also*
   initiation of marijuana use
   in college, vii
   in Colorado, 3
   duration and, 45
   in given populations, 43
   tolerance and, 200
Fixing America's Surface Transportation
   Act (FAST Act), 196, 198
Florida, medical marijuana laws in, 261*t*
Food, Drug, and Cosmetic Act, 273
Food and Drug Administration (FDA),
   2, 8, 249*b*, 271–274
Foundation for Advancing Alcohol
   Responsibility, 194, 200
France, epidemiological field survey
   estimates for, 58, 59*f*, 62
functional compensation hypothesis, 107

gender
   central nervous system development
      and, 93, 95–96
   CIP differences in international
      trends, 62*f*, 63*t*
   CUD symptoms and, 80
   differences in abuse symptoms, 80
   differences in international
      trends, 60–64
   in explanation of behavioral
      patterns, 105
   lifetime prevalence rates by, 19*t*
   past 12-month prevalence by, 21*t*, 27*t*
   past 30-day prevalence by, 23*t*, 25*t*,
      26*t*, 28*f*
geographic division
   lifetime prevalence rates by, 19*t*
   past 12-month prevalence by, 21*t*
   past 30-day prevalence by, 23*t*, 26*t*
Georgia, DWI courts in, 209
Germany, epidemiological field survey
   estimates for, 58, 58*f*
glaucoma, treatment of, 6, 256, 265, 266,
   275–276, 300*t*
global intellectual neurocognitive
   functioning. *See also* neurocognitive
      profile, during adolescence
   decision-making, 102–103
   inhibitory control, 101–102
   less commonly studied domains, 103
   literature summary, 97–98, 97*t*
   memory/memory impairment, 98–99
   processing speed and attention, 99–100
   working memory, 100–101
Government Accountability Office
   (GAO), 298
Governors Highway Safety Association
   (GHSA), 194, 196, 207
Griffith-Lendering study, 125
Guam, medical marijuana laws in, 261*t*
GW Pharmaceuticals, 273

Harm Reduction Journal, 265
Hawaii, medical marijuana laws
   in, 261*t*
health risks, as dose-dependent, 4, 5, 166,
   170, 277
highway safety. *See* marijuana-impaired
   driving

HIV/HIV patients, 15, 175, 256, 265–266, 275, 300*t*

Illinois, medical marijuana laws in, 261*t*
impaired driving. *See* marijuana-
impaired driving
implied consent, 203–204
independent oversight, guidelines for, 302
individual domain, in substance use, 224.
See also risk and protective factors
inhibitory control, 97*t*, 100–102
initiation of marijuana use. *See also* first-
time marijuana use
in adolescence, 74
availability and, 225
neurocognitive functioning and,
96–97, 109
onset of dependence and, 81
past 12-month initiation, 27*t*
psychotic symptoms and, 124
suicidal ideation and, 147
survey estimates, 26–27
use trajectories and, 75
Institute for Behavior and Health, 195,
207, 299
Institute of Medicine, 268
Integrated Project DRUID (Driving
under the Influence of Drugs,
Alcohol and Medicines), 205
International Association of Chiefs of
Police (IACP), 194, 195, 206
International Cannabis Products Safety
Commission, 40, 65–66
International Journal of Drug Policy, 282
international trends. *See also*
epidemiological field survey
estimates
conclusions on, 64–66
gender differences in CIP, 60–64, 62*f*, 63*t*
19th c. comparisons, 46
region-specific prevalence estimates, 42*t*
terms used, 40
UN Office on Drugs and Crime, 40–41
validity of data, 41–46
interpretation, of publish data, 7–8
interventions
motivational interviewing (MI),
243, 244*b*

in non-clinical settings, 242–244
technology-delivered, 245–246
web-based, 246
investors, targeting of, 303
Ireland, epidemiological field survey
estimates for, 56, 57*f*

*Journal of the American Medical
Association*, 275
*Joy of Quitting Cannabis: Freedom From
Marijuana* (Sullivan), 236

King, Maryland v., 204

Lancet/Lancet Psychiatry, 268, 282, 283
laws/legislation
federal laws, 1–2, 208, 297–298, 303
on implied consent, 203–204
on legal limits, 202–203
state laws, 197–202, 200*f*, 260–261*t*,
302–303
on testing rates, 204–205
legalization
legislation about, viii
of medical marijuana, vii
movement toward, 1
perception of risk/harm and, 4, 219
policy confusion/discussion, 2, 8
state laws on, 260–264*t*
license removal, administrative (ALR),
207–208
lifetime prevalence, 18–20, 19*t*, 44. *See
also* prevalence rates
Lithuania, 62
"Lucid Act," 197
lung cancer, 136, 149, 172, 173–175, 173*t*
lung function. *See also* chronic
obstructive pulmonary disease
(COPD); respiratory cancer
acute effects of marijuana on, 165–166
airway pathology, 171–172
chronic bronchitis symptoms, 167*t*
chronic effects of marijuana on, 166–170
cross-sectional/longitudinal studies
of, 167–168
HRCT imaging of, 170
respiratory tract infection/disorders,
174–176

MADD (Mothers Against Drunk
    Driving), 181, 194, 196
Maine, medical marijuana laws in, 261t
MAMMA (Mothers Advocating Medical
    Marijuana for Autism), 269
marijuana-impaired driving
    administrative remedial measures,
        207–208
    vs. alcohol impairment, 186–187
    effective sanctions, 209–210
    enforcement policies and, 205–207
    federal laws on, 197–198
    highway safety and, 188–191
    implied consent and, 203–204
    improved data collection and,
        208–209
    legal limits on, 202–203
    literature review, 186–188
    other substances and, 191–193, 192f
    public education strategies, 194–197
    state laws on, 198–202, 200f
    strategies for reduction of, 193–194
    testing rates, 204–205
marijuana industry
    business of, 298–299
    data collection and, 302
    as rapidly evolving, 1
    regulation of, 303
marijuana-infused products, 2. See also
    edibles/concentrates
marijuana plant
    components of, 2
    medicinal properties of, 269–275
Marijuana Tax Act (1937), 258
Marinol (dronabinol), 8, 247–248, 271
Maryland, medical marijuana laws
    in, 262t
Maryland v. King, 204
Massachusetts, medical marijuana laws
    in, 262t
McNeely, Missouri v., 204
media coverage, on marijuana's health
    effects, 144
Medical College of Calcutta (Indian), 257
medicalization, vii, 229, 279, 281,
    285–286
medical marijuana

adverse effects of, 268–269
for chronic pain, 266–268
dispensary locations, 283
effects of laws on, 279–283
evidence of effectiveness, 275–277
history of, 257–259
interpretation of published data, 7–8
laws/increased use relationship,
    279–280
legalization of, 7–2
methodological issues, 283–284
other substance use and, 284
placebo control difficulties, 278
political controversy over, 259, 265
self-regulated dosing, 277–278
state laws on, 260–264t
term use/meaning, 2
use of, 32–33
users of, 265–266
medical vs. therapeutic distinction, 8
Medicare, medical marijuana and, 268
medicinal properties. See also medical
    marijuana
    cannabinoid receptors and, 269–270
    of CBD, 272–274
    dosage issues, 274
    effectiveness of, 275–277
    of THC, 271–272
    of whole plant marijuana, 270–271
memory/memory impairment
    in adolescents, 98–99
    working memory, 100–101
mental health/mental health disorders,
    4–6. See also bipolar disorder;
    psychotic outcomes, from
    marijuana use; schizophrenia/
    schizophrenia spectrum disorders
metabolism, of marijuana, 185–186
methodological limitations (in study of
    adolescence)
    aberrant brain structure and, 107
    age inclusion, variability in, 103–104
    cannabis exposure thresholds,
        104–105
    causation inference and, 107–108
    control group comparisons, 106
    domains of neurocognition and, 107

examination of residual effects,
    105–106
future research recommendations,
    108–109
high-risk populations, 105
potency of cannabis and, 106
Mexico
    CUD cross-national comparisons, 80
    epidemiological field survey estimates
        for, 50–51, 50f
Mexico Addiction National Survey, 51
Miami–Dade County State Attorney's
    Office, 204
Miami–Dade Police Department, 191
Michigan, medical marijuana laws in,
    209, 262t
Minnesota, medical marijuana laws in,
    262t, 295
minors, sales to, 303
Missouri v. McNeely, 204
Monitoring the Future (MTF), 15, 17,
    24–25, 25t, 29, 34, 39, 64, 195, 219,
    221, 222, 280, 282, 284
Montana, medical marijuana laws
    in, 262t
Montana v. Egelhoff, 202
Mothers Advocating Medical Marijuana
    for Autism (MAMMA), 269
Mothers Against Drunk Driving
    (MADD), 183, 194, 196
motivational enhancement therapy
    (MET), 237–239, 240b, 241–242,
    245–246

Nabilone (Cesamet), 272
nabiximols (Sativex), 8, 248, 273, 277
National Academies of Sciences,
    Engineering, and Medicine, 211,
    266, 268, 296, 299
National District Attorneys Association,
    194, 196
National Epidemiologic Survey on
    Alcohol and Related Conditions,
    32, 281
National Highway Traffic Safety
    Administration (NHTSA), 187, 188,
    191, 194, 196, 205, 206, 209, 281

National Household Surveys on Drug
    Abuse, 222
National Institute of Mental Health
    (NIMH), 47
National Institute on Drug Abuse, 35,
    66, 166, 187, 194, 196, 267, 280, 299
National Institutes of Health (NIH), 6
National Longitudinal Study of
    Adolescent Health, 224, 225
National Monitoring of Adolescent
    Prescription Stimulants
    (N-MAPSS), 17–18
National Organization for the Reform
    of Marijuana Laws (NORML),
    195, 259
National Roadside Survey (NRS), 183,
    184, 188, 196, 208
National Sheriffs Association, 194, 196
National Survey on Drug Use and Health
    (NSDUH), 3, 15, 19t, 21t, 23t, 25t,
    27t, 77, 219, 237, 280
National Transportation Safety Board
    (NTSB), 194, 196, 209, 247–248
nausea
    cannabinoid use for, 275–276
    from chemotherapy, 256, 258
    Dronabinol for, 271
    hemp extract for, 257
    marijuana's effect on, 6, 7
    Nabilone for, 272
Netherlands, 73, 79t, 80, 221
neurocognitive profile, during
    adolescence
    aberrant brain structure and, 107
    age inclusion, variability in, 103–104
    cannabis exposure thresholds,
        104–105
    causation inference and, 107–108
    control group comparisons, 106
    domains of neurocognition and, 107
    examination of residual effects,
        105–106
    future research recommendations,
        108–109
    high-risk populations, 105
    potency of cannabis and, 106
Nevada, medical marijuana laws in, 262t

New Hampshire, medical marijuana laws
in, 263*t*
New Jersey, medical marijuana laws
in, 263*t*
New Mexico, medical marijuana laws
in, 263*t*
New York, medical marijuana laws
in, 263*t*
NIMH Epidemiologic Catchment Area
surveys, 47
nonendogenous cannabinoids, 6
North Dakota, medical marijuana laws
in, 263*t*
North Dakota, Birchfield v., 204
Northern Ireland, epidemiological field
survey estimates for, 56
Norway, 62
"number needed to prevent" data, 138*f*,
136–140

Obama administration, 199
Obamacare, 133
Ohio, medical marijuana laws in, 264*t*
ONDCP (White House Office on National
Drug Control Policy), 187, 194, 196
on-site collection tests, 205
oral cannabis/cannabinoids, 7, 276
oral fluid testing, 202, 204, 205
oral solution cannabidiol (Epidiolex), 8,
272–273
Oregon, medical marijuana laws in,
264*t*, 266
Oregon Health Authority, 266

Pacific Institute for Research and
Evaluation, 190
palliative vs curative treatment, 7
panic attacks, 142–143
past 12-month prevalence. *See also*
prevalence rates
among adolescents/adults, 20–22, 27*t*
comparison of rates of marijuana use,
24, 25*t*
of heavy marijuana use, 30–31
region-specific estimates, 42*t*
past 30-day prevalence. *See also*
prevalence rates

among adolescents/adults, 22–23, 26*t*
comparison of rates of marijuana use,
24–25, 25*t*
of heavy marijuana use, 30–31
trends over time in, 27–29, 28*f*
peer domain, in substance use, 224. *See
also* risk and protective factors
Pennsylvania, medical marijuana laws
in, 264*t*
perception of risk/harm, vii, 4, 34–35, 219
Peru, epidemiological field survey
estimates for, 51–52, 53*f*
pharmacotherapy, for CUD, 246–249
placebo control, of marijuana
studies, 278
point of collection tests, 205
policy implications
accountability and, 299–300
Big Marijuana claims, vs. scientific
facts, 300–301*t*
for business interests, 299–300
changing cultural attitudes, 296
for drug policy reform, 299
for federal prosecutions, 297–298
for marijuana as medicine, 297
for states with legalization, 302–303
Positive and Negative Syndrome Scale
(PANSS), 125–126
posttraumatic stress disorder (PTSD),
143, 266, 272
potency, of cannabis
in artisanal preparations, 272–273
in chronic psychosis, 136
in cognitive functioning, 187–188
DSM-based cannabis symptoms
and, 81
increase in, 1, 65, 73, 91, 104, 106,
237, 285
lung health and, 176
plant breeding for, 276
in psychoactive effects, 185
in psychotic disorders, 268
regulation of, 302–303
in suicide risk, 146
traffic safety and, 184
in treating chronic pain, 266
variability of, 170

prevalence rates
  comparison of, 24–26
  for drug-impaired driving, 204
  lifetime prevalence, 18–20
  of marijuana use, vii
  past 12-month prevalence, 20–22, 21t, 27t
  past 30-day prevalence, 22, 23t, 24–25, 25t, 26t, 27–29, 28f, 30–31
  of US schizophrenia, 129–130
prevention science, 219, 227. *See also* risk and protective factors
processing speed and attention, in adolescents, 99–100
product liability laws, 303
protective factors. *See* risk and protective factors
psychotic outcomes, from marijuana use
  age of onset for, 127
  chronic psychosis risks, 127–128
  dose-response curve, 124
  recovery time following psychotic breaks, 128–129
  reports of serious side effects, 122–123
  self-medication/reverse causation in, 124–125
  THC in clinical subjects, 125–128
PTSD (posttraumatic stress disorder), 143, 266, 272
Puerto Rico, medical marijuana laws in, 264t
pulmonary function. *See* lung function

race/ethnicity
  cannabis use prevalence and, 73–74
  CUD prevalence and, 77–78
  heavy marijuana use by, 30f
  lifetime prevalence rates by, 19t
  past 12-month prevalence by, 21t
  past 30-day prevalence by, 23t, 25t, 26t
randomized control trials
  on antipsychotics, 249
  on marijuana's effectiveness as medicine, 275
  on marijuana's effect on cognition, 4
  on PTSD treatments, 272
  on smoked vs. non-smoked cannabis, 267

of technology-delivered interventions, 245
of THC and psychotic symptoms, 126
on THC/CBD, 4
on treatment approaches, 239
recovery. *See also* interventions; treatment
  from cannabis use disorder (CUD), 82–83
  following psychotic break, 128–129, 149
  from substance use disorders, 210
recreational laws, 34
remission
  of cannabis-dependent adolescents, 102
  from cannabis use disorder (CUD), 73, 82–83
Research Domain Criteria, 83
research/future research needs
  on cannabis use disorder (CUD), 83, 237–238, 249–250
  on marijuana use/negative health effects, vii–viii
  on risk and protective factors, 226–229
  in study of adolescents, 108–109
respiratory cancer, 165, 172–174, 176
respiratory tract infection/disorders, 174–176
Rhode Island, medical marijuana laws in, 264t
risk and protective factors
  community, 221–222
  conceptual issues in, 220–221
  family, 223–224
  individual, 224
  longitudinal studies on, 219–220
  peers, 224
  research directions for, 226–229
  school, 222–223
  society, 221
Rocky Mountain High Density Trafficking Area, 280
Romania, 62
Russian Federation, 62, 64

sanctions, effective, 209–210
San Diego Suicide Study, 147

Sativex (nabiximols), 8, 248, 273, 277
schizophrenia/schizophrenia spectrum
    disorders
    age of onset for, 127
    dose-response effect in risk for, 124
    family history of psychosis in, 133–135
    marijuana popularity vs psychosis
        rates, 130–132
    marijuana use and, 5
    marijuana use/psychotic disorders
        association, 132–133
    marijuana use rates vs. psychosis rates,
        129–130
    "number needed to prevent" data,
        138f, 136–140
    symptom rarity among average users,
        137–138
school domain, in substance use, 222–223.
    See also risk and protective factors
school settings, delivery of services
    in, 243
The Science of Marijuana (Iversen), 257
Scientific Committee to Monitor
        the Effects of Marijuana Policy
        Changes, 299
scientific debate, on marijuana's health
    effects, viii–ix
scientific facts, vs. Big Marijuana claims,
    300–301t
Scotland, epidemiological field survey
    estimates for, 56, 56f
sobriety checkpoints, 194, 207
societal domain, in substance use, 221.
    See also risk and protective factors
Society of Forensic Toxicologists,
    194, 196
South Dakota, sobriety program in,
    209–210
Standardized Field Sobriety Test
    (SFST), 206
state laws
    guidelines for, 302–303
    on marijuana-impaired driving,
        198–202, 200f
    on medical marijuana, 260–264t

Substance Abuse and Mental Health
    Services Administration
    (SAMHSA), 16
Substance Abuse Module, 18
substance use disorder (SUB), 72, 75–77,
    83, 237, 239, 240–244, 246–250
suicide, marijuana and risk for, 145–148
Syndros (dronabinol), 8, 271

technology-delivered interventions
    (TDIs), 245–246
Teen Marijuana Checkup (TMCU),
    243–244, 246
tetrahydrocannabivarin (THCV), 275
THC (delta-9-tetrahydrocannabinol). See
    also cannabinoids
    addiction/addictive properties, 176
    contents/properties of, 2
    impact on cognitive function/mental
        health, 4–5
    medicinal properties of, 271–272
    metabolism of, 185–186
    psychoactive effects of, 2–3
    psychotic symptoms in clinical
        subjects and, 125–128
    therapeutic applications, 6–7
    therapeutic vs. medical distinction, 8
tobacco/tobacco use. See lung function
traffic safety. See marijuana-impaired
    driving
treatment. See also cannabis use disorder
    (CUD), treatment of; glaucoma,
    treatment of; interventions
    access to, 242, 244b, 247b
    for alcohol abuse, 209, 243, 245
    of chronic pain, 266–268
    palliative vs curative, 7
    psychosocial treatment literature,
        238–239, 240b, 242b
Treatment Episode Data Set, 283
24/ 7 Sobriety Program, 209–210

United Kingdom (Britain)
    epidemiological field survey estimates
        for, 56, 57f

MI-based interventions in, 243
  schizophrenia incidence in, 131
  suicide attempts in, 147
United States
  CUD cross-national
    comparisons, 80
  CUD prevalence in, 77
  effects of legalization in, 221
  epidemiological field survey estimates
    for, 49–50, 50f
  marijuana as controlled substance
    in, 1–2
  onset/progression of use in, 74
  real-world experimentation in, 295
  shift in laws/regulations in, 237
  study of marijuana's impact on
    psychotic disorders in, 123
University of Michigan, 3–4
University of Mississippi, 258
UN Office on Drugs and Crime,
  40–41, 46
Uruguay, epidemiological field survey
  estimates for, 53, 54f, 55
U.S. Bureau of Narcotics and Dangerous
  Drugs, 40
US Drug Enforcement Agency
  (DEA), 272
US National Mortality Followback
  Survey, 145

vaping/vaped marijuana, 4
Vermont, medical marijuana laws
  in, 264t

Virginia Association of Chiefs of
  Police, 206

Washington
  medical marijuana laws in, 264t
  postlegalization traffic safety data,
    188–191, 192t
  recreational laws in, 34
Washington Traffic Safety Commission
  (WTSC), 190, 192
Washington University Risk Behavior
  Assessment, 18
Web-based interventions, 246. See also
  interventions
We Save Lives, 196
White House Office on National Drug
  Control Policy (ONDCP), 187,
  194, 196
withdrawal symptoms, 76, 144–145, 238,
  247–248, 268. See also cannabis
  withdrawal
working memory, in adolescents, 100–101
World Drug Report (UN; WDR),
  40–41, 46
World Health Organization (WHO),
  46–47, 143
World Mental Health Surveys (WMHS),
  44, 48, 51

youth, impact of marijuana policy
  on, 3–4
Youth Risk Behavior Surveillance System
  (YRBSS), 16, 25t, 281